Vertebral Musculoskeletal Disorders

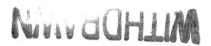

To Monica and Anne

Vertebral Musculoskeletal Disorders

Brian Corrigan
MB, BS, FRCP, FRCPE, FRACP, FACRM, DPhysMed
Head, Department of Rheumatology, Concord Hospital, Sydney, Australia

G. D. Maitland
MBE, AUA, FCSP, FACP, FACP (Specialist in Manipulative Physiotherapy), MAPPLSci
Specialist Lecturer, University of South Australia

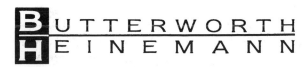

OXFORD   BOSTON   JOHANNESBURG   MELBOURNE   NEW DELHI   SINGAPORE

Butterworth-Heinemann
Linacre House, Jordan Hill, Oxford OX2 8DP
225 Wildwood Avenue, Woburn, MA 01801-2041
A division of Reed Educational and Professional Publishing Ltd

℞ A member of the Reed Elsevier plc group

First published 1998

British Library Cataloguing in Publication Data
A catalogue record for this book is available from the British Library

Library of Congress Cataloguing in Publication Data
A catalogue record for this book is available from the Library of Congress

ISBN 0 7506 2965 7

Data manipulation by David Gregson Associates, Beccles, Suffolk
Printed and bound in Great Britain by The Bath Press plc, Avon

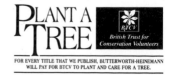

Contents

Preface

This book is mainly intended as an introductory text to spinal disorders. Spinal pain is an extremely common problem in the community, and will involve 80 per cent of all adults at some time during their lives. It is the most common form of musculoskeletal problems and the second leading cause of worker absenteeism in industry. Patients with this problem are usually first seen by their general practitioners and may then be referred to a variety of different specialists, including those in orthopaedic medicine, orthopaedic surgery, casualty, sports medicine, rheumatology or physiotherapy departments. There is no consensus among these practitioners as to what constitutes the best management of these problems. However, most would agree that the role of surgery for prolapsed disc has diminished so rapidly that it is no longer considered to be primarily a surgical condition, and that almost always a trial of conservative treatment is necessary before any surgical treatment is undertaken.

In this book we have taken as our starting point our highly successful text, *Practical Orthopaedic Medicine*. Although the format remains the same, it has now been completely rewritten, a new chapter on the spine and sport added, and a review of the vast literature concerned with spinal disorders undertaken. The amount of information published in the past 10 years or so with all the new technology is truly incredible The aim is also to introduce the controversial subject of manipulative therapy, how it is assessed clinically and its role in the overall management of spinal problems. Accordingly, emphasis is on physical methods of treatment and how manipulative techniques fit into the overall scheme of management. The relationship between the musculoskeletal system and the nervous system is so intimate that it is more appropriately entitled 'the neuromusculoskeletal system'. The techniques described are all derived from the teachings of Geoff Maitland and further details describing these techniques are to be obtained in his book *Vertebral Manipulation*, 5th edition (1984). The line drawings demonstrating the various techniques are also taken from this book.

Special thanks go to the following. Dr Bain Shenstone at Concord Hospital for all of his most valuable help with suggestions and reading (and rereading) of the text; Dr Barry Oakes, who was the very first person to suggest that this book needed to be written; Ms Kaye Lee and all her staff in the library at Concord Hospital, who taught us how to surf the Net; Ms Janeen Jardine and her staff in the Clinical Photography Department of Concord Hospital; Anne Maitland and Kate Ward for their help with the illustrations; and Caroline Makepeace, publisher of medical books at Butterworth-Heinemann in Oxford, who deserves special thanks as she has helped with suggestions and has been very understanding of our many problems.

1 Form and function

The spine consists of a complex, flexible system that is built up with successive levels of segmental intervertebral joints. The intervertebral joint, at each segmental level below the second cervical vertebra, is shaped as a three-pronged structure comprising one anterior and two posterior joints, all acting as single functional unit, known as the mobile segment (Figures 1.1 and 1.2).

The anterior joint is formed between two vertebral bodies separated by the fibrocartilaginous intervertebral disc, and strengthened by the anterior and posterior longitudinal ligaments. The disc is the largest avascular cartilaginous structure in the body and its thickness varies in each of the spinal areas, being normally thickest in the lumbar region and thinnest in the cervical. The two posterior synovial zygapophyseal joints that form the posterior parts of this intervertebral joint complex are formed by the articular processes, one process descending from the superior vertebra and one process ascending from the inferior vertebra. The mobile segment is supported by surrounding ligaments and muscles to provide movement and shock-absorbing properties (Oegema, 1993).

The spine is well adapted for its three major functions:

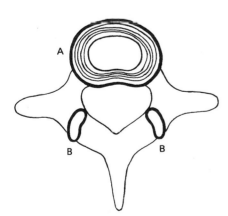

Figure 1.1 The mobile intervertebral joint, seen from above, is composed of the intervertebral disc (A) in front and the two apophyseal joints (B) behind

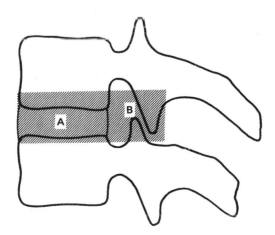

Figure 1.2 The mobile intervertebral joint (shaded) seen from the side, with the intervertebral disc (A) in front and the apophyseal joint (B) behind

Support. The rigid support necessary to support body weight and transmit compressive forces is achieved through the vertebral bodies, which have a thick outer rim that contains thin inner bony trabecular struts for added support.

Protection. The neural arch is made up of laminae, pedicles, and superior and inferior articular processes. These short bony processes enclose the spinal cord, cauda equina and the emerging nerve roots with their dural investments, providing protection for them.

Movement. Spinal movements comprise a summation of synchronized movements that take place at each intervertebral level. Bony projections, the transverse process and the spinal processes allow muscle and ligament attachments to help control movement. Normal spinal function requires that spinal movements can take place without encroaching upon the vertebral canal or the numerous nerve fibres that pass with their blood supply through the intervertebral foramen.

The intervertebral discs

The vertebral bodies are linked by 23 intervertebral discs, which are no longer looked upon as inert washers. Their chemical composition, which determines their functions, is complex. Despite the lack of any major blood supply, the discs have a high metabolic activity with a system of fluid and nutrient exchange. As with all other connective tissues, they are composed of cells, the chondrocytes and an extracellular matrix, or ground substance, containing varying proportions of collagen fibres and proteoglycans.

Chondrocytes

Chondrocytes in the adult disc have a similar structure and function to those present in articular cartilage. Although they only constitute about 5 per cent of the disc by volume, they play an essential role in maintaining its health and controlling its activity (Ohshima and Urban,

1992). The chondrocyte, embedded in the extra-articular matrix, is metabolically very active, and is responsible for both the synthesis and degradation of collagen and proteoglycans. This is mediated by its contained enzyme systems, collagenases, cathepsin and proteinases, which are themselves under the control of both activators and inhibitors.

Collagen

Collagen fibres arise from Sharpey's fibres embedded in the cranial and caudal confines of the vertebrae. They are randomly orientated to form a three-dimensional lattice network that is immersed in the ground substance. They have a high tensile strength (Ebara et al, 1996), although there is a marked regional variation throughout the disc (Skaggs et al, 1994). The fibres are able to support and distribute loads within the disc (Best et al, 1994) by becoming reoriented upon compression or during movement (Oegema, 1993). Several different types of collagen fibres have been described, but the annulus fibrosus is composed mainly of type I collagen fibres (Kaapa et al, 1994), and their orientation produces the lamellar arrangement of the annulus.

Proteoglycans

Proteoglycans are large molecules comprised of protein and polysaccharides that vary markedly in size and may exist as single units or monomers, or be shaped into large aggregates, aggrecan (Oegema, 1993; Johnstone and Bayliss, 1995). In the monomer, the protein present is formed into a core protein which acts as a backbone, and to which side chains containing glycosaminoglycans (GAGs) are linked, each GAG formed from repeating chains of disaccharides (Ghosh, 1990a). The disc has four such GAGs: keratan sulphate; chondroitin 4 sulphate; chondrotin 6 sulphate, plus the linear non-sulphated hyaluronic acid. The core protein is linked to the hyaluronic acid by a link protein, and the GAGs are spread out at right angles to the core protein. The shorter keratan sulphate is located nearest to the core protein and the chondroitin sulphate at a further distance.

Disc structure

Each disc is made up of three components: (1) the annulus fibrosus; (2) the nucleus pulposus; and (3) the cartilage endplates.

1. The annulus fibrosus forms the largest component of the adult disc, and makes up its outer elastic fibrocartilaginous layer. It is formed into layers, or lamellae, which resemble the skin of an onion (Figure 1.3), and are separated by loose connective tissue. The fibres in each lamella run spirally from one vertebra to its neighbour, so that in each successive layer the fibres run obliquely in alternate directions, criss-crossing at angles to each other (Marchand and Ahmed, 1990). In the lumbar spine there are some 12–15 lamellae, arranged in two distinct zones; an outer ligament zone which joins the vertebral rims, and an inner zone whose fibres are continuous with the cartilage endplate enveloping the nucleus (Finch and Taylor, 1996) (Figure 1.4). In the lumbar region the disc is thicker anteriorly than posteriorly, and its shape also varies. It becomes concave posteriorly, so that there is a greater concentration of fibres in this area (Bogduk and Twomey, 1991), which allows them to withstand forward flexion better and so prevent injury (Bogduk and Twomey, 1991). The elastic annulus is resilient, so that after being stretched, it can recoil and springs back to recover after mechanical deformation.

2. The nucleus pulposus is a hydrated gel that represents the adult remnant of the embryonic notochord, and accounts for nearly half of the cross-sectional area of the adolescent disc (Oegema, 1993). It has a dull, semigelatinous appearance, and in the lumbar spine it lies towards the posterior region of the disc. It has a large content of proteoglycans, with few, more delicate type II collagen fibres.

    The function of the proteoglycans is to retain water (Ghosh, 1990a; Boos et al, 1994; Paajanen et al, 1994). They do this very efficiently, for they contain a large fixed negative charge that keeps the chains stiff, attracting fluid into their domain (Ghosh, 1990a). As the fluid swells, the proteoglycans become constrained and immobilized by the surrounding prestressed collagen network, allowing the nucleus to act as a sealed hydraulic system. When the disc is compressed, fluid is forced out of the nucleus; as the compression is released, fluid is imbibed, and so the pressure rises until equilibrium is reached.

3. Cartilage endplate. In childhood, this thin plate of cartilage, which also functions as an epiphysis, covers the upper and lower surfaces of the vertebrae. After puberty, secondary ossification centres appear in the peripheral areas of the cartilage, hence its title of 'ring epiphysis', which then fuse with

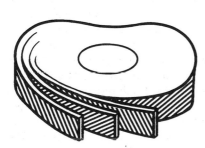

Figure 1.3 The annulus is composed of lamellae in which the fibres of each successive layer run at right angles to each other

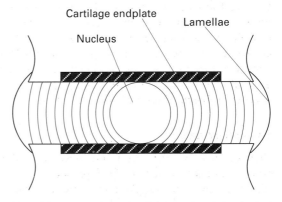

Figure 1.4 The fibres of the annulus are embedded in the cartilage end-plate and the vertebrae. The anterior fibres are embedded in the anterior aspect of the vertebra

the vertebral bone after the age of 21 years. The central portion of the endplate remains cartilaginous, forms the cartilage endplate, approximately 0.6 mm thick, and envelops the nucleus pulposus. Countersunk beneath its surface lie the vertebral endplates, which contain numerous small perforations for vascular channels extending from the cancellous bone of the vertebral body. If the human spine is experimentally loaded to failure in compression, the vertebral endplate will fracture before the disc (Ranu, 1990).

Disc nutrition

Disc nutrition is mediated through an interchange of fluid and solutes derived from the vascular channels in the bone, and transported via perforations in the adjacent cartilage endplate in and out of the disc. Fluid exchange is enhanced by the intermittent loading and unloading, which is also responsible for each individual disc's daily variation in height (Adams and Hutton, 1983; Adams et al, 1987, 1994; Tyrrell et al, 1985; Krag et al, 1990; Boos et al, 1994; Botsford et al, 1994). The interchange is regulated in part by proteoglycans present in the cartilage endplate (Roberts et al, 1996), and if it becomes calcified, the movement of solutes becomes restricted (Roberts et al, 1996).

Functions of the intervertebral discs

The structural components of the discs act as a unit to form a hydrostatic cushion (Adams et al, 1996) which is capable of being deformed, while at the same time providing the necessary stability for the disc to transmit loads, allow spinal movement and provide nutrition.

The discs need to resist the relatively large compressive loads that come not only from the weight of the body and viscera, but also from muscle action. The increasing size and thickness of the vertebrae and discs from the cervical to the lumbar spine is some evidence of its role in resisting compressive forces. The compressive loads are able to distort the nucleus pulposus,

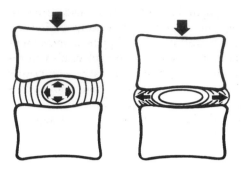

Figure 1.5 Mechanical stress is transmitted radially in all planes by the nucleus and is absorbed by the annulus

which is fluid, and hence is incompressible. The pressure within the nucleus is increased and the vertical forces are redistributed in a radial manner, where it is absorbed by the elasticity of the surrounding annulus fibrosus (Figure 1.5). The tensile strength of the annulus, of the order of 2 kg/mm^2, is considerably greater than is normally required, so that in a healthy intact disc these forces can be easily absorbed. As pressure is also distributed in part to the superior and inferior vertebral endplates, weight can then be transmitted from one vertebra to the next.

The discs are also responsible for allowing movement between the vertebrae, but human movement is much more complex than any simple model can portray. Spinal movements are of three types: physiological or cardinal movements; combined movements, e.g. lumbar flexion to the left combined with rotation to the right; and accessory movements. The normal physiological movements are flexion, extension, lateral flexion to each side and rotation to each side. At each spinal level their range of movement might be small, but their summation can result in producing a considerable range. Forward bending is a two-part movement involving the lumbar spine and the pelvis, although it is still not certain whether they move simultaneously or sequentially (Nelson et al, 1995). In the saggital plane, flexion in the three-pronged intervertebral joints involves a synchronized motion that takes place in both the anterior cartilaginous discs and the posterior synovial joints. In the anterior joint, the vertebral bodies roll over the essentially incompressible gel structure of the disc nucleus, comparable to that of a ball-bearing, so stretching the annulus posteriorly and compressing it anteriorly. The opposite movement takes place on extension. The nucleus also moves correspondingly posteriorly and anteriorly (Beattie et al, 1994). Simultaneous movements take place in the zygapophyseal joints as their superior articular processes move in a superior direction on flexion.

Zygapophyseal joints

The synovial posterior zygapophyseal joints are formed from the articular processes, one of which descends from the superior vertebra and the other ascends from the inferior vertebra (Figure 1.6). The joint processes are short and

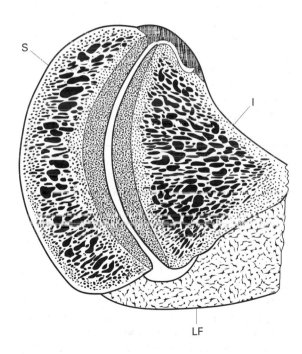

Figure 1.6 A transverse (horizontal) section through a lumbar zygapophyseal joint. Note how the posterior capsule is fibrous and attaches to the inferior articular process (I) well beyond the articular margin, but at its other end it attaches to the superior articular process (S) and the margin of the articular cartilage. The anterior capsule is formed by the ligamentum flavum (LF). Reprinted from *Clinical Anatomy of the Lumbar Spine* by N. Bogduk and L. Twomey with kind permission of Churchill Livingstone

stout and the concave articular surface of the superior process appears to embrace the slightly convex inferior process. The facets on these articular processes are lined by articular cartilage, and the synovial membrane, which extends over their superior and inferior margins (Bogduk and Twomey, 1991), is enclosed by a capsule. The capacious synovial joint so formed contains large superior and inferior recesses, into which synovial folds project, containing vascular adipose tissue (Giles and Taylor, 1987), fibro-adipose meniscoid bodies (Engel and Bogduk, 1982; Bogduk and Engel, 1984; Bogduk and Jull, 1985; Jones et al, 1989) and maybe osseous or cartilaginous bodies (Jensen et al, 1994a). The anteromedial part of the capsule merges with the ligamentum flavum, which can exert a pull on the capsule that can prevent its entrapment within the joint (Mooney and Robertson, 1976). The joints have a rich neural supply (Yamashita et al, 1990) which includes nociceptive fibres (Bogduk and Long, 1980). The medial branch of the dorsal ramus runs medially around the base of the superior articular process to send branches to the joint and to the joints above and below it (Mooney and Robertson, 1976; Bogduk et al, 1982). The synovial folds projecting into the joint cavity are also richly innervated (Giles and Taylor, 1987) and may possibly become entrapped (Giles and Taylor, 1987; Jones et al, 1989).

The zygapophyseal joints are well adapted to their role in assisting movement, resisting forward displacement of the vertebral body, controlling rotation and maintaining stability (Stokes, 1988; Bogduk and Twomey, 1991; Patwardhan, 1994). At each spinal level they play an important role in allowing spinal movements, while at the same time limiting their range and maintaining spinal stability. In the lumbar spine they permit the physiological movements of forward flexion, lateral flexion and extension, but they limit rotation. The physiological movements are aided by the accessory movements in controlling the amplitude, range and direction of movement at each intervertebral joint by a sliding motion of approximately 6 mm between the two plane surfaces of the joints

The sagittally orientated joints protect against axial rotation, and the coronally orientated joints protect against shearing forces (Bogduk and

Twomey, 1991). Opposition of the facet surfaces prevents overdisplacement and so prevents any potential injury to the discs and surrounding ligaments in torsion and shear and to a lesser extent in axial compression and bending (Andersson, 1983; Stokes, 1988; Kahmann et al, 1990).

The shape and orientation of the joint facets determine the degree to which each joint contributes to these various functions (Bogduk

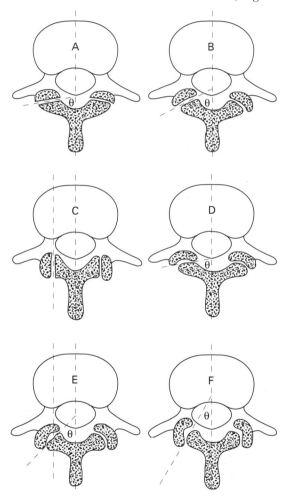

Figure 1.7 The varieties of orientation and curvature of the lumbar zygapophyseal joints. **A:** Flat joints orientated close to 90° to the sagittal place. **B:** Flat joints orientated at 60° to the sagittal plane. **C:** Flat joints orientated parallel (0°) to the sagittal plane. **D:** Slightly curved joints with an average orientation close to 90° to the sagittal plane. **E:** 'C' shaped joints orientated at 45° to the sagittal plane. **F:** 'J' shaped joints orientated at 30° to the sagittal plane. Reprinted from *Clinical Anatomy of the Lumbar Spine* by N. Bogduk and L. Twomey with kind permission of Churchill Livingstone

and Twomey, 1991). In the lumbar spine, the joints show marked variation in their shape and orientation (Figure 1.7), and in the upper lumbar spine they may be curved so that either forward displacement or rotation will be better resisted (Bogduk and Twomey, 1991). Their orientation at the lumbosacral joint also varies, although in general the facets on the inferior articular process of L5 face forward and downward, while those of the sacral facet face backward and upward to prevent any forward slipping.

Aging changes occur in these joints, as they do in the rest of the lumbar spine (Twomey and Taylor, 1985; Taylor and Twomey, 1986; Bogduk and Twomey, 1991). Articular cartilage steadily increases in thickness with maturity. Focal degenerative changes, which begin in the fourth decade and are more marked in the superior process, can be related to the stresses usually applied to these joints. Subchondral bone thickness increases until the age of 50 years and then gradually thins (Twomey and Taylor, 1985; Bogduk and Twomey, 1991).

Spinal nerves

The spinal cord with its dural investment lies within the confines of the vertebral canal, normally ends at about the level of L2 (Figure 1.8), and can usually adapt well to the considerable alterations that need to take place in it during spinal movements. The dorsal and ventral nerve roots emerge from the spinal cord to run a course in close proximity to the bony posterior structures and the intervertebral discs, where they can be easily compressed, before emerging through the intervertebral foramen. The nerve roots are invested by root pouches, funnel-shaped extensions of the spinal dura and arachnoid, which prevent angulation of the nerve roots at their exit from the dural sac and protect them during movement. The nerve root is capable of movement within the intervertebral foramen, and the lower lumbar nerve roots undergo an excursion of approximately 0.5 cm when the leg is passively elevated.

The intervertebral foramen is a short, funnel-shaped opening through which pass the spinal nerves, formed by the union of the ventral and dorsal nerve roots, the sinuvertebral nerve, which is coursing back into the spinal canal, blood vessels, arteries, veins and lymphatics, all cushioned by epidural fat. The foramen is bounded anteriorly by its adjacent vertebral bodies and disc, superiorly and inferiorlly by pedicles, and posteriorly by the superior and inferior articular processes, which have a zygapophyseal joint between them (Figure 1.9). Both the anterior and posterior joints of the mobile intervertebral joint complex help to form the boundaries of this foramen, and degenerative changes in these joints can reduce the foramen's cross-sectional area.

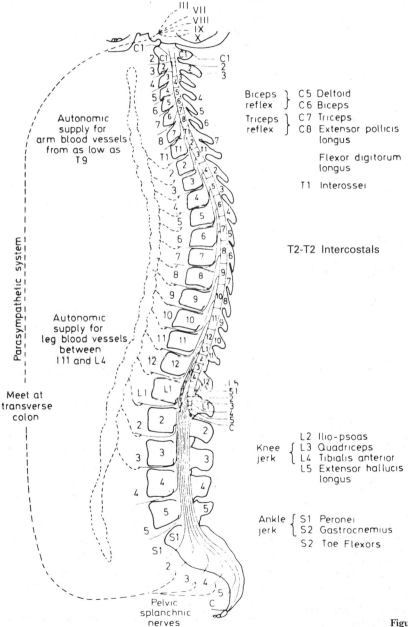

Figure 1.8 Nerve roots and the spine

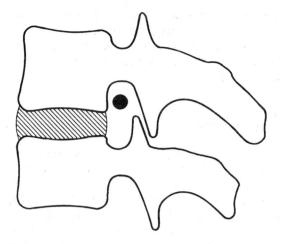

Figure 1.9 The intervertebral foramen with its nerve root is bounded in front by the intervertebral disc and vertebral bodies, above and below by the pedicles, and behind by the apophyseal joint

The ventral and dorsal nerve roots join to form the spinal nerve that divides outside the foramen into anterior, or ventral, and posterior, or dorsal, rami. The posterior primary ramus of L1–L4 travels approximately 5 mm from its origin (Bogduk and Twomey, 1991), and then divides into medial, lateral and intermediate branches (Bogduk and Twomey, 1991). The medial branch is of importance as it innervates the zygapophyseal joint at the same level, together with the one above and the one below (Bogduk, 1983), and also supplies the medially arranged small muscles of the spine. The lateral branch of the posterior primary ramus passes laterally, close to the transverse process, and penetrates the sacrospinalis muscle, which it supplies.

The sinuvertebral nerve arises from the ventral rami, just distal to the dorsal root ganglion. This slender filament is joined by a branch from the sympathetic trunk, and enters the spinal canal through the intervertebral foramen. It divides into an ascending and a descending branch and ends as a fine, arborizing network of free nerve filaments (Figure 1.10). It anastomoses with the

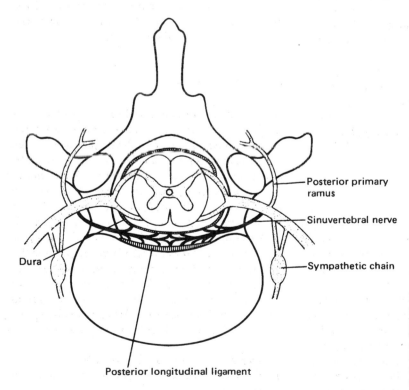

Posterior primary ramus

Sinuvertebral nerve

Sympathetic chain

Dura

Posterior longitudinal ligament

Figure 1.10 The sinuvertebral nerve arises from the spinal nerve and passes back through the intervertebral foramen to supply the dura and posterior longitudinal ligament. The posterior primary ramus is also shown dividing into a medial and a lateral branch

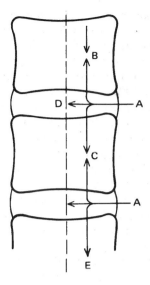

Figure 1.11 The sinuvertebral nerve (A) anastomoses with the nerve above (B) and below (C). It also anastomoses with the nerve from the opposite side (D). It may also pass downwards over several intervertebral segments (E)

sinuvertebral nerve at adjacent levels and also with its contralateral nerve, before being widely distributed (Figure 1.11). It supplies the outer half of the annulus of the disc at its own level (Yoshizawa et al, 1980; Cavanaugh, 1995), and also the one above (Bogduk et al, 1981), the posterior longitudinal ligament, the dura, periosteum and blood vessels (Bogduk and Twomey, 1991). Mechanoreceptors are also present in the disc and longitudinal ligaments (Roberts et al, 1995).

Muscles

The muscles are necessary for movement, provide stability and protection to the joints, assist in shock absorption and aid in the nutrition of the joints. They may be divided into posterior and anterior groups. The posterior group has three layers: a superficial layer, the erector spinae, a large torque producing group that links the pelvis and thoracic cage and acts to stabilize the trunk; a middle layer, the bipennate multifidus; and a deep layer that includes the rotators responsible for segmental stability. Anteriorly placed are the anterior and lateral abdominal

muscles and the psoas muscle. Richardson and Jull (1995) have drawn attention to the role of the transversus abdominis in stabilization of the lumbar spine and its role in rehabilitation in back pain.

Ligaments

The longitudinal ligaments, anterior and posterior, are firmly attached to the of the annulus fibrosus, itself a ligamentous structure, to reinforce it. They act to prevent excessive motion, and are provided with mechanoreceptors to aid in posture and movement (Roberts et al, 1995). The posterior longitudinal ligament diminishes significantly in size the more caudal it becomes (Ohshima et al, 1993), which is of relevance since it has the ability to contain a prolapsed disc (Ohshima et al, 1993).

The ligamentum flavum contains elastic fibres which assist with spinal movements such as standing up from a forward bending position. It forms part of the smooth posterior wall of the spinal canal and of the anterior capsule of the zygapophyseal joint, and helps to maintain that joint in its position (Figure 1.6).

Spinal curves

Before birth, the spinal column is present as a single curvature with its concavity directed forward. The subsequent development of three compensatory curves allows two of them to be curved anteriorly, one in the cervical and one in the lumbar spine, and two of them to be curved posteriorly, one in the thoracic and one in the sacral spine (Figure 1.12). The cervical lordosis develops after the infant is capable of raising the head, and the lumbar lordosis develops after the infant assumes the erect posture and the hips and pelvis are extended. These reciprocal curves allow efficient energy absorption by the spinal column and increase the efficiency of the spinal muscles (Gelb et al, 1995). Other functions are:

- To maintain the upright posture
- To allow ease of movement and increased flexibility

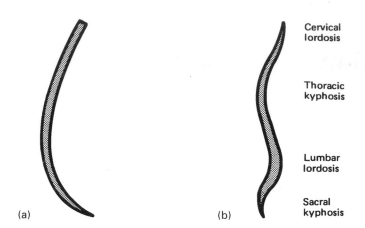

Cervical
lordosis

Thoracic
kyphosis

Lumbar
lordosis

Sacral
kyphosis

(a)   (b)

Figure 1.12 (a) In the fetus the spine has a simple c-shaped curve. (b) In the adult, compensatory curves are formed

- To increase the inherent strength of the spine and resist axial compression
- To increase shock-absorbing properties
- To help spinal stability
- The thoracic and sacral curves are necessary to help contain the thoracic and pelvic contents.

Aging changes

Disc changes are inevitable with aging (Buckwalter et al, 1993), and their structure and chemical composition alter from infancy to old age (Twomey and Taylor, 1985).

At birth, the nucleus has a low collagen content, whereas its proteoglycan content, mainly chondroitin sulphate, and accordingly its water content, is high. The water content, approximately 88 per cent of its total weight, is responsible for the disc turgescence so that the disc will bulge if its gelatinous surface is cut.

With increasing maturity (Urban and McMullin, 1988), the cell content will gradually decrease, the water content also decreases, and the proteoglycan composition varies as the chondroitin sulphate becomes replaced by keratosulphate. Approximately 65 per cent of its content will be made up of proteoglycans, 20 per cent of collagen, and the rest of elastin and other minor components (Fujita et al, 1993). The tensile properties of the annulus fibrosus become lost as the collagen content increases (Acaroglu et al, 1995), with an increase in the ratio of its type I to type II fibres, and it becomes more hyalinized and fragmented. The elastic content falls and there is an increase in the non-collagenous proteins (Ghosh, 1990a; Buckwalter, 1995).

In old age, it is not possible to determine the exact boundaries between the nucleus and the annulus (Buckwalter, 1995). The water content falls to about 70 per cent, and the nucleus has a more solid structure so that it appears dry and granular and has lost its turgescence. The nucleus, devoid of its fluid content, is unable to fulfil its role of translating vertical pressure into horizontal pressure, and these pressures are not applied to the annulus. The markedly reduced incidence of acute disc prolapse in elderly people may be explained by these changes.

Other aging changes that take place in the lumbar spine include: the vertebrae and discs undergo remodelling; ligaments and muscles lose strength and the zygapophyseal joint articular cartilage may fibrillate. There is a significant decrease in the range of all lumbar movements, due to an increase in disc stiffness of up to 40 per cent (Twomey and Taylor, 1985).

2 Disc degeneration

The problem with intervertebral discs is that they are liable to degenerate. Normally, chondrocytes, proteoglycans and collagen function as a unit, and dysfunction or damage to any one of the components from any cause can ultimately result in disc degeneration (Fujita et al, 1993; Jensen et al, 1994a). Also, each component has been implicated as the initiating factor in causing disc degeneration: the annulus fibrosus (Marchand and Ahmed, 1990); cartilage endplate (Sandover, 1983; Miller et al, 1988; Roberts et al, 1989; Modic, 1994); subchondral bone (Modic et al, 1988a; Lenz et al, 1990); and nucleus pulposus (Ohshima and Urban, 1992; Jensen et al, 1994a; Erkintalo et al, 1995). However, which part of this unit actually initiates the process remains unknown (Yu et al, 1989a; Osti et al, 1990). The changes associated with disc degeneration may have some similarities to those of aging, but there are important differences and they result from a different mechanism from that of the aging changes (Kraemer, 1995).

Macroscopically, the early stages of disc degeneration are characterized by progressive fraying and dehydration of the nucleus. Alterations in disc structure develop with tears in the annulus fibrosus (Yu et al, 1989a; Osti et al, 1990; Gordon et al, 1991; Ellenberger, 1994), which are in turn able to initiate further degenerative changes (Yu et al, 1989a; Jensen et al, 1994b; Latham et al, 1994). Three types of tear have been described: radial; rim (transverse or peripheral); and circumferential (or concentric) (Vernon-Roberts and Piric, 1977; Modic et al, 1988a,b; Yu et al, 1989a,b; Osti et al, 1990; Gordon et al, 1991; Bogduk and Twomey, 1991; Modic and Ross, 1991; Latham et al, 1994), which may be filled with vascularized granulation tissue (Ross et al, 1989). Radial tears, which are consistently associated with disc degeneration (Yu et al, 1989a,b), involve all layers of the annulus between the nucleus and the surface of the disc, while transverse tears involve rupture of collagen fibres (Yu et al, 1989a,b; Modic and Ross, 1991).

The end result of disc degeneration is a progressive fibrosis with loss of the distinction between the annulus and the nucleus, the lamellae lose their organization, the cartilage endplate thins out and the disc becomes fissured and crumbling, developing a brown discoloration (Modic et al, 1988a; Modic and Ross, 1991; Jensen et al, 1994a, Francois et al, 1995). As the disc becomes thinner, the changes may be mirrored on X-ray as a loss of disc height (Vernon-Roberts and Pirie, 1977).

Mechanisms

The basic cause of disc degeneration remains unknown, and the two major theories currently described, which are not mutually exclusive, relate to alterations in biochemical and biomechanical factors.

Biochemical factors

Alteration in chondrocyte function probably plays a major role in determining the onset of disc degeneration. There may be a decline in cell nutrition, together with accumulation of lactate and fall in pH, or with an increase in cell senescence and loss of concentration of viable cells (Buckwalter, 1995). The chondrocyte contains enzyme systems which can lead to an increased rate of matrix degradation and alteration (Fujita et al, 1993; Francois et al, 1995). The enzymes include neutral proteinases, such as metalloproteinases and serine proteinases, which can degrade the matrix at neutral pH, plus collagenases (Fujita et al, 1993). The proteoglycan aggregates are degraded, becoming smaller and non-aggregating (Jensen et al, 1994a), the chondroitin sulphate and water contents are decreased, keratan sulphate is increased and collagen fibre types are altered (Vanharanta, 1994). As a result, the rate of matrix synthesis is unable to keep pace with its rate of degradation. However, whether there is any correlation between the biochemical and the histological changes has been questioned (Schiebler et al, 1991; Raininko et al, 1995).

Alteration in the collagen and proteoglycan composition leads to loss of the normal mechanical properties of the disc, which then becomes unable to withstand normal pressures. When the nucleus is damaged, further stress is placed on the annulus, resulting in degeneration of its fibres (Brown, 1971) and ultimately disc degeneration may lead to disc prolapse (Erkintalo et al, 1995) with or without nerve compression.

Biomechanical factors

The discs are normally subjected to flexion, extension, rotation and compression stresses throughout life. In animal experiments (Kaapa et al, 1994), these stresses can lead to disc injury, but its mechanism of production in humans remains conjectural (Jensen et al, 1994a). Two major forces, compression and torsion, can ultimately result in damage to chondrocytes, proteoglycans and collagen fibres (Farfan et al, 1970; Vanharanta et al, 1988a,1989; Bogduk and Twomey, 1991; Vanharanta, 1994).

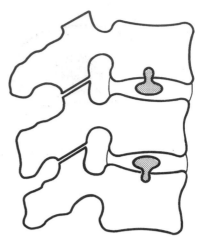

Figure 2.1 A Schmorl's node is formed by a prolapse of the nucleus into the superior or inferior vertebral body

Compression injury follows a fall or heavy lifting that can lead to fracture of the vertebral endplate (Farfan et al, 1972; Bogduk and Twomey, 1991). This may heal, but if not, a Schmorl's node (Figure 2.1), a mushroom-shaped protrusion that is contained by a thin layer of compact bone visible on X-ray, may form (Figure 2.2). Alternatively, a process of nuclear

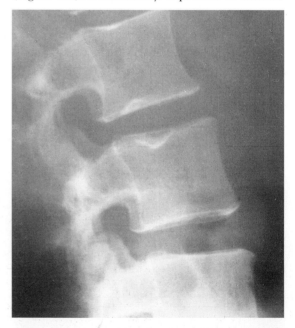

Figure 2.2 Schmorl's nodes

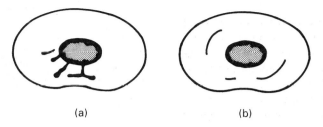

Figure 2.3 (a) Radial fissures in a degenerated annulus; and (b) concentric fissures

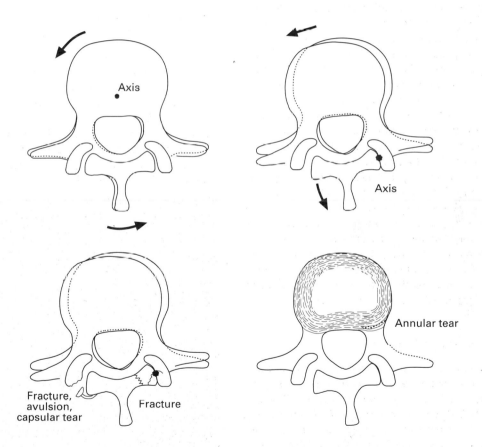

Figure 2.4 Rotation injuries of the lumbar spine. Axial rotation of a lumbar segment is initially limited by impaction of a zygapophyseal joint, but further rotation may occur about a new axis in the impacted joint, resulting in the disc being exposed to a lateral shear force and the contralateral zygapophyseal joint swinging backwards. The impacted zygapophyseal joint may suffer fractures of its articular processes or of the pars interarticularis. The contralateral joint may suffer fracture avulsions or tears of its capsule. The anulus fibrosus of the intervertebral disc may suffer peripheral, circumferential tears. Reprinted from *Clinical Anatomy of the Lumbar Spine* by N. Bogduk and L. Twomey with kind permission of Churchill Livingstone.

degeneration with proteoglycan denaturation, plus loss of proteoglycan aggregation and function, is initiated. The annulus fibrosus is not designed to withstand compression forces, and will ultimately start to fail and buckle, producing disc bulging and annular tears in the process known as internal disc disruption. Radial fissures develop from the nucleus into the annulus (Figure 2.3). They may be asymptomatic at first, but ultimately they may reach the outer annulus, which contains nerve. They can also allow a track through which the nucleus can escape its confines and produce a disc herniation (Modic et al, 1988b, Yu et al, 1989a,b, Ross et al, 1990).

Rotational stresses can produce a posterolateral circumferential tear in the peripheral fibres of the annulus fibrosus (Farfan et al, 1970, 1972; Bogduk and Twomey, 1991) (Figure 2.4). Potentially, these tears could occur with everyday activity such as twisting, and especially twisting and flexion, and ultimately lead to degenerative changes in the other disc components. During rotation, the zygapophyseal joints provide protection to the annular fibres of the disc until the facets become impacted. With further movement, while these same forces are applied, the joint or its contralateral one may be damaged (Bogduk and Twomey, 1991). The annulus is strained in torsion and a peripheral tear can result (Bogduk and Twomey, 1991). The presence of any pre-existent zygapophyseal joint disorder could exacerbate this problem.

Pathophysiological factors

No single factor is known to be responsible for the initiation of disc degeneration (Heliovaara et al, 1991), although some of the known associated features have been identified.

Age and sex

The process of disc degeneration usually commences at a relatively early age, during the second decade in men (Miller et al, 1988; Jensen et al, 1994b; Erkintalo et al, 1995), and reaches its peak during the fourth decade. One or more lumbar discs were degenerated in 57 per cent of

20-year-old patients who had low back pain and in 35 per cent of asymptomatic controls of the same age (Paajanen et al, 1989). It may occur in either sex (Videman et al, 1984, Pope, 1989), but it begins to develop later in women (Jensen et al, 1994a). In men, discs may be more susceptible to degeneration than in women because of the larger size of the disc and hence longer avascular pathways (Miller et al, 1988). In men, the prevalence of disc degeneration decreases after the age of approximately 60 years (Kelsey et al, 1990; Laslett et al, 1991) and it is not common for a first attack of disc prolapse to occur after that age (Heliovaara, 1989; Kelsey, et al 1990; Laslett et al, 1991). Accordingly, disc prolapse is uncommon in juveniles or in elderly people.

Trauma

Trauma was originally assumed to be the sole cause of disc prolapse, a view that was later modified to its being considered the single most important factor. It is now apparent that trauma is rarely implicated as the initiating factor in disc prolapse (Gordon et al, 1991), and a disc prolapse can only be precipitated in an already degenerated disc (Brinkman, 1986). The ability of normal discs to resist direct pressures is such that the force necessary to produce a nuclear prolapse is greater than that required to fracture a vertebra.

Posture

The load imposed on certain areas in the spine may contribute to the increased incidence of disc degeneration at these sites. This applies particularly to the lumbosacral junction, where the fixed sacrum articulates with the flexible lumbar spine so that, as body weight is transferred from the spine to the sacroiliac joints, a shearing force is applied across the lumbosacral disc. Similarly, the lordotic curve in the cervical spine results in an increased load on the C5 and C6 discs at the centre of that curve.

Besides the static loads, dynamic loads are imposed during movement or lifting. When the spine is acting as a first-class lever system, the intradisc pressure can be estimated. In lifting a 90-kg load with the hips and knees locked and the

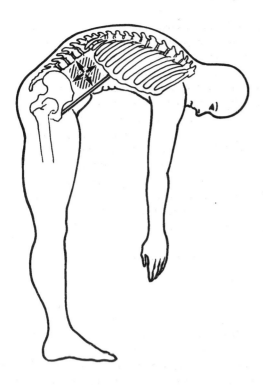

Figure 2.5 The protective role of the intra-abdominal contents in reducing pressure on the spine

back arched, the effect of leverage on the lumbosacral disc can be estimated to produce a load of approximately 1000 kg. Since the spine cannot withstand such great forces, it seems that some compensatory in-vivo mechanism must be present (Dietrich and Kurowski, 1985). Bartelink (1957) proposed that a raised intra-abdominal pressure turned the semi-fluid abdominal contents into a partially solid pillar, so protecting the lumbar spine from some of the effects of weight bearing (Figure 2.5). A similar mechanism was proposed during bending and lifting, when the rise in intra-abdominal pressure again played a role in protecting the spine. Subsequently, this theory had to be modified (Gracovetsky et al, 1985), as it was considered that the role of the abdominal muscles was to brace or extend the lumbar spine by pulling on the thoracolumbar fascia (Bogduk and McIntosh, 1984). Accordingly, the compensatory mechanism still remains to be explained adequately (Bogduk and Twomey, 1991), as there is little consensus as to

the biomechanical role of intra-abdominal pressure during lifting, and the understanding of it remains poor (Marras and Mirka, 1996).

Nachemson and Morris (1964) conducted in-vivo experiments to measure the lower lumbar intradiscal pressures and total loading when volunteers adopted certain standardized positions. Pressure was found to be highest in the sitting position, when the average intradiscal pressure varied from 10 to 15 kg/cm^2, corresponding to a total load of 100–175 kg. Readings in standing subjects were 30 per cent lower than in the sitting subjects, presumed to be due to the effect of an increase in the intra-abdominal pressure. When the subjects were lying down, the readings were 50 per cent lower than when they were sitting. When the subjects wore an inflated abdominal corset, the pressure on the discs was decreased by 25 per cent, possibly due to the effect of increasing compression on the abdominal wall, thereby increasing its protective role. Intradiscal pressure is highest in the sitting position, and this postural problem may be exacerbated by the poor design of most modern chairs. Car seats are often poorly adapted to normal spinal mechanics, and may be associated with the reported increased prevalence of back disorders in motor-vehicle drivers.

It has been customary to lay blame on humankind's upright stance, and consider that the human spine has not evolved to an appropriate degree for it to compensate, as the basic cause of disc degeneration (Evans, 1982). Rats that are made to walk on their hindlegs develop disc degeneration in the lumbosacral disc (Cassidy et al, 1988). Alternatively, Putz and Muller-Gerbl (1996) found the spine to be ideally adapted to its role in stability and movement in the upright posture. In addition, some four-legged animals develop disc degeneration with subsequent disc prolapse. These include some breeds of dogs, cats (Ghosh, 1990b), rodents (Ziran et al, 1994) and experimental animals in whom the discs have the same basic structure as human discs (Osti et al, 1990; Moore et al, 1996).

Other postural abnormalities that have been proposed include: an increase or decrease in lumbar lordosis; scoliosis; unequal leg length; hamstring tightness; weak abdominal and back musculature; pregnancy (Ostgaard et al, 1991);

or use of incorrect footwear, any of which may play some part in producing abnormal spinal mechanical stresses. Radiological surveys have been undertaken to attempt to confirm the relationship between these abnormalities and disc disorder. La Rocca and Macnab (1970) described two groups, each of 150 people aged between 35 and 40 years, who had been engaged in heavy work all of their adult lives. The members of one group had no back symptoms, while those in the other were having treatment for low back pain. The radiological anatomical variants, especially lordosis and the lumbosacral angle, were similar in both groups. Similarly, Hult (1954) was unable to demonstrate any correlation between the presence of lumbar lordosis and disc degeneration.

Occupation

Some occupations or sporting activities (Howell, 1984; Sward et al, 1990a; Videman et al, 1995a) involve heavy workloads with extremes of bending or twisting or prolonged standing or sitting, which are important aetiological factors for disc degeneration (Videman et al, 1990, 1995a). Labourers, especially those who are required to handle heavy weights (Sandover, 1983; Svensson and Andersson, 1989; Frymoyer et al, 1983; Kelsey et al, 1984a; Bigos et al, 1986; Heliovaara, 1989; Riihimaki et al, 1989, 1990; Hsu et al, 1990; Holmstrom et al, 1992; Videman et al, 1995b), and members of the nursing profession (Kumar, 1990) have an increased incidence of disc degeneration. Battie et al (1995) found that heavy lifetime workload was associated with increased disc degeneration in the upper lumbar discs, but that leisure time heavy loading was the sole factor associated with increased degeneration in the lower lumbar discs.

An increased incidence of disc degeneration may be related to the sustained disc loading, especially at or towards the limit of lumbar flexion in some occupations, with the result that a considerable amount of fluid is expressed from the disc (Twomey and Taylor, 1995). Alternatively, it may be a function of the cumulative biomechanical load over the exposure time (Kumar, 1990). Problems may be exacerbated if lifting methods are incorrect (Biering-Sorensen et al, 1989), or if bending and lifting are undertaken in awkward positions. Correct lifting techniques are important (Mundt et al, 1983, Kelsey et al, 1984a), and improper lifting techniques are perhaps the most frequent cause of back injury (Bigos et al, 1986). Risks are increased by lifting heavy weights at an average of over five times a day, or twisting while lifting and with the knees kept straight (Kelsey et al 1984a). Driving (Frymoyer et al, 1983; Pope, 1989; Malchaire and Masset, 1995), especially driving heavy vehicles (Pope, 1989; Burdof and Zondervan, 1990), may cause added strains, and drivers may also be required to perform increased bending and lifting tasks (Howell, 1984). However, psychosocial factors, such as boredom resulting from monotonous work tasks, may also have a role (Vallfors, 1985; Frymoyer et al, 1983).

Vibration

Vibration is regarded as a common problem in disc degeneration (Sandover, 1983; Bongers et al, 1988, 1990; Wilder et al, 1982, 1985; Burdof and Zondervan, 1990; Videman et al, 1990; Hansson and Holm, 1991; Johanning, 1991; Boshuizen et al, 1992; Bovenzi and Zadini, 1992; Pietri et al, 1992; Pope and Hansson, 1992), and vibration in the range of 4–5 Hz is implicated, as it corresponds to the resonating frequency of the seated human spine (Wilder et al, 1985). Drivers of heavy vehicles (Kelsey, 1975; Pope, 1989), and crane operators have increased levels of disc degeneration over controls (Bongers et al, 1988).

Sedentary living

Lack of activity and exercise are known to play an important role in some disease processes, such as coronary heart disease. All elements of the musculoskeletal system react adversely to inactivity, with loss of tissue (Twomey and Taylor, 1995). The spine requires movement and exercise at all stages of life to maintain function (Twomey and Taylor, 1995), so a sedentary occupation may be an increased hazard for disc degeneration (Kelsey and Ostfield, 1975; Evans et al, 1989; Salminen et al, 1993), and it may be enhanced by the increase in disc pressure that occurs when sitting (Nachemson and Morris, 1964; Nachemson and Elfstrom, 1970). Spinal intervertebral joint motion and the action of the surrounding muscles aid the nutrition of the normal disc, which is dependent on fluid exchange. Lack of exercise results in a loss of these normal forces, so that disc nutrition could become disturbed, leading to degenerative changes (Cox and Trier, 1987; Evans et al, 1989). Much of the productivity lost in industry due to back pain may be related to the physical changes that result directly from bedrest and inactivity (Deyo and Bass, 1989).

Activity

Activity is helpful and plays a prophylactic role in aiding disc nutrition (Cady et al, 1979; Porter et al, 1989; Burton et al, 1989; Burton and Tillotson, 1991; Leino, 1993; Videman et al, 1995a). Vigorous exercise has been shown to increase disc nutrition in animals (Holm and Nachemson, 1988; Ghosh, 1990b) and, by inference, immobilization would have an opposite effect (Ghosh, 1990b). Although the role of activity has been questioned (Battie et al, 1989), regular participation in exercise and sports is associated with less back pain in later adulthood (Videman et al, 1995a), despite any increase in X-ray degenerative changes in some sports (Videman et al, 1995a). There are no apparent benefits from vigorous exercise as compared with light to moderate levels of exercise (Videman et al, 1995a).

Congenital anomalies

Congenital anomalies in the lumbosacral spine are a common finding (Tini et al, 1977), and their relevance to degenerative disc disease remains controversial. Some conditions, such as variations in the numbers of lumbar vertebrae, spina bifida occulta (SBO) or transitional vertebrae have been considered as being of no clinical significance. However, a higher incidence of disc prolapse in patients with SBO at the lumbosacral junction was found by Avrahami et al (1994), who argued that it was not a benign condition, but that it was a cause of vertebral instability and disc degeneration.

A considerable degree of anatomical interchange is possible between the last lumbar and

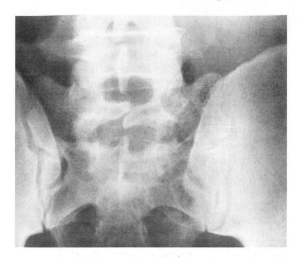

Figure 2.6 Congenital anomalies at L5 and S1

first sacral segments, so that one may have the physical characteristics of the other (Figure 2. 6). Transitional vertebrae, such as sacralization and lumbarization, were found on CT or MRI to be associated with disc degeneration at the level above it (Elster, 1989). Transitional vertebrae, particularly if there is fusion on one side and a false joint on the other side, or lumbosacral facet asymmetry, may lead to increased mechanical strains with consequent disc degeneration. In most cases these anomalies are asymptomatic, but symptoms may arise in two situations. First, the lower lumbar joints may be subjected to an increased and asymmetrical stress, leading to accelerated disc degeneration. When the lower lumbar segment is completely sacralized, disc degeneration may occur at the spinal level immediately above it. If sacralization is unilateral, disc degeneration tends to occur on the contralateral side at the same level. Second, the pseudarthrosis formed between the lumbar transverse process and the sacrum may undergo degenerative changes and may be associated with localized back pain.

The lumbosacral zygapophyseal joints may lie in asymmetric planes, called tropism, so that one or both lies in the sagittal rather than the coronal plane. Although not significant in itself, it may contribute to disc degeneration (Farfan et al, 1970, Farfan, 1984). Some correlation between asymmetric joints and disc degeneration has been described (Noren et al, 1991; Hagg and Wallner, 1990), although it has not been confirmed (Cassidy et al, 1992a; Vanharanta et al, 1993). The obliquely oriented joint may be less capable of resisting rotation, so predisposing to a loss of normal rhythmic movement and ultimately to disc degeneration or vertebral instability (Farfan et al, 1972).

Heredity

Hereditary factors are known to be important in some breeds of animals, including certain breeds of dogs and cats (Ghosh, 1990b), which are more prone to the development of disc degeneration. For some time it has also been considered that heredity may play a role in humans, since it is not uncommon to find some families with a high familial incidence. However, this could be due to environmental rather than hereditary factors. Studies in humans have been conducted to support the role of heredity versus environmental risk factors in disc degeneration (Porter and Thorp, 1986; Postacchini et al, 1988; Kelsey et al, 1990; Battie et al, 1991, 1995; Varlotta et al, 1991). Battie et al (1995) investigated 115 pairs of identical twins with MRI and using multivariate analysis. They concluded that the general concordance of disc degeneration in twins could be explained primarily on the basis of genetic influences, and that environmental factors played only a minor role. In a cohort study of 640 schoolchildren followed for 25 years (Harreby et al, 1995), the two risk factors discovered for back pain in adulthood were a family history and pain during the adolescent growth spurt. Also, in one

trial, the first-degree relatives of teenage patients had more disc degeneration than did controls (Kelsey et al, 1990).

Obesity

It seems most reasonable to advise overweight patients with low back pain to reduce their weight. But it is not so easy to prove that obesity, or rather an increased body mass index, plays a causal role in disc degeneration (Battie et al, 1990a). Two large series (Bostman, 1993; Makela et al, 1993) found an increased body mass index to be associated with low back pain and disc degeneration, although it seems that the greatest risk occurs in women who are at least 20 per cent overweight (Deyo and Bass, 1989).

Smoking

Numerous studies have addressed the relationship between disc degeneration and smoking (Frymoyer et al, 1983; Svensson et al, 1983; Kelsey et al, 1984b; Cady and Trier, 1987; Holm and Nachemson, 1988; Deyo and Bass, 1989; Biering-Sorensen and Thomsen, 1986; Biering-Sorensen et al, 1989; Battie et al, 1989; Frymoyer, 1992; Boshuizen et al, 1993). Causative factors that have been suggested include reduction in the blood supply (Frymoyer et al, 1983), or that smokers may live more sedentary lives, or cough more (Kelsey et al, 1984b). After quitting smoking, the increased risk still remains for some time (Deyo and Bass, 1989). However, one paper found no correlation between smoking and disc degeneration (Boishuizen et al, 1993).

3 Low back pain

Low back pain is the most common complaint among patients who present with musculoskeletal disorders. It may be:

1. Vertebrogenic, arising from vertebral column disorders
2. Arising from visceral structures
3. Vascular in origin
4. Psychogenic in origin.

Vertebrogenic disorders

Vertebrogenic disorders, disorders of the vertebral column, are the most common causes of low back pain, and any of the innervated structures in the back may produce somatic pain. Their classification has always been difficult and the lack of any practical, widely accepted classification is one reason why their management remains a problem. Classifying spinal pain would be straightforward if the underlying pathology were always known, but in a large proportion of patients it is not. Most classifications consist chiefly of lists, such as the anatomical or neural structures involved and their lesions, but are of no practical value in a clinical setting.

A practical approach clinically is to diagnose those disorders in which the pathology has been well described. This first category comprises two main groups: one group is the rheumatological vertebral disorders (*see* Chapter 7); and the other

is those with intervertebral disc degeneration and its sequelae (*see* Chapter 5). Diagnosis of these disorders can usually be made clinically according to their symptoms and signs together with ancillary tests, such as X-rays and laboratory tests, or more extensive investigations if necessary.

The problem is that after identifying all those causes with a known pathological basis, a considerable number of patients with low back pain remain, but in whom no demonstrable pathological basis for their symptoms can be identified. Classification in this second category remains a problem and it can be made only on a clinical basis by describing certain clinical syndromes. Many patients in this category have a mechanical derangement of movement in the spinal intervertebral joint complex, associated with alterations in the normal pattern and range of spinal joint movements The mechanical derangement may be due to several causes, including zygapophyseal joint disorders, and is discussed in Chapter 6.

Some clinical features of mechanical low back pain include: back pain is worse as the day goes on, and is usually made better with rest and night pain is absent; pain varies from day to day or even by the hour and is made worse by heavy activity although it may not be felt until some time after the activity has ceased; there may be some stiffness after rest, although it is usually of a minor degree and eases again on movement; pain may be associated with a sensation of catching and constitutional symptoms and signs are lacking. These mechanical symptoms are to be contrasted with those of the inflammatory spinal disorders in which pain and stiffness are usually worse first thing in the morning, are often severe, are made worse with rest and constitutional signs may be marked.

Pain in disc degeneration

The early stages of intervertebral disc degeneration are painless, since at this stage the innermost fibres of the annulus fibrosus or the cartilage endplate, which lack any nerve fibres, are involved. Also, the disc is normal in appearance, and clinical diagnosis at this stage is not possible. Moreover, some patients, even after disc degeneration has developed, still may remain asymptomatic (Powell et al, 1986; Boden et al, 1990a; Vanharanta, 1994; Erkintalo et al, 1995). Pain becomes evident when radial tears associated with internal disc disruption develop and neural fibres in the outer annulus become involved (Bogduk et al, 1981; Coppes et al, 1990; Bogduk and Twomey, 1991). Pain is usually felt as a deep, dull ache, usually localized at first, but it may be referred more widely, especially to the buttock area. Pain tends to be relieved by rest and is exacerbated by activities that stress the disc, including bending. Nerve root pain and neurological symptoms do not occur. Plain X-rays are usually normal at first or may show indirect changes such as some evidence of loss of disc height. Subsequently, the clefts that develop in the disc will become visible as the vacuum phenomenon (Francois et al, 1995), and after some time, marginal osteophytes will start to be formed (Francois et al, 1995). MRI (Pevsener et al, 1986; Tertti et al, 1990; Ellenberger, 1994; Jensen et al, 1994a,b; Herzog et al, 1995; Simmons et al, 1995; Videman et al, 1995b; Boden, 1996) is the best imaging modality since it can measure any alteration in the water content of the nucleus, and it may show other changes, including an annular tear, at an early stage. However, it may also be positive in an asymptomatic patient (Boden et al, 1990a; Boden, 1996). In one study (Boden et al, 1990a), MRI was performed on 67 individuals who had never had low back or leg pain and about one-third had a substantial abnormality. Of

those aged under 60 years, 20 per cent had a herniated disc, and disc bulging was also a common finding. MRI may also be normal in the presence of an abnormal discogram (Zucherman et al, 1988; Osti and Fraser, 1992; Gunzberg et al, 1992; Brightbill et al, 1994; Boden, 1996).

Provocative discography and CT-discograhy (Vanharanta et al, 1987; Bogduk, 1991; Bogduk and Modic, 1996) have also been used. To be considered positive, discography must reproduce the patient's pain, while the discs at adjacent levels do not reproduce the pain (Vanharanta et al, 1987, 1988b; Bogduk and Modic, 1996). The greater the degree of disc disruption, the more likely it is that the pain will be reproduced. Local anaesthetic injected into the affected disc should then abolish it for a time.

The natural history of disc degeneration at this stage remains unknown (Rhyne et al, 1995), although the outcome in discogram-positive, unoperated patients has been reported as being good (Rhyne et al, 1995). Surgery is not often undertaken, although a fusion may be performed, but the results are usually disappointing.

Sciatica

Sciatica is pain in the distribution of the sciatic nerve or its branches, resulting from direct nerve root pressure or irritation. It does not include leg pain referred from the spinal joints. The vast majority of cases of sciatica follow an entrapment neuropathy of a lumbosacral nerve root either in the spinal canal or in the intervertebral foramen, the most common cause being a prolapsed intervertebral disc. Prolapse of nuclear material through an already weakened annulus fibrosus produces a space-occupying lesion in the spinal canal with compression of the nerve roots and their dural sleeves. Bony entrapment may occur laterally along the course of the nerve root as it traverses the inner border of the superior articular facet, where the nerve lies in a gutter before passing around the pedicle to emerge through the intervertebral foramen. Less common forms of extradural space-occupying lesions (Transfeldt et al, 1993) include a tumour, abscess, haematoma or synovial cyst (Figure 3.1). A synovial cyst is a diverticulum (Francois et al,

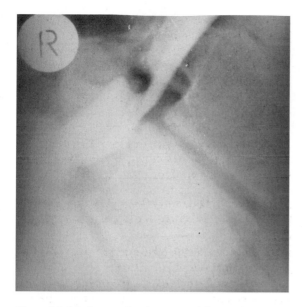

Figure 3.1 Myelogram showing a synovial cyst arising from the zygapophyseal joint

1995) that arises when zygapophyseal joint synovium prolapses through the medial margin of the recess, especially the cranial one (Jensen et al; 1994a; Francois et al, 1995; Hsu et al, 1995; Kornberg, 1995). It may calcify or else erode the adjacent bone (Francois et al, 1995).

The usual history in patients with sciatica is one of intermittent attacks of low back pain that can recur over some years. In one such attack sciatic pain develops and the back pain may be relieved (Deyo et al, 1990a). Pain is usually described as severe, sharp and having an unpleasant nagging quality, with sensory changes distributed along the corresponding dermatome (Figure 3.2). However, among the majority of patients who have low back pain, nerve root compression is not a particularly common symptom (Mooney, 1987; Bogduk, 1991), and the mechanism of its production is not completely understood (Rydevik et al, 1984; Mooney, 1987; Hasue, 1993; Kawakami et al, 1994a,b; Garfin et al, 1995; Olmarker et al, 1995). Compression of a normal peripheral nerve produces sensory and motor changes, but not pain (Olmarker and Rydevik, 1991; Kuslich et al, 1991). Similarly, compression

alone of a lumbosacral nerve root does not cause pain (Olmarker and Rydevik, 1991; Kuslich et al, 1991; Kawakami et al, 1994a,b; Garfin et al, 1995). The lumbar spinal nerve roots have unique structural, vascular and metabolic regions in the nervous system, as they have no epineurium and are dependent upon the cerebrospinal fluid for nutrition and so could react differently to spinal nerves (Parke and Watanabe, 1985; Mooney, 1987). However, compression of an inflamed nerve root does produce pain (Rydevik et al, 1984; Garfin et al, 1995). In an in vivo experiment at operation, Kuslich et al (1991) found that a normal nerve root was insensitive to pressure, whereas stretching produced mild paraesthesia only, but that stimulation of a compressed or stretched nerve root produced marked pain. The pain was eliminated when local anaesthetic was instilled. In addition, pressure over the posterior longitudinal ligament and the annulus at operation was found to produce back pain but not leg pain.

Accordingly, mechanical compression of a nerve root is not sufficient to cause pain and is further evidenced by the findings at myelography, CT and MRI in which 20–30 per cent of disc prolapses remain asymptomatic (Hitselberger and Witten, 1968; Holt, 1968; Weisel et al, 1984; Deyo et al, 1990a; Hasue, 1993). That an inflammatory component is required to produce pain has been demonstrated experimentally (Kawakami et al, 1994a,b), and in humans (Smyth and Wright, 1958; Marshall et al, 1977; McCarron et al, 1987; Greenbarg et al, 1988; Kuslich et al, 1991; Olmarker et al, 1993, 1995; Hasue, 1993; Willburger and Wittenberg, 1994; Saal, 1995; Takahashi et al, 1996). At operation, the deformed nerve root is stretched over the disc, and is found to be inflamed (Dilke et al, 1973; Greenbarg et al, 1988; Kuslich et al, 1991). Injection of 10 ml of saline around the nerve root produces an increased inflammatory change (Dilke et al, 1973), and caused an exacerbation of pain. The successful use of extradural corticosteroid injections in patients with disc prolapse most likely acts by relieving this inflammatory oedema (Dilke et al, 1973; Olmarker et al, 1994, 1995).

Many agents, inflammatory, biochemical and vascular, are potential initiators of the inflamma-

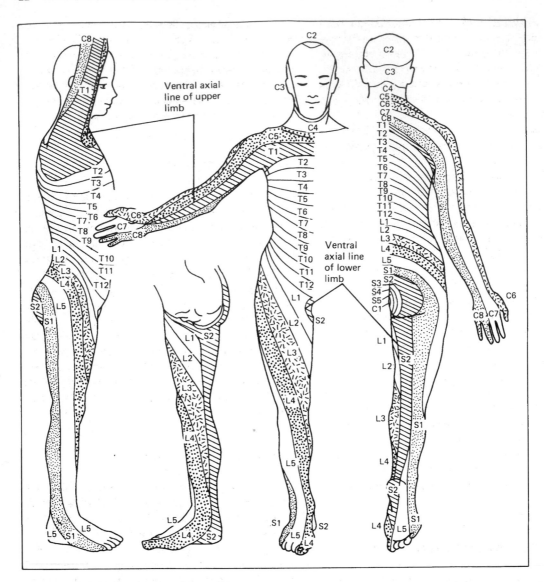

Figure 3.2 Dermatome chart based on embryological segments

tory change, including phospholipase A2 (PLA2) (Saal et al, 1992; Hasue, 1993; Saal, 1995), a variety of cytokines (Hasue, 1993; Wehling et al, 1996) such as interleukin 1 (Wehling et al, 1996), nucleus pulposus, substance P (Beaman et al, 1993; Cavanaugh, 1995), and calcitonin gene-related peptide (CGRP) (Weinstein, 1991). Phospholipase A2, an inflammogen (Franson et al, 1992) is released from the discs in high concentrations (Saal et al, 1992, Willburger and Wittenberg, 1994) and is responsible for the

release of prostaglandins, themselves potent inflammatory mediators, from cell membranes. Prostaglandin E2 is also produced by the cytokines interleukin 1α and tumour necrosis factor α, which are produced by chondrocytes and found in increased numbers in disc tissue taken at operation (Takahashi et al, 1996). Several neuropeptides, including substance P and CGRP (Weinstein, 1991), released from the dorsal root ganglion, are involved in nociception transmission and the sensitization of nerve fibres (Kawakami et al, 1994a,b), and produce vasodilatation, plasma extravasation and histamine release (Cavanaugh, 1995). Autologous nucleus pulposus (McCarron et al, 1987; Olmarker et al, 1993, 1995; Cavanaugh, 1995) has also been used experimentally to produce an inflammatory reaction.

Inflammation may follow chemical irritation from degraded disc material spilling into the extradural space (Marshall et al, 1977). Marshall et al (1977) reasoned that some of the pain from disc prolapse results from the local chemical irritation of nerve roots from these substances at the site of disc injury. Lactic acid, produced under the anaerobic conditions of disc metabolism (Ohshima and Urban, 1992), may be another source of chemical irritation (Nachemson, 1969). Vascular changes may also play a role (Jayson et al, 1984; Cooper et al, 1995; Olmarker and Rydevik, 1991; Olmarker et al, 1993; Garfin et al, 1995). Arterial lesions that result from stretching the nerve root may lead to ischaemia. Venous congestion may also play a role, which may help to explain the exacerbation of pain that occurs with coughing or straining. Venograms of the vertebral plexus show abnormal patterns due to venous obstruction that result in dilatation of the epidural and subarachnoid venous plexuses.

Spinal pain that occurs in other conditions, including other disc disorders and zygapophyseal joint pain, are considered later in their appropriate chapters.

Pain from visceral structures

Pain in the back may be referred from retroperitoneal, pelvic or intra-abdominal structures. Retroperitoneal causes include disorders of the abdominal aorta or kidneys. Intra-abdominal lesions include peptic ulcer, pancreatitis, gall bladder disease and endometriosis. In the thoracic region, pleurisy, aortic aneurysm, coronary heart disease or bronchial carcinoma may produce back pain.

For the correct diagnosis of any of these disorders an accurate history and general examination is needed. Most cases of visceral pain will have associated features that should provide the necessary clue, and pain should not be made worse by spinal movements. In some patients who have a visceral disease, such as gall bladder disease, an associated area of referred pain and muscle spasm may be found in the paravertebral muscles. Pressure over this area may reproduce the pain, and local anaesthetic injected into these locally tender areas may relieve the pain.

Vascular lesions

Back and buttock pain may occur in patients with an aneurysm of the abdominal aorta or a lesion of the abdominal aorta at its bifurcation, due to atherosclerosis or trauma. Pain may be either constantly present or of a typically claudicant variety that follows exertion and is relieved by rest. Diagnosis is made by finding an abdominal swelling or alterations in the peripheral pulses in the lower limbs, together with a normal spinal examination. Diagnosis of an abdominal aneurysm is confirmed on ultrasound (LaRoy et al, 1989) or abdominal CT. Vascular disorders in the limbs need to be differentiated from spinal canal stenosis, which also causes a claudicant type pain.

Psychogenic factors

Assessment of patients with back pain is not complete after establishing a physical diagnosis alone, for psychological and emotional reactions may also need to be assessed. A person's body image is derived from the sensory input from the outside world, postural reactions and emotional and subconscious influences. The importance of the back in this image is reflected in many everyday expressions and in the patient's belief that the back is a complex, easily damaged structure. In patients with chronic low back pain, in whom a structural diagnosis can be made with confidence in only about 50 per cent (Frymoyer, 1988), it is inevitable that psychogenic or psychosocial factors should be considered as being of some significance (Frymoyer, 1988). Their prevalence remains uncertain. One problem is to avoid overlooking their diagnosis on the one hand and overdiagnosing them on the other. Accordingly, considerable expertise may be needed to prevent a patient with an organic disease from receiving an incorrect diagnostic label, while examples abound of patients with an organic disease, including even secondary deposits, who have been incorrectly diagnosed as having a psychosomatic disorder.

Developing adequate research tools has also been a problem. The Minnesota Multiphasic Personality Inventory (MMPI) is the most commonly used (Block et al, 1996), and others that have been developed include AGPAR, Health Locus of Control, and work profiles. Pain drawings can be a most useful tool (Mann et al, 1993; Vucetic et al, 1995; Ohlund et al, 1996).

Patients who present with solely psychogenic low back pain are uncommon (Kanner, 1994), although the influence of psychological factors, such as anxiety and tension, on a patient's reactions and pain are more common. Some patients present a picture of smouldering resentment concerning their circumstances and it becomes much easier to blame a painful back as the cause of all their trouble. A patient with an inadequate personality may be unable to formalize conflict after a stressful situation by appropriate action or expression. Alternatively, some are able to find sympathy and attention from their family with their complaint of backache, especially if the back needs to be visibly supported in a brace. For these patients, pain and suffering may become a way of life. Others may have a low pain tolerance, sometimes associated with an inability to accept any form of bodily discomfort, and may make excessive use of their hands, both in their description of pain and in the demonstration of its site.

Some problems may be iatrogenically determined, exacerbated by the lack of a firm, accurate medical diagnosis or prognosis, or because of an incorrect use of a diagnostic label such as 'arthritis' or 'spondylitis'. These patients often present with aged X-rays on which minor osteophytic lipping has been highlighted with arrows drawn by the radiologist and are convinced that their ultimate fate is to be crippled in a wheelchair. It is impossible to cure arrows.

Diagnosis

When assessing musculoskeletal disorders, an accurate history of the site of pain, its quality,

degree, rate of onset, periodicity and modification by such external factors as rest, movement, physical activities and diurnal variations, help to establish an organic pattern to the symptoms. Musculoskeletal pain is usually described as being dull and aching, made worse with movement; its site, radiation and behavioural patterns are also consistent. The detection of signs is based on knowledge of anatomical relationships so that besides eliciting any positive, confirmatory signs it is also important to record relevant negative findings. Thus the presence of organic disease is confirmed by finding signs that are consistent with the symptoms and by the absence of inconsistent signs.

A typical problem patient who complains of low back pain, on the other hand, often describes pain as being variable and diffuse (Leavitt et al, 1982), and uses terms such as 'throbbing', 'burning', 'numbing', 'a pressure' or 'knife-like'. Pain is generalized and not localized to recognized anatomical sites, its site and radiation are often inconsistent, may be constantly present ('day and night'), and is unrelieved by most medications ('nothing ever works with me'). A first reaction during the history taking is to offer a detailed history of how an accident happened at work or some perceived psychological insult. Symptoms are often only vaguely described, often with the use of the hands to indicate areas of involvement, or they may be conscious of symptoms being exacerbated at times of increased stress. At times, patients are content to rely on old X-rays or reports to justify their claim about the severity of pain rather than on a detailed history of current problems.

Great difficulty may be experienced in assessing a patient who has, or has had, an organic back lesion, but whose symptoms are exacerbated or prolonged by psychological factors. Knowledge of psychological stresses or conflict that the patient has undergone, such as loss of a relative, recent domestic trauma, impending litigation proceedings can then be of benefit. In patients who have a psychogenic overlay, symptoms are usually out of proportion to signs. Pain is often described as 'agonizing' without the patient exhibiting any obvious degree of suffering. They show inconsistency in either the anatomic relationship ('pain radiates up and down the spine'), its reaction to external factors or in a prolongation of normally expected rates of healing.

Examination may reveal a lack of consistently positive signs, or there may be inconsistent signs such as a discrepancy between the reported degree of pain and the ability to move the affected parts, or complaints of marked tenderness. While testing, the knowledge of anatomy is utilized to assess the consistency of the patient's responses, of pain patterns with inconsistent joint findings, and finding abnormal postures or gait. Some patients report that pain is produced during formal clinical testing, but may not show any discomfort later while performing natural movements such as dressing. Alternatively, another test may be performed without the patient realizing that the same joints and muscle groups are again being stressed. For example, while standing a patient may report that back pain is made worse by spinal extension, yet no pain is reported while lying prone with the legs extended or weakness may be complained of in the absence of any muscular atrophy. Waddell et al (1980) reported five non-organic tests to identify those who amplified their pain. These are: tenderness is often non-anatomical; pressure on the vertex causes pain; discrepancies in the straight leg raising test between sitting and supine; stocking distribution of hyperesthesia; and over-reaction to the examination. These tests were corroborated by Werneke et al (1993) in patients who did not return to work. Two other useful tests were added by Kummel (1996), who found that in these patients, neck movements or limitation of shoulder movements were able to produce back pain.

Management

The management of a patient with psychogenically determined symptoms may be difficult, if for no other reason than it takes a deal of time explaining to them where their real problem lies. The first requirement should always be to obtain the patient's confidence (often said, but in practice so often overlooked), and accept that their symptoms are real to them. The patient should never be told that there is nothing wrong or that the symptoms are imaginary. An accurate diagnosis is the next requirement to enable a firm reassurance about the origin of the symptoms. Considerable time needs to be taken explaining their origin and significance (Lacroix et al, 1990). Often such patients have been diagnosed as having arthritis, and have been treated unsuccessfully for this presumed diagnosis, so some time must be spent in reassuring them that that diagnosis is not correct. If symptoms are sufficiently disabling, a pain clinic or a psychiatrist's help should be enlisted at an early stage (Altmaier et al, 1992).

Anti-inflammatory drug therapy does not produce any great benefit, and in most cases these patients have already gone through the gamut to no avail. Simple analgesics such as paracetemol are to be preferred. Antidepressant tablets taken in a sufficient dosage are usually of marked benefit in those who are depressed, and can also help sufferers of chronic pain.

Physical methods of treatment are contraindicated as they tend to confirm the patient's fears of having an underlying organic basis, while at the same time being most unlikely to provide any benefit.

Other well-described psychological states have been associated with low back pain. Of these, anxiety states and depression are relatively common and hysteria and malingering, are decidedly uncommon.

Anxiety states

Tension associated with an underlying anxiety state is perhaps the most common psychogenic problem and can be associated with pain (Arntz et al, 1994). Symptoms of an anxiety state are the musculoskeletal expression of the underlying tension. Prolonged contraction of back muscles, ultimately leading to pain and fatigue, can be used to explain to patients the proposed mechanism of their symptoms. Contributory factors include a patient's family or social situation and, at times, an underlying depression may also be present. There may be a family history of arthritis or spondylosis, so a patient's anxiety that he or she will also eventually become crippled is very real. Patients complain of back and other musculoskeletal aches and pains, usually present over a long period of time, and have usually been given several unhelpful diagnostic labels. Symptoms usually include: stiffness, weakness and clicking in the spine; a feeling of exhaustion; lack of well-being; and, often, poor sleep patterns. Previous treatment will usually have been with a wide variety of tablets, all singularly unsuccessful.

Depression

Overt depression is usually easy to diagnose as it presents with sustained lowering of mood or loss of interest in pleasurable events. It consists of: (1) Cognitive changes with faulty thinking patterns; (2) vegetative disturbances in biological rhythms with loss of appetite and sleep; and (3) psychomotor slowing in physical activity, speech and thought. Symptoms need to be present for at least three weeks. If the patient becomes agitated or restless, it may be difficult to differentiate depression from an anxiety tension state.

Depressed patients often present with various somatic symptoms, among which musculoskeletal symptoms, especially low back pain (Magni et al, 1994), are common (Craufurd et al, 1990). The problem with many patients is to determine which comes first: whether the low back pain is causing depression (Wesley et al, 1991) or whether depression is causing back pain. No easy answer to this question is possible, as it will often be impossible to determine in any one particular patient, since pain promotes depression and

depression promotes pain (Magni et al, 1993, 1994).

Back pain tends to be described as being deep, centred in the lumbar midline, is severe and often unremitting, and is often worse during the early hours or first thing in the morning. Patients feel tired and exhausted and need to lie down frequently, although their fatigue is not relieved. Disturbances of sleep pattern, either an inability to get to sleep, or more commonly, waking early in the morning, aid in the diagnosis. Inevitably, the patient will blame the sleep problems on his or her low back pain.

Management may require psychiatric assessment and includes the use of the newer anti-depressants, the reversible monoamine oxidase inhibitors and serotonin reuptake inhibitors which are usually well tolerated and effective.

Hysteria

In some patients, this reaction may be an expression of a psychological need or conflict (Kanner, 1994). There may be a secondary gain to be obtained, either as a financial reward or as an emotional advantage in their interpersonal relationships, usually within the family. However, the secondary gain may not be readily obvious.

The typical hysterical reaction in back patients is camptocormia, derived from the Greek word for 'bent trunk'. There is an exaggerated back

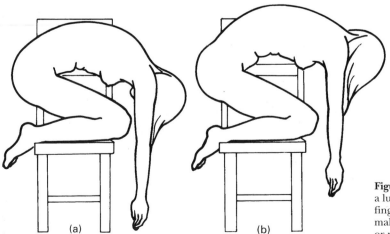

Figure 3.3 Burn's test. (a) A patient with a lumbar disc prolapse can still touch the fingers to the floor. (b) A patient who is malingering often cannot touch the floor or may overbalance

stiffness, usually associated with complaints of diffuse lumbar pain, and an acutely flexed back, with the arms hanging loosely and eyes directed downwards. The deformity often disappears when the patient adopts a different position, such as lying down, or on distracting his attention, or on suggestion. Gait may also be bizarre. This condition may often follow minor trauma, or may occur in young men such as army recruits or in workers seeking compensation.

Malingering

Malingerers are conscious of the fact that their complaint of pain is untrue, and so it is not truly a psychological disorder (Kanner, 1994). The condition is rare, the diagnosis may be difficult to prove, and medicolegal litigation and secondary gain may be involved. There is often a great discrepancy between the nature of the original injury, the patient's description of pain and his or her length of disability. Examination may reveal a diffuse and inconsistent tenderness, known as the migratory pointing test. In the Burn's test, the patient kneels on a chair and is asked to bend over to touch the floor with the fingers. Patients who have sciatica almost always can do it or at least attempt it. If the patient is malingering, he or she announces an inability to attempt it because of 'the great pain' it causes, or else may tend to overbalance off the chair (Figure 3.3).

4 Examination of the lumbar spine

An accurate history is first essential for diagnosis, and some points to take note of in a history of back pain include:

1. The type of pain, its severity and characteristics
2. Its distribution
3. Its onset, whether gradual or sudden
4. Whether pain is constant, intermittent or progressive
5. Factors that aggravate or relieve pain: rest; sitting; posture; certain activities; exercise; coughing; sneezing; straining
6. Whether pain is present at night or at certain times of the day
7. Whether movement is restricted, its relation to pain and any diurnal variation in stiffness
8. The presence of any neurological symptoms, such as pins and needles or numbness, and their distribution.

The past medical and surgical history, any history of past spinal symptoms or injury, the patient's occupation and the effect of the back trouble on this occupation, any sporting or unaccustomed activities, any family history of spinal troubles, the effect of any treatments such as medication, physiotherapy or surgery and any side effects produced from these treatments should then be elicited.

Associated spinal symptoms

Other symptoms may provide a clue to the correct diagnosis. In inflammatory conditions such as spondyloarthritis, pain associated with stiffness is typically worse early in the morning or at night. Sleep may be disturbed, so that the patient has to get up and walk about. Stiffness eases after a variable period during the day, its duration being dependent on the degree of inflammation that is present. Stiffness usually eases during the day, although it may return after a bout of heavy exercise. Extra-articular features may be present (*see* Chapter 7).

In patients with a spinal malignancy, pain is severe, often present at night, so that patients may have to try to sleep sitting up, and typically it becomes progressively worse. It may also present as a pathological fracture with a sudden onset of pain, usually severe and localized, which needs to be differentiated from other causes of fracture such as osteoporosis.

Pain may be aggravated or relieved in certain positions, thus offering a clue to diagnosis. Pain caused by intervertebral disc prolapse is usually made worse by sitting or straining, and may be relieved by rest. Pain that intensifies on standing, but eases when sitting is more characteristic of spondylolisthesis. Pain made worse by walking and eased by resting occurs in lumbar spinal canal stenosis.

Nocturnal pain that prevents sleep occurs in two separate circumstances. It may indicate inflammatory changes associated with spondyloarthritis, disc prolapse or tumours, but it is also common with depression. With organic lesions, pain tends to lessen with rest. Patients with psychogenic problems usually report that pain is constantly present and is unrelieved by most therapies, including rest.

Patients with back pain and a fever always require urgent and intensive investigations to ascertain its cause, which may be infection, discitis or osteomyelitis, subacute bacterial endocarditis, tumour, particularly lymphoma, or a leaking abdominal aortic aneurysm. Fever is often associated with an elevated erythrocyte sedimentation rate and an increased white blood cell count.

The patient's age may also provide a clue. Up until the age of 10 years, an infective discitis would be the most likely problem; 10–20 years, Scheuermann's disease or a juvenile disc syndrome; 20–30 years, intervertebral disc prolapse, spondyloarthritis or spondylolisthesis; 40–50 years, a mechanical spinal disorder; 50 years and over, malignancy; and 60 years and over, osteoporosis, lumbar canal stenosis or DISH (diffuse idiopathic spinal hyperostosis).

Examination of the lumbar spine

The patient's posture, build, gait and ability to move freely should be observed and the following assessed: pelvic level; leg length; spinal curves; other deformities and muscle changes.

Test flexion, extension and lateral flexion, and observe: range; rhythm; reproduction and behaviour of pain; and presence of an arc of pain.

Auxiliary tests can be carried out: overpressure; rapid movements; sustained pressure; quadrant position; and slump test.

Test passive movements: passive physiological range at each spinal level; and accessory movements at each spinal level.

Palpation can be performed. Neurological testing involves testing for: power, sensation and reflexes; straight leg raising; and femoral nerve stretch.

Sacroiliac joint tests, a general medical examination and ancillary tests (radiology, CT, MRI, discography, bone scanning and laboratory investigations) are all relevant.

Inspection

Inspection should begin as soon as the patient is first met, as considerable information may be gained by observing the patient's body build, gait and whether or not any limp is present. An assessment of whether spinal movements are free or restricted may be obtained by observing him or her getting into or out of a chair, or the position that is adopted while sitting. The patient should then be asked to stand with the back, shoulders and legs exposed for inspection. Good lighting is necessary, so that those features such as pelvic level, disturbances of spinal curves or other deformities, and intervertebral movements may be observed.

Pelvic level

The pelvic level is first estimated with the examiner standing behind the patient, noting any discrepancy between shoulder and scapular levels on each side, and the level of skin creases in the back, buttock folds or posterior knee joints. The thumbs are then placed over the patient's posterior superior iliac spines, with the fingers placed along the iliac crest, to compare the relative heights of these two landmarks (Figure 4.1). If

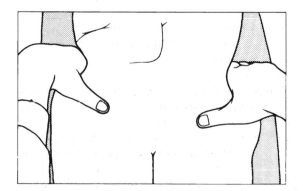

Figure 4.1 Determining the pelvic level in a patient with scoliosis. The fingers are placed along the iliac crests and the thumbs over the dimples of Venus

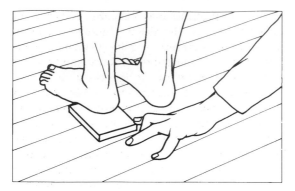

Figure 4.2 The use of blocks of varying sizes in a patient with a shortened left leg

any discrepancy between the two levels is noted, wooden blocks, graduated in height from 0.5 cm, are placed under the heel of the shorter leg until the pelvis and the skin creases are on the same levels (Figure 4.2). The test should then be repeated with the patient sitting and the levels and symmetry of the anterior and posterior iliac spines checked.

Compensation for the short leg may take place by tilting of the pelvis, which results in a scoliosis to the same side as the short leg, and the shoulder becomes tilted to the opposite side.

Leg length inequality

The measurement and clinical significance of leg length inequality remain controversial, but nonetheless should be incorporated into the routine examination. Opinions vary widely as to the significance of leg length inequality (Giles and Taylor, 1982; Subotnick, 1981; Wooden, 1981; Dieck et al, 1985). Leg shortening of 6 mm or less should never be regarded as a cause of symptoms, and many asymptomatic patients have a difference of up to 12 mm in their leg lengths. True and apparent leg length inequalities need to be differentiated.

True leg length

This is measured using bony landmarks from the anterior superior iliac spine to the tip of the medial malleolus of the ankle with the patient supine, the pelvis level and the hips in the neutral position. The theoretically ideal measurement from the centre of the normal axis of hip movement is impractical, since it is sited in the centre of the acetabulum, and so the nearby iliac spine is used. As this site is lateral to the axis of movement, any discrepancy will produce a difference in measurement, hence the importance of first ensuring that the pelvis is level, with neither hip in an adducted or abducted position. Normally, with the patient lying supine and both legs in line with the trunk, a line drawn across the two iliac crests is level, and indicates that a line bisecting the hips would be at right angles to the pelvis. In addition, with the legs extended, the medial malleoli of both ankles should lie at the same level. These measurements can readily be made by inspection and palpation of the bony landmarks.

The measurement of leg length may be inaccurate, especially if any pelvic rotation or asymmetry or hip deformity is present. If the pelvic level appears to be tilted, an attempt should be made to set the pelvis square by moving the legs so that they lie in line with the trunk. The pelvis may then be seen to rotate. However, it is impossible to correct this pelvic tilt if a fixed adduction or abduction deformity of the hip is present. Accordingly, if one hip lies in a position of fixed adduction or abduction, the other hip must then be placed at a similar angle before making the measurement. Having established that a true shortening is present, the knees are then flexed to a right angle, and the upper and lower legs of both legs inspected to determine whether to not the shortening is above or below the knee.

Apparent shortening

This is estimated by measuring from the umbilicus to the medial malleolus of each ankle and noting the difference between the two distances. Apparent shortening may arise from an abnormality of the hip joint, such as a flexion or adduction deformity, or else from a pelvic tilt. X-rays have been used to assess leg length (Clarke, 1972; Giles and Taylor, 1981; Friberg, 1983), but it is a research tool that does not help clinically.

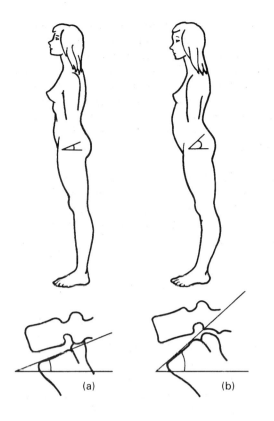

Figure 4.3 (a) The normal degree of lumbar lordosis is determined by the angle formed at the lumbosacral joint, the lumbosacral angle. (b) Excessive lordosis is associated with an increase in the lumbosacral angle above 30 degrees

Spinal curves

The development of the normal curves in the lumbar, thoracic and cervical spines is observed with the patient standing. The degree of lumbar lordosis is determined by the lumbosacral angle, normally about 30 degrees (Figure 4.3a), which is the angle of inclination that the upper border of the sacrum forms with the horizontal plane. In the lumbar spine, lordosis may be increased, decreased or reversed (kyphosis). An increased lordosis results from an increase in the normal lumbosacral angle to greater than 30 degrees. This causes the pelvis to tilt forwards, and to compensate the lumbar lordosis is increased (Figure 4.3a,b). A decrease in the normal lumbar lordosis is usually associated with the presence of marked paravertebral muscle spasm.

Lumbar kyphosis may be either localized or generalized. A localized lumbar kyphosis produces a posterior angular deformity, most often due to a localized bony abnormality such as a collapsed vertebra. A generalized lumbar kyphosis is rare (Larouche et al, 1995), is usually associated with a protective muscle spasm, and lumbar extension becomes restricted. Scheuermann's disease is characterized by the presence of a smooth thoracic kyphosis, accentuated on forward flexion. In older patients, a lumbar kyphosis may be due to spondylosis, ankylosing spondylitis or metabolic bone diseases such as osteoporosis.

Scoliosis is a lateral curvature of the spinal column, assessed by noting any lateral deviation from a line drawn between the spinous processes of T1 to the midline of the sacrum. It may be structural, compensatory or protective. With structural scoliosis, the lateral curvature is associated with a vertebral rotation, and both the curve and the rotation become more accentuated on forward flexion. A compensatory scoliosis commonly develops in patients with a discrepancy in the pelvic level as the result of leg length inequality (Figure 4.4).

Scoliosis may be either ipsilateral or contralateral, according to the relationship of the displacement of the patient's thorax to the painful side. An ipsilateral scoliosis is a lateral displacement of the patient's thorax towards the painful side. The scoliosis associated with a disc prolapse represents an attempt to decrease the tension on the nerve root, and so is protective in nature, and is called protective, antalgic or sciatic scoliosis. Sciatic scoliosis is really a misnomer, since a similar deformity may be present in a patient with central back pain without leg pain, due to an acute mechanical derangement of an intervertebral joint without any definite evidence of a disc prolapse. For these reasons, the term 'protective list' has also been used to describe the deformity. The relationship of these deformities to spinal movements will be considered later.

Other deformities

In cases of advanced osteoporosis, the patient loses height and the costal margins may impinge on the pelvic rim. A severe degree of

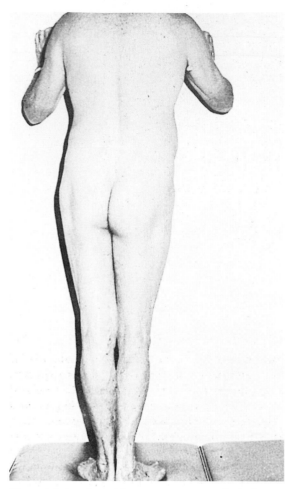

Figure 4.4 A patient with a compensatory scoliosis due to a short right leg. Note also the asymmetry of the buttock

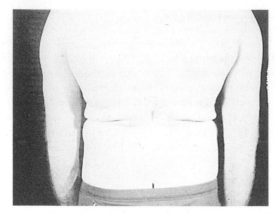

Figure 4.5 Abnormalities in the skin folds in a patient with spondylolisthesis

Active movement

The patient, while standing as relaxed as possible with the feet together and the hands by the side, is first asked whether any symptoms are felt in this position. Active lumbar spinal movements should then be performed to assess:

- The range of movement
- Any disturbances of rhythm
- Reproduction and behaviour of pain
- The presence of an arc of pain.

These factors are usually assessed simultaneously during movement. For example, while testing vertebral movements, the examiner should also watch the body contours and spinous processes carefully to observe whether the spinal joints unroll rhythmically and evenly, or whether there is any localized restriction of the movement in the spinous processes between two or three vertebrae. However, for ease of description, these factors will be considered individually.

spondylolisthesis may be suspected if any disparity in the skin creases, an increased lumbar lordosis or a palpable 'step' in the lumbar spine is found (Figure 4.5). Paravertebral muscle spasm may be either unilateral or bilateral, and is usually present as a reflex protective mechanism. The spasm may be obvious on inspection, when it stands out as a prominent muscle band to the side of the spinous processes. Muscle spasm that is present on standing may increase, decrease or disappear during active spinal flexion or extension movements. At times spasm may become evident only during these movements.

In patients with nerve root pressure and lower motor neurone lesions, muscle wasting and fasciculation may be seen in the buttock or leg.

The patient is asked first to flex the spine by bending forwards in an attempt to touch the toes with the knees kept straight and the feet together. However, much of this forward movement takes place in the hips. Active movement into spinal extension is next tested, followed by active lateral flexion to each side. Active rotation is not routinely tested in the lumbar spine, as most of this movement takes place in the thoracic spine.

Range of movement

The range of forward flexion may be assessed by measuring the distance that the patient's fingertips reach from the floor. Although a patient may be able to compensate for lumbar stiffness by flexion of the hips, the lumbar spine in this position will nevertheless have been flexed to the limit of its available range of flexion. The normal range of flexion shows wide individual variation but is usually taken to be 75–90 degrees.

Extension is tested next by asking the patient to arch the spine backwards, increasing the normal lumbar lordosis. The range of this movement is approximately 20 degrees.

The range of lateral flexion is assessed by asking the patient to slide the fingers down the leg and noting the position of the fingers in relation to the knee. The examiner must be careful to ensure that the patient does not move the spine into slight flexion or extension during this manoeuvre. The normal range of this movement is approximately 25 degrees.

Alteration in range

The range of movement may be normal, decreased or increased. The normal range depends on the patient's age and build, so it is always necessary to establish the usual distance that the patient could flex before the onset of his or her disorder.

Restriction in range may be due to pain or stiffness, and may be associated with muscle spasm. In intervertebral disc prolapse, flexion, and less often extension, is usually painful and limited, whereas lateral flexion usually remains normal. In lumbar spondylosis, ankylosing spondylitis or osteoporosis, movement may be diminished in all directions. Hypomobility syndromes may be suspected if there is limitation of movement in only one or two directions, and their usual pattern in the lumbar spine is a reduced lateral flexion associated with limitation of either extension or flexion.

The range of movement may also be increased. In spinal hypermobility, the patient may be able to flex sufficiently to place the back of the hands on the floor or the head on the knees.

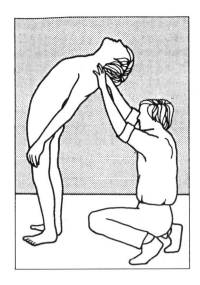

Figure 4.6 Observing lumbar extension

Rhythm

Movements are repeated again while watching for any disturbance of the normal smooth rhythm. The pattern of spinal movement in flexion and lateral flexion is best viewed by standing behind the patient. While observing lumbar extension, it is best to kneel behind the patient and support the shoulders to prevent overbalancing (Figure 4.6). If pain is not severe, repeated movements can also be used to demonstrate any disturbance in their normal rhythm, detected by a loss of intervertebral joint movement, or else as a change in the normal contour.

Normal rhythmical lumbar movement during forward flexion comprises a synchronous unrolling of each intervertebral level. At the same time, the normal lordosis becomes flattened until, on full flexion, there is a slight reversal of this curve, resulting in a continuous smooth convex lumbar and thoracic curve (Figure 4.7). Simultaneously, a synchronous movement of the pelvis produces an increase in the lumbosacral angle, posterior displacement of the hips and rotation of the pelvis around the hips.

During lateral spinal flexion, the normally mobile spine develops a C-shaped curve. Any restriction of intervertebral joint movement sufficient to produce a flattening of the normal

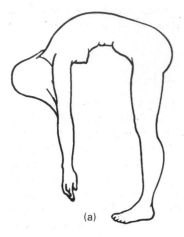

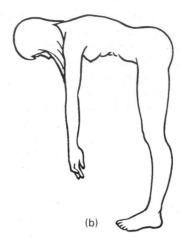

Figure 4.7 (a) Forward flexion is normally accompanied by a loss of the normal lumbar lordosis and a smooth curve between the lumbar and thoracic spines. (b) Forward flexion in a patient with restricted movement in the lumbar joints accompanied by persistence of the lumbar lordosis and loss of the normal smooth curve

C-shaped curve may be of significance, especially if it is associated with reproduction of pain (Figure 4.8).

The contours of a scoliosis or kyphosis that are present on standing may be altered on movement. Several different patterns of spinal deformity may be produced and detected during active spinal flexion and extension:

- A scoliosis present on standing may become more marked during forward flexion
- A scoliosis may only become evident during forward flexion
- A scoliosis present on standing may disappear on forward flexion
- An alternating scoliosis may appear on forward flexion

- An arc in the middle range of flexion may occur, during which scoliosis appears, only to disappear on further movement
- On flexion, the extensor muscles on both sides may display marked spasm, holding the spine rigid in a position of lordosis.

Reproduction of pain

If no pain is present while standing, the patient is asked to move into the various directions being tested until pain is felt. If pain is present while standing at rest, the patient should be asked to bend only until the pain begins to increase. The range of this movement is noted. However, if pain is not severe, and no distally referred pain is produced, the patient is asked to move further

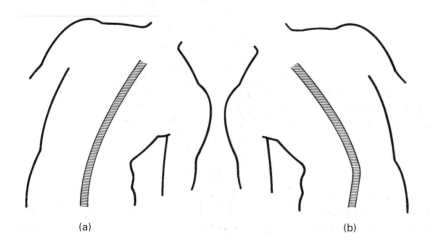

Figure 4.8 (a) Lateral flexion to the right is normal and accompanied by a smooth spinal curve. (b) Lateral flexion to the left is abnormal due to a limitation of movement at one lumbar spinal segment

into the range and report any difference in severity, site or distribution of symptoms, such as an increase in severity of pain or an increase in the area of referral. Should pain become too severe or be referred distally, the movement is stopped and the patient returned to the upright position. Otherwise, the patient continues to move to the limit of the available range and reports any changes in symptoms.

An arc of pain

An arc of pain, which may only be experienced at one point in the range, usually indicates an organic lesion of the intervertebral joint segment, such as vertebral instability. The typical pattern is that the patient stands without pain, but during flexion, pain may be experienced at the mid-range of the movement and then disappears on further flexion. Alternatively, pain may be appreciated only when standing up from the forward flexed position. Commonly a scoliosis develops at this same point in the range, although at times this may occur but be painless.

Auxiliary tests

Five additional tests used to assess the spinal origin of pain may be extremely useful.

Overpressure

Overpressure is applied to the spine at the limit of its painless range by the examiner producing small oscillatory movements. This may reproduce the symptoms, and allow the examiner to determine the end-feel of the movement.

Rapid movements

If pain is not provoked during the normal spinal movements, it may help to repeat the test movements quickly to determine if pain and spasm are reproduced.

Sustained pressure

Sustained pressure is applied for approximately 10 seconds, first in extension and then in lateral flexion towards the painful side, to determine if

this position can reproduce back or leg pain. Pain may also be brought on when the pressure is released.

The quadrant position

This is a most useful passive movement test to reproduce pain by positioning the lumbar joint under maximum stress and reducing the size of the intervertebral foramen (Maitland, 1986). In the lumbar spine, it is found by passively moving the patient first into full lumbar extension, followed by lateral flexion and rotation towards the side of pain. The test is particularly useful in being able to reproduce pain in patients who have leg pain without back pain, for example, in patients with a lateral canal stenosis.

The examiner stands behind and to one side of the patient. The lumbar spine is first moved to the limit of its extension, without the patient bending the knees. The examiner holds the patient's right shoulder with his left shoulder positioned near the patient's occiput to take the weight of the head (Figure 4.9). Overpressure is then applied at the limit of this range and the patient is guided into the quadrant position by laterally flexing and then rotating the spine towards the painful side. This movement is continued until the limit of this range is reached, and overpressure is again applied. It is ceased if pain is reproduced.

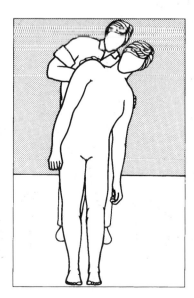

Figure 4.9
Quadrant test for the lumbar spine

The slump test

This is a very useful test for patients with back or leg pain, for it applies tension to pain-sensitive structures, such as the nerve root, dura and nerve root sleeve, in the vertebral canal or intervertebral foramen, by putting them at maximal stretch (Maitland, 1979). Attention to detail is necessary, as the aim of the test is to provoke pain, and asymptomatic patients might also experience some degree of pain or stiffness, especially in the knees or thoracic spine. The patient is asked to report any symptoms, especially pain, at all stages of the test and if they become evident the test is discontinued.

A positive test reproduces the patient's pain, which should then be alleviated when the test movement is released. The value of this test rests in its value of being able to assess the site of origin of pain, although it does not indicate any specific diagnosis. It is particularly helpful in patients with posterior thigh pain, which may have been attributed to a hamstring problem, but is really a referred pain from a lower spinal joint. In addition, it can be used as a treatment technique to stretch the involved spinal structure (Maitland, 1985).

The patient sits erect, knees flexed against the edge of the couch, hands behind the back. The patient then slumps, fully flexing the thoraco-lumbar spine but not the neck. Overpresssure to the shoulders fixes the lumbar spine. The head and neck is then fully flexed. Overpressure is maintained by the examiner placing his or her chin on the patient's head, so leaving the left hand free to palpate the spine. The patient extends the knee, and the ankle is fully actively dorsiflexed. Neck flexion is reduced gradually so that the head is lifted gradually. The test is repeated with both knees extended and the neck flexed, and finally, neck flexion is released.

Passive movements

There are two distinct passive movements tested at each one of the intervertebral joints: the passive range of physiological movements at each spinal joint; and the accessory movements at each level.

Passive physiological movements

The passive range of physiological movements at each individual spinal joint is tested by the examiner producing the physiological spinal movements with one hand and feeling the movement between adjacent bony spinous processes with the fingers of the other hand. In the lumbar spine, the physiological movements of flexion and extension, lateral flexion and rotation are tested by passive movements, while palpating them to appreciate the passive movement of each individual joint. This is achieved by the examiner moving the intervertebral joint through a full range while palpating between adjacent bony prominences and comparing the movement obtained at each level. The ability to assess normal or abnormal movement by these means requires considerable practice to obtain a proper sense of 'feel' for the movement.

Flexion–extension

These movements may be tested using either one or both of the patient's legs, but as it is generally easier to use only a single leg, this method will be described.

The patient lies on the right side with the right leg underneath in a position of slight flexion at the hip and knee. The examiner stands in front of the patient's upper chest facing towards the hips. The left forearm is placed across the thorax so that the fingers of the left hand can palpate between the lumbar spinous processes, and the

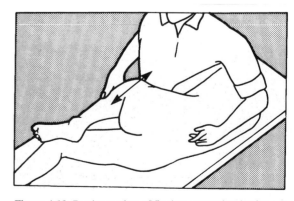

Figure 4.10 Passive testing of flexion–extension in the lumbar spine

thorax is stabilized between the left arm and the left side. The patient's upper (left) leg is then grasped below the knee with the examiner's right hand (Figure 4.10).

Flexion and extension of the lumbar spine are produced by flexing and then releasing the patient's left leg at the hip. The middle finger of the examiner's left hand in the interspinous space can feel the movement of flexion and extension as an opening and closing of the interspinous gap.

Lateral flexion

The patient lies on the right side with hips and knees flexed so that the lumbar spine is relaxed midway between flexion and extension. The examiner, standing in front of the patient, reaches across to the patient's left side, his or her left forearm along the spine pointing towards the feet, and his or her right forearm under the patient's ischial tuberosity. The pad of the examiner's left middle finger is placed facing upward in the underside of the interspinous space to feel the bony margins of the adjacent vertebrae (Figure 4.11).

By grasping the patient's pelvis and upper thigh with his or her right forearm and right side, the examiner laterally flexes the patient's lumbar spine from below upward by rocking the pelvis. This is achieved by pulling with the right forearm so that the patient's left ilium moves cephalad. The pelvis is then returned to its mid-position by the examiner pushing against the patient's upper

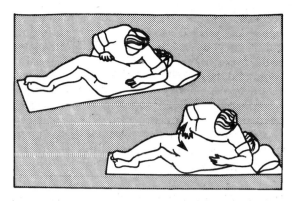

Figure 4.12 Passive testing of rotation in the lumbar spine

left thigh with his or her right side. This oscillatory movement rocks the pelvis around the fulcrum of the underside hip and femur so that lateral flexion is easy to produce and palpate.

Rotation

Although testing the active range of lumbar rotation does not provide much information, testing the small range of passive rotation is often of value.

The starting position is similar to that for lateral flexion, and the examiner makes sure that the patient's top knee can slide freely forwards over the knee underneath. The examiner leans across the patient and places his or her left forearm along the spine to palpate the interspinous space from underneath, while twisting slightly to face the patient's hips. The patient's left trochanter is held over the examiner's right hand, the heel of his or her hand anterior to the trochanter with all fingers spread out behind it (Figure 4.12).

The examiner stabilizes the patient's thorax with his or her left arm and then pulls the patient's pelvis towards him or her with the right hand so that the left side of the pelvis and the lumbar spine rotate forwards. The palpating finger keeps pace with this movement so that the displacement of the distal spinous process from the proximal one can be felt easily. The pelvis is then returned to its original position by the heel of the examiner's right hand and forearm.

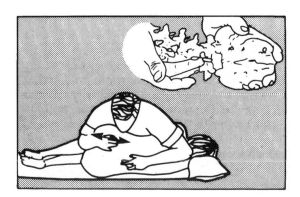

Figure 4.11 Passive testing of lateral flexion in the lumbar spine

Accessory movements

Accessory movements are produced at each intervertebral spinal joint by pressure applied by the examiner against the patient's bony vertebral processes. The type and range of movement normally present can be appreciated after some practice. The tests are used to assess the accessory movements, the range of movement, the reproduction of pain, the behaviour of the pain throughout the range of movement, the presence of any muscular spasm, and the end-feel of the movement.

Attention to detail is mandatory if the correct movement is to be achieved. Posteroanterior and transverse pressures are applied by the examiner with the thumb or through the pisiform bone, firstly over the spinous process, and next the transverse process. This produces an oscillatory movement, which needs to be applied at the correct speed to appreciate the movement of a single vertebra in relation to the adjacent one: too quick or too slow and the vertebral movement will not be appreciated. Light pressure is applied and relaxed two or three times per second. Provided no pain is produced, the amplitude and depth of movement is increased further and repeated another two or three times. The movement should then be repeated to a greater depth until either a painless normal range or pain with or without any restriction of the movement is demonstrated.

The patient lies prone, with the arms by the side and the head turned to one side. The three basic manoeuvres are:

1. Posteroanterior pressure against the spinous process, which can also be inclined either at the inferior margin of the spinous process towards the patient's head or at the superior margin towards the feet (Figure 4.13a).
2. Transverse pressure against the lateral surface of the spinous process, which can also be inclined towards the patient's head or feet (Figure 4.13b). The transverse direction can be inclined in varying directions and degrees until it becomes applied in a posteroanterior direction.
3. Posteroanterior pressure against the transverse process, which may be varied either by

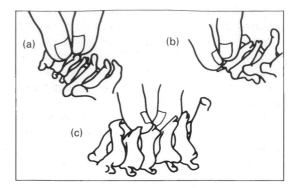

Figure 4.13 Passive intervertebral movement. (a) Posteroanterior pressure over the spinous process may be inclined in a cephalad or caudal direction. (b) Transverse pressure against the spinous process may be directed either laterally or inclined until it becomes a posteroanterior pressure. (c) Posteroanterior pressure over the transverse process may be inclined either medially or laterally

directing the direction of the pressure towards the patient's head or feet, or else by directing it in a medial or lateral direction (Figure 4.13c).

Testing the passive intervertebral joint movements is essential in assessing intervertebral joint lesions, and, especially if movements are restricted, symptoms may be reproduced by testing at an appropriate joint. The movements may elicit pain, restricted movement and/or spasm. Pain usually increases in intensity and distribution with increasing movement, and may be felt at any stage in the range or at the limit of the range. If the range of movement is limited, the type of resistance, due to either a sense of tightness or muscle spasm, is then assessed. This is particularly relevant in hypomobility syndromes, where the essential clinical finding is a loss of these movements. The finding of a restricted movement will also indicate the type of mobilization therapy to be used.

Palpation

The spinous processes are most readily palpable, especially on flexion of the spine; Ll and L2 are often the most readily identified because of their shape. The transverse processes can usually be palpated if the patient lies prone and relaxed, unless the overlying muscles are too thick. The line joining the tops of each iliac crest usually lies over the spinous process of L4. Palpation here may detect any alteration in the bony alignments, such as spondylolisthesis.

On each side of the body, the subcutaneous iliac crest ends at the posterior superior iliac spine and may be identified by an overlying skin dimple ('the dimple of Venus'). A line joining both posterior spines lies over S2. The sacroiliac joint is not accessible to palpation at all, as it lies too deeply and is overhung by the posterior iliac spine. Its midpoint lies some two fingers lateral to the posterior superior iliac spine at approximately the level of the second sacral segment.

Muscle spasm may be felt with the patient lying prone and relaxed, using a gentle transverse movement of the examiner's finger over the paraspinal muscles. Any areas of tenderness are usually felt over the interspinous ligament of the involved intervertebral joint or to one side of the joint. A feeling of thickening in the soft tissue in the interspinous spaces may be found in chronic disorders, its degree and quality being proportional to the duration of the disorder. Areas of tenderness in muscles or in relation to the iliac crest and posterior iliac spines are usually non-specific, and the area over the transverse process of L1 and L2 is often tender in normal patients. Pain may be provoked over the painful joint if each spinous process is tapped sharply with a tendon hammer or the fingertips. Finally, the examiner palpates over the course of the sciatic nerve from the sciatic notch to the popliteal fossa.

Neurological testing

Power, sensation and reflexes

A neurological examination to detect the presence of any sensory, motor and reflex change is necessary, as a patient may sometimes be unaware of a neurological deficit, and also to act as a baseline when determining any future changes. Note is made of any gait disturbance, fasciculations and muscle wasting by measuring the circumfer-ence of the thigh and calf. Sensory disturbances are sought in the dermatome distribution of the lumbosacral nerves. Isometric tests are generally used to test for any muscle weakness that may result from nerve root compression. Although each nerve root supplies more than one muscle, and most muscles have more than one nerve root supply, nonetheless, most muscles are supplied predominantly by one root. Those of clinical significance are listed in Table 4.1. However, plantar flexion of the foot cannot be tested adequately by an isometric contraction. Instead, weakness of plantar flexion will become evident if the patient stands on one leg, and, with the knee in full extension, raises him- or herself up onto the toes some six times. Similarly, weakness of ankle dorsiflexion will become evident if the patient attempts to walk on his or her heels, and then has difficulty in raising the foot or balancing. The girth of the limbs above and below the knee is measured by a tape measure to record any muscle wasting. Reflexes include the knee jerk (L3 and L4) and ankle jerk (S1 and S2), and plantar responses are tested for any evidence of an upper motor neurone lesion. Straight leg raising and the femoral nerve stretch are important tests and will be considered in detail.

The straight leg raising test

Straight leg raising tests the free movement of the lower lumbar (L4 and L5) and the upper sacral (S1 and S2) nerve roots, together with their dural sleeves, within the spinal canal and their intervertebral foramen. This is fortuitous since L4, L5 and S1 are the nerve roots that are most commonly involved in disc prolapse (Supik and Broom, 1994). During the test, the pelvis rotates slightly at first, followed by a movement in the lumbar joints. Hence, lesions of these joints, as in ankylosing spondylitis, may produce pain or limitation of the range of straight leg raising. The restriction in range may be even more pronounced by any back muscle or hamstring spasm. After the first few degrees of passive elevation of the leg, the sciatic nerve begins to move in the sciatic notch. During the first 30 degrees of movement, the lumbosacral cord is moving but the nerve roots are still stationary. Beyond 30 degrees, the hip acts as a pulley to apply traction

Table 4.1 Isometric tests of the lumbar spine

Movement	Muscle	Nerve root	Isometric tests
Hip flexion	Iliopsoas	L2	The patient lies supine and holds the flexed hip and knee at 90 degrees while resistance is applied just above the knee
Knee extension	Quadriceps	L3	The examiner threads one arm under the patient's lower thigh to place his or her hand on the opposite thigh. While the patient holds the leg just short of the fully extended position resistance is applied against the front of the leg, just above the ankle
Ankle dorsiflexion and inversion	Tibialis anterior	L4	The patient holds the foot in dorsiflexion and inversion while the examiner applies resistance against the dorsomedial surface of the proximal end of the first metatarsal
Great toe extension	Extensor hallucis longus	L5	The patient holds the foot and toes dorsiflexed whilst resistance is placed against the nail of the big toe
Extension of toes	Extensor digitorum longus	L5 and S1	The patient holds the foot and toes dorsiflexed whilst resistance is applied against the dorsal surface of all toes
Ankle eversion	Peroneus longus and brevis	S1	The patient is asked to keep the heels together with the soles of the feet twisted away from each other. Resistance is applied against the lateral borders of the feet, pushing them together
Knee flexion	Hamstrings	L5 and S1	The patient holds the knee flexed to 90 degrees while resistance is applied behind the patient's heel
Hip extension	Gluteus maximus	L4 and L5 S1 and S2	The patient lies prone and holds the hip extended with the knee bent while the examiner applies a downwards resistance just above the knee with one hand, palpating the gluteal mass with the other hand to assess firmness
Plantar flexion	Gastrocnemius	S1	The patient stands on one leg and raises himself up onto the toes through a full range up to six times
Flexion of toes	Flexors digitorum and hallucis longus	S2	The patient holds his toes fully flexed whilst resistance is applied against the palmar surface of all toes

to the sciatic nerve, and from about 30 to 70 degrees the nerve roots will move in the intervertebral foramen. The range of movement of the spinal nerves in the neural foramen during this test is 2–5 mm (Smith et al, 1993).

When a disc prolapse impinges on one of these nerve roots and their dural sleeve, traction on the nerve root during the test will reproduce sciatic pain. Moreover, the test correlates strongly with the severity of symptoms due to stretching of an affected nerve root (Charnley, 1951; Hakelius and Hindmarsh, 1972; Edgar and Park, 1974; Brieg and Troup, 1979; Waddell, 1987a; Kosteljanetz et al, 1988; Deyo et al, 1992a; Supik and Broom, 1994; Jonsson and Stromqvist, 1995; Karbowski and Dvorak, 1995). The test is also an objective sign in that the decrease in the range of the leg movement may correlate with the degree of nerve root involvement (Charnley, 1951). It is also the most sensitive preoperative physical diagnostic sign that correlates with the intraoperative findings (Supic and Broom, 1994). As a general rule, the more positive the test, the larger the disc prolapse (Kortelainen et al, 1985; Shiqing et al, 1987; Jonsson and Stromqvist, 1995). In almost all patients with intervertebral disc prolapse that results in L4, L5 or S1 nerve root pressure, the range of straight leg raising is reduced.

For a test to be considered positive, it must also reproduce the patient's pain. While the patient is lying supine, or if he or she raises the affected leg by flexing the hip and knee, the nerve root is not subjected to any increase in tension. However, when the affected leg is passively elevated with the knee extended, the inflamed nerve root is put under increasing tension as it moves in its intervertebral foramen.

A set clinical routine should always be followed (Cameron et al, 1994), and extreme gentleness is required at all times.

The patient lies supine and each leg is tested separately. The hips should be tested to ensure that their movements are normal. The straight leg raising test is always performed first on the painless side.

The patient's hip is placed in a slight degree of adduction and medial rotation. The leg is then passively lifted by the heel with one hand, while the knee is maintained in extension with the other hand, and the range of the movement is estimated. It is usually up to 90 degrees, but may vary from 70 to 120 degrees, as it may vary with age, joint mobility and the natural degree of hamstring tightness. This movement is normally painless, except for a possible sensation of tightness behind the thigh or knee, although pain may at times be experienced in the contralateral, affected leg (see below). The height that the leg is raised is usually measured by estimating the angle that the leg forms with the horizontal; the distance of the malleolus from the bed may also be measured. Measurement with an instrument does not add much further information (Hsieh et al, 1983; McCombe et al 1989; Goeken and Hof, 1994).

The leg on the affected side is then lifted by the heel, while the knee is kept fully extended with the hip in a slight degree of adduction and slight medial rotation (Figure 4.14a). The pelvis should not be allowed to rise or rotate. The test movement is continued until pain and/or paraesthesia commence, and they should reproduce the symptoms. The range of this movement is then estimated.

If the foot of the affected leg is now passively dorsiflexed, the nerve root is further stretched and so pain should be exacerbated (Figure 4.14b).

Other tests that increase tension on the nerve root and other pain-sensitive structures in the vertebral canal and reproduce pain include:

1. Neck flexion: the affected limb is elevated, as described above, to a position just short of that producing pain. If the patient now flexes the neck, leg pain may be reproduced (Figure 4.14c).
2. Popliteal fossa compression, also known as the bowstring sign: the limb is elevated to an angle just short of producing pain. The knee is then slightly flexed and supported on the shoulder of the examiner, who then applies pressure over the popliteal fossa with both of his thumbs. Pain should again be reproduced (Figure 4.14d).
3. With the patient supine and the hip and knee flexed to 90 degrees, the knee is passively extended until pain is reproduced (Figure 4.14e)

A normal straight leg raising test is found only rarely in the presence of a lumbar intervertebral disc prolapse, with a lateral disc prolapse into the intervertebral foramen, in canal stenosis, rupture of a root, or after migration of loose disc fragments into a different region of the neural canal.

The crossed straight leg raising test

Pain may at times be exacerbated in the affected leg when the opposite, non-painful leg is being lifted. This occurs with a large central disc prolapse, when stretching the normal nerve root pulls on the dural sac, so increasing tension on the affected nerve root and producing sciatic

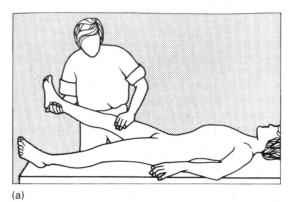

(a)

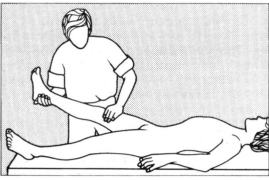

(b)

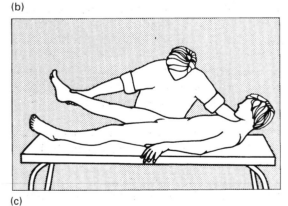

(c)

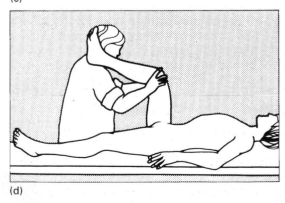

(d)

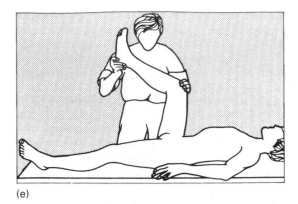

(e)

Figure 4.14 (a) The straight leg raising test. Straight leg raising is reduced in the right leg. (b) Pain is increased by passive dorsiflexion of the foot. (c) Pain may also be reproduced by lowering the leg and passively flexing the neck. (d) Popliteal compression test. (e) Lasègue's test

pain (McCombe et al, 1989; Deyo et al, 1992a). Of 351 patients with back pain who came to surgery, 58 had a positive 'well-leg raising test' of whom 56 proved to have a prolapsed disc (Hudgins, 1979). False positive and false negative results have also been described (Auld et al, 1969; Vaz et al, 1978).

Femoral nerve stretch test

In this test, passive hip extension is used to place tension on the femoral nerve roots, especially L3, to reproduce pain. The normal leg should always be tested first. The patient lies prone with the knee flexed to 90 degrees. The examiner places one hand under the thigh to extend the hip,

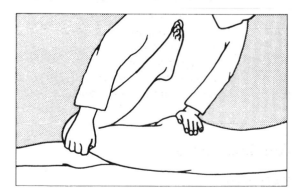

Figure 4.15 Normal femoral nerve stretch test. The hip is passively extended with the knee flexed

while the other hand steadies the patient's pelvis. With femoral nerve root pressure, the range of hip extension is restricted and thigh pain is reproduced (Figure 4.15). By comparing the degree of decreased movement in the affected leg when compared with the normal side, an estimation of the degree of nerve root compression may be obtained.

As with the straight leg raising test, the degree of nerve compression should correlate with the degree of restricted movement. In the most severe degrees of nerve root involvement, the patient may experience pain even when lying prone with the hip fully extended, or on stretching the thigh by flexing the knee. As the degree of nerve root pressure improves, the range of movement is correspondingly increased. As this test reproduces pain from any of the structures being stretched, a similar result is found in a lesion of the quadriceps muscles, such as contusion injury or its complication, myositis ossificans. These conditions are easily differentiated clinically from nerve root compression.

Sacroiliac joint tests

The sacroiliac joints are tested routinely in patients with back or leg pain; these tests are described in Chapter 11.

General medical examination

A general physical examination, including the abdomen and chest, is necessary. In cases of suspected pelvic lesions, a rectal or vaginal examination is necessary, and no case of sciatica has been properly investigated until such an examination has been performed. Arterial supply to the legs is assessed by palpating the femoral, popliteal, posterior tibial and dorsalis pedis arteries.

Ancillary tests

Radiology

The role of radiology in the assessment and diagnosis of back pain remains strongly debated, especially since the advent of highly expensive modern technology. X-rays need not, and should not, be taken routinely in all patients with back pain when seen for the first time, or used as a general screening procedure (Boden, 1996). Judgement is needed in ordering and interpreting them, lest the end result is treating the X-rays and not the patient. Also, the demonstrated changes may not be the cause of the patient's pain. Moreover, some X-ray changes, such as congenital anomalies, may be of no clinical significance, and the early stages of many spinal conditions, such as tumours or osteoporosis, may not be evident on X-rays.

Disc prolapse has been described in up to 30 per cent of asymptomatic patients with CT (Wiesel et al, 1984), MRI (Powell et al, 1986; Weinreb et al, 1989; Boden et al, 1990a; Greenberg and Schell, 1991; Jensen et al, 1994b) and myelography (Hitselberger and Witten, 1968), while it has long been known that plain X-rays do not correlate with low back pain or its outcome (McRae, 1956; La Rocca and MacNab, 1970; Magora and Swartz, 1976; Biering-Sorensen et al, 1985; Pope, 1989; Seidenwurm and Litt, 1995). Considerations with their use include radiation exposure, cost effectiveness, medicolegal implications, variations in interpretation and terminology, who is to order it, whether it will improve management, and the expectations of individual patients (Deyo, 1994; Enzmann, 1994; Kent et al, 1992; Modic and Herzog, 1994; Seidenwurm and Litt, 1995; Brant-Zawadzki et al, 1995, Simmons et al, 1995, Taylor et al, 1995)

X-rays are indicated if back pain is severe, recurrent or persistent, mainly to show bony changes. They should include anterior–posterior (AP), lateral and oblique views of the lumbar spine, and an X-ray of the pelvis to show the sacroiliac joints. The standard AP view is usually taken with the patient lying down and is centred on the body of L3. Lateral views are taken in two positions, one centred over L3 and the other over L5 to demonstrate the lumbosacral joint. A pelvic X-ray should be ordered if malignancy, metabolic bone disease, Paget's disease or sacroiliitis is suspected.

The vertebrae are inspected for any abnormalities in shape, size, bony texture, and their alignments. The shape of the bones is usually altered due to wedging, which indicates either a fracture after trauma, secondary deposits or osteoporosis, or Scheuermann's disease. The vertebral bodies in osteoporosis or osteomalacia may be biconcave due to bone softening and ballooning of the discs. The size of the vertebral body is increased in Paget's disease, associated with abnormalities of the trabecular pattern. This pattern is also altered with a haemangioma, but the vertebral body is not increased in size. Bony projections such as the pedicles, transverse processes or spinous processes are then inspected. They should be easily visible and equal; if one is missing, a secondary malignant deposit is most likely.

Oblique X-rays are useful for demonstrating a spondylolysis or, possibly, degenerative changes in zygapophyseal joints. Lateral views taken in the upright position with the spine in flexion and extension may be needed to demonstrate vertebral instability. Normally, in full flexion, the vertebral endplates or adjacent vertebrae from T12 to L5 should remain parallel. X-rays may demonstrate a loss of the normal alignment and backward or forward vertebral movement.

The intervertebral discs are radiolucent, and although changes of disc disorders may be seen on X-rays, it usually takes some time for the appropriate changes to develop. Narrowing may involve the whole or part of the disc; a partly narrowed disc produces a wedge-shaped disc deformity. The disc is inspected for the presence of any gas or calcification.

Computed tomography (CT)

This non-invasive technique uses a computerized X-ray display to recreate a three-dimensional image of the spine, and outline any structural changes. Soft tissue or bony window settings can be used, so it is of particular help in delineating bone structures (Herzog et al, 1995). Images can be accurately localized, and the plane and number of sections determined, so that excellent visualization of each disc and its relationship to the surrounding soft tissues is possible. It is especially useful in cases of trauma, disc prolapse, lumbar canal stenosis, vertebral rheumatic diseases, and zygapophyseal joint abnormalities (Carrera et al, 1980a,b; Carrera and Williams,

1984; DeLauche-Cavellier et al, 1992; Maigne et al, 1992; Dullerud and Nakstad, 1994).

Limitations include radiation exposure and a slightly restricted field of view (Herzog et al, 1995). It is not a very good technique for visualizing the spinal cord or dura, so that if a diagnosis remains uncertain, it has been combined with a myelogram (CTM) or discogram (CTD), although they have been superseded by MRI, which is a more appropriate test.

Magnetic resonance imaging (MRI)

This modality is based on different physical properties, and has no ionizing radiation. It utilizes the protons in hydrogen nuclei, which are exposed to a huge magnetic field and pulsed radio waves of a predefined frequency, causing excitation and spinning of the protons, a fraction of which are induced to a higher energy level. When the pulse is discontinued, energy in the form of oscillating radiofrequency waves is detected as a signal that can be reconstructed and manipulated. The signal strength, density of protons, their state of motion and their relaxation times (TR) and excitation times (TE) are used in image formation. Using a spin-echo technique, a short relaxation time will result in a T1-weighted image, and a long relaxation time in a T2-weighted image. The normal disc shows white on a T2-weighted spin echo sequence, while disc degeneration is seen as a dark signal on heavily T2-weighted images (TR >2000 m/s, TE 60–90 m/s).

MRI has advantages over other forms of imaging in the diagnosis of low back pain, especially in detecting disc hydration and disc degeneration. Because it bonds to hydrogen ions, a high signal intensity occurs in the presence of water, as found in normal discs, while disc degeneration, with its low water content, appears as a dark signal. Accordingly, it has proven most useful in providing a non-invasive technique to evaluate the changes taking place with disc degeneration, and may show a tear in the annulus (Schiebler et al, 1991; Modic and Ross, 1991; Osti and Fraser, 1992; Modic, 1994; Deyo, 1994; Ellenberger, 1994; Jensen et al, 1994a,b; Videman et al, 1995; Brant-Zawadzki et al, 1995; Wipf and Deyo, 1995; Seidenwurm and Litt, 1995; Raininko et al, 1995; Erkintalo et al, 1995; Herzog et al, 1995). It is most useful in patients with disc prolapse and radiculopathy (Jensen et al, 1994b), and its ability to show resolution of soft tissue allows it to determine whether a disc is contained by the posterior longitudinal ligament or whether it has been extruded (Herzog et al, 1995). It can also show spontaneous resolution of a prolapsed disc (Bozzao et al, 1992; Herzog et al, 1995). There is a high correlation between the findings of disc degeneration on MRI and on discography (Linson and Crowe, 1990), and, since MRI is less painful than discography, it is taking over the role in its diagnosis. MRI is also of considerable help in the diagnosis of other spinal conditions, including soft tissue or disc disorders such as prolapse and extrusion, canal stenosis, and zygapophyseal joint disorders (Jensen et al, 1994a; An et al, 1995; Herzog et al, 1995).

Problems with the use of MRI include: its cost; the fact that an abnormal MRI may be found in asymptomatic people (Powell et al, 1986; Boden et al, 1990a); the time taken to perform the examination, which can make patients feel claustrophobic; the fact that patients with metallic implants, although not orthopaedic ones, cannot be scanned, and the impossibility of fitting very obese people into the machine (Powell et al, 1986; Boden et al, 1990a).

Discography

Discography uses a water-soluble radio-opaque dye injected under X-ray control directly into the nucleus pulposus. The technique itself can provide some useful information, such as the volume and ease with which the injection is given, as degenerated discs admit a larger volume of dye more easily than do normal discs. For the test to be considered positive, the injection must reproduce the patient's pain and injection into the other discs not do so. Injection of local anaesthetic should then abolish the pain. Its usefulness has been compared with that of MRI (Linson and Crowe, 1990; Simmons et al, 1994).

The main indication is in the diagnosis and assessment of internal disc disruption (Adams et al, 1986; Walsh et al, 1990; Bogduk, 1991; Moneta et al, 1994; Rhyne et al, 1995) when it may be best combined with CT (CT-discography)

(Vanharanta et al, 1987, 1989; Bernard, 1990; Moneta et al, 1994). However, its indications and usefulness remain controversial (Nachemson, 1989; Heggness and Doherty, 1993; Guyer and Ohnmeiss, 1995; Schwarzer et al, 1995a; Bogduk and Modic, 1996).

Myelography

Myelography using non-ionic water-soluble agents carries a sufficient morbidity to ensure that the procedure is never undertaken lightly. With disc prolapse, the column of dye should be indented or distorted with evidence of compression or shortening of the nerve root's dural sheath. It lacks both sensitivity and specificity, and has been largely superseded by MRI. It may still be used for preoperative assessment in patients with spinal canal stenosis or spinal tumour, or it may be used at times with a CT scan.

Bone scanning

This non-invasive technique is more sensitive than conventional radiography, although it is not overly specific, since a number of bone disorders can show the same appearances on scan (Holder, 1990). It employs a radionuclide such as technetium 99m-labelled methylene diphosphonate (Tc99m MDP), which, when taken up by bone, is bound to hydroxyapatite crystals. Its initial accumulation is dependent upon the blood supply, and it is used to show alterations in blood flow, or a later blood pool phase to show altered bone metabolism. The major role for scanning is in delineating metabolically active, pathological changes, especially infections, discitis, tumours (except for lytic lesions such as multiple myeloma), inflammatory diseases or metabolic bone disease. It is especially useful in stress fractures, and so is the best investigation to detect spondylolysis.

Laboratory investigations

Standard laboratory tests to investigate spinal disease include a full blood count: the haemoglobin concentration may be low in inflammatory diseases or tumours, the white cell count may be increased in infections or discitis. The erythrocyte sedimentation rate (ESR) or C-reactive protein (CRP) is a useful guide in inflammation or tissue destruction. It is always dangerous to ignore an unexplained elevated ESR, as it may have resulted from inflammatory lesions or tumours. Very high levels may be associated with discitis, polymyalgia rheumatica or multiple myeloma. A biochemical profile should include serum protein, creatinine, calcium, phosphorous and alkaline phosphatase levels, and prostate-specific antigen and acid phosphatase activity if prostatic secondaries are suspected. Blood cultures are needed if infection is suspected. Urine analysis should be performed routinely on all patients.

Electromyography may be used to localize the level of a spinal lesion with nerve root pressure, and evidence of denervation may be found two weeks after the onset of nerve damage. A lumbar puncture is rarely indicated, but should be performed if infection or a spinal tumour is suspected. In a lumbar disc prolapse, the cerebrospinal protein concentration is usually normal or slightly increased, although with a large prolapse the value may rise. Bone marrow examination or bone biopsy may be indicated for the diagnosis of generalized disorders, especially multiple myeloma or tuberculosis.

Other investigations are described in the appropriate sections.

5 Lumbar intervertebral disc syndromes

Disc degeneration is the underlying basis for several different clinical syndromes. These include:

- Intervertebral disc prolapse
- Spondylosis
- Lumbar canal stenosis
- Vertebral instability
- Isolated disc resorption
- Acute cauda equina syndrome
- Juvenile disc syndrome.

Disc prolapse

The nuclear material of the disc may escape from the confines of the annulus and prolapse in an anterior, superior, inferior or posterior direction (Figure 5.1).

- An anterior prolapse is generally asymptomatic as no nerves are compressed.
- In adolescents, prolapse in an anterosuperior direction through the developing epiphyseal ring may be associated with Scheuermann's disease.
- A superior or inferior prolapse bulges through the vertebral endplates into the vertebral body, producing a Schmorl's node (*see* Figure 2.1). This prolapse is contained by a thin layer of compact bone, visible on X-ray (Takahashi et al, 1995) (*see* Figure 2.2).

- Nuclear material can prolapse through the weakened posterior aspect of the annulus until it is restrained posteriorly only by the integrity of the posterior longitudinal ligament, which determines to some extent the final direction it takes. If the ligament remains intact, the disc may prolapse in a posterolateral direction, but if the ligament is ruptured, disc material may become sequestered within the spinal canal (Figure 5.2). The prolapsed disc is composed mainly of nuclear material, but also of varying mixtures of annular and separated cartilage endplate material. If the prolapse stretches and compresses the nerve root against the bony canal or thickened ligamentum flavum, it produces back and leg pain, or back pain alone, or it may be asymptomatic in 20–30 per cent of cases (Hitslberger and Witten, 1968).

Disc prolapse occurs at the L4–L5 or L5–S1 levels in more than 95 per cent of patients (Frymoyer, 1988; Deyo et al, 1992a; Kanner, 1994; Wipf and Deyo, 1995), and at the L3–L4 and L2–L3 levels in up to 5 per cent (Wipf and Deyo, 1995). The age of onset ranges usually from 20 to 50 years (Frymoyer, 1988), with a peak at about 40 years. Accordingly, the diagnosis should be critically reviewed when symptoms appear for the first time in patients below the age of 16 or over 50, as other diagnoses are more common at these ages. Either sex may be involved, although males are

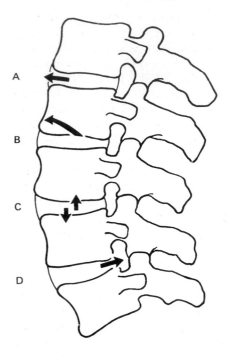

Figure 5.1 Direction taken by a nuclear prolapse. An anterior prolapse (A) does not impinge on any neural structures. (B) An anterosuperior prolapse associated with Scheuermann's disease. (C) A vertical prolapse producing Schmorl's nodes. A posterior prolapse (D) may produce neural compression

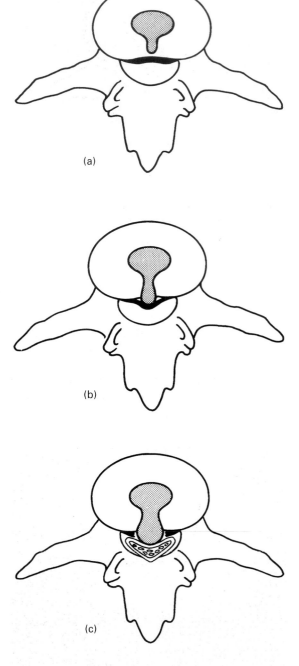

generally considered to be the more commonly affected.

The clinical picture will depend upon the interrelationship between the anatomical and pathological features involving the disc, the spinal canal and the neural elements.

The size of the disc prolapse, the direction it takes, which may be into a central, posterolateral or a lateral, intraforaminal, position (Figures 5.3 and 5.4); and its relation to the nerve root, which may lie either medially, laterally or under the prolapse, are important considerations. The spinal canal may vary in size, shape and capacity. It is normally oval in shape, but it may vary from triangular to trefoil shape if it becomes narrowed in congenital or pathological canal stenosis. Anatomical considerations also determine which nerve root is involved. In the spinal canal, the nerve roots on either side pierce the dura, run obliquely downwards at the back of the vertebra,

Figure 5.2 Lumbar disc prolapse. (a) In the first stages of prolapse the nuclear material bulges posteriorly through defects in the annulus. (b) The prolapsed nuclear material is contained by the posterior longitudinal ligament. (c) Disruption of the posterior longitudinal ligament allows disc material to prolapse into the spinal canal

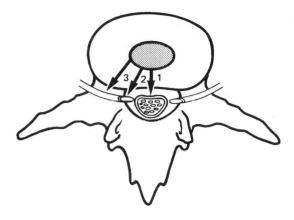

Figure 5.3 A disc prolapse may proceed: (1) in the central midline and compress the dura; (2) posterolaterally and compress the nerve root; or (3) laterally and compress the nerve root in the intervertebral foramen

curve around the pedicle and cross the inferior disc before emerging through their intervertebral foramen. At the L4 disc level, the L4 nerve root runs through its intervertebral foramen and the L5 and sacral nerve roots are still contained within the dural sac. At the lumbosacral level the L5 nerve root is contained within its intervertebral foramen and the dural sac contains only the sacral nerve roots.

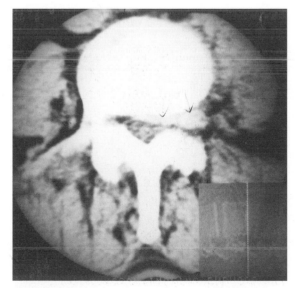

Figure 5.4 Posterolateral and intraforaminal disc prolapse

The nerve root compressed by prolapse of the L4–L5 intervertebral disc depends on the direction taken by the prolapsed material. The L5 nerve root may be involved by a posterolateral disc prolapse (Figure 5.5); with a lateral prolapse the L4 nerve root is involved in its intervertebral foramen, whereas a central disc prolapse may compress the L5 nerve root. Similarly, a posterolateral lumbosacral disc prolapse usually compresses the S1 nerve root, but a laterally directed prolapse will compromise the L5 nerve root in its intervertebral foramen. Other changes in the neurological presentation may occur because of anomalous spinal segmentation, and rarely are two nerve roots involved with a disc prolapse.

Clinical findings

Pain may be initially confined to the lower back, and its onset is usually sudden and severe, although it may develop more gradually. Pain is described as deep, dull and aching or severe, knife-like ('like a hot poker') in the low back, either in the midline or to one side or in the buttock. It may be intermittent at first, relieved by rest or changes in position, but is usually made worse by sitting or sudden straining, such as coughing or sneezing. It is usually made worse by certain movements that produce compressive, tensile or shear stresses on the disc. Pain may be brought on for no apparent reason, although

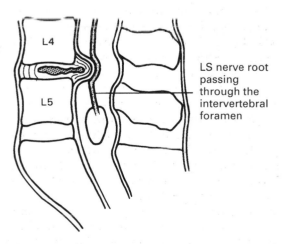

LS nerve root passing through the intervertebral foramen

Figure 5.5 A prolapse of the L4–L5 intervertebral disc may compress the L5 nerve root

many patients relate it to some minor traumatic incident or after a strain such as bending, lifting or twisting, when it may be associated with a tearing sensation. There may be a history of attacks of back pain, sometimes associated with a sensation of back-locking. Back pain may be followed some later time by leg pain, almost always unilateral and usually severe. Back pain may disappear when the leg pain begins. Associated symptoms may include neurological symptoms such as paraesthesia, hyperalgesia, leg cramps or weakness.

Examination

Signs consist of varying combinations and degrees of mechanical lumbar spinal joint derangement plus nerve root involvement. The mechanical derangement is evidenced by alterations in posture, muscle spasm, alterations in the spinal contours and disturbance of movements.

Mechanical derangements

Alterations in posture

The patient may be unable to bear weight on the painful leg, and so stands with the hip and knee flexed and the back held rigid. The gait may also be antalgic, with as little weight as possible being transferred to the painful side.

Muscle spasm

The paravertebral muscles are nearly always found to be in spasm due to a reflex muscular contraction, a protective reflex that limits movements of the spine and the inflamed nerve root. Spasm may be bilateral or unilateral, and usually extends over several lumbar spinal segments. It is usually easily palpable, and should be assessed with the patient standing, moving and lying prone.

Alterations in spinal contour

Alterations in the normal lumbar curvature may be present either as scoliosis or loss of the normal lordosis. Scoliosis may be observed with the patient standing, or on flexion or extension of the lumbar spine. The scoliosis is contralateral in 85 per cent of cases, and ipsilateral in approximately 15 per cent. It has been considered to be protective in nature, in an attempt to alter the relationship of the nerve root to the prolapsed disc (Figure 5.6). Scoliosis may be quite marked,

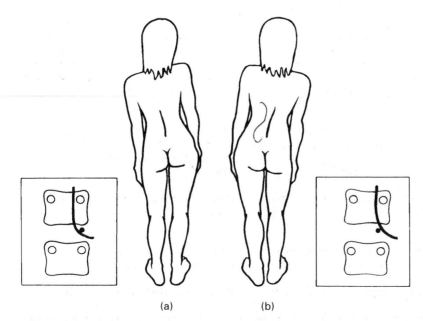

(a)   (b)

Figure 5.6 Relationship between a protective scoliosis and the site of nerve root pressure. (a) A contralateral protective scoliosis is usually associated with a disc prolapse on the lateral side of the involved nerve root. (b) An ipsilateral scoliosis is usually associated with a disc prolapse on the medial side of the involved nerve root most commonly with an L5 intervertebral disc prolapse. In juvenile disc lesions, a marked degree of scoliosis may occur with marked muscle spasm, but with relatively little pain.

Disturbance of active movement

Forward flexion is the movement most commonly reduced in range, and its degree of restriction usually reflects the severity of the prolapse. It may also be associated with a scoliosis. In a severe attack, only a small range is possible before being limited by pain and muscle spasm. In a moderate attack, the patient may be able to flex to approximately half the normal range. Loss of extension is less common, but when lordosis is lost, extension will usually be markedly limited and painful. Lateral flexion is usually of full and painless range to each side, although it may at times be painfully limited to one side, more commonly towards the side of pain.

Passive movements

The passive ranges of physiological and accessory movements are also limited because of pain, stiffness and muscle spasm.

Nerve root involvement

Nerve root involvement, associated with a loss of freedom of movement of the nerve root in the spinal canal or its intervertebral foramen, is indicated by the presence of a neurological deficit. Neurological assessment determines the nerve root involved and its degree of compression. Motor changes including muscle weakness and wasting provide a good indication of the involved neurological level. Muscles are tested by inspection, isometric contraction and functional movements. Sensation and knee and ankle reflexes are tested in both legs (Table 5.1). Straight leg raising and femoral nerve stretching are tested next (*see* Chapter 4).

Palpation

The affected spinal level is usually tender to palpation in the midline, or in the paravertebral area on the same side as the disc prolapse. The sciatic nerve may also be tender, particularly over the sciatic notch or in the popliteal fossa.

Clinical variations

The most common pain pattern is back pain

Table 5.1 Nerve root involvement in intervertebral disc prolapse

Involved root	Pain distribution	Sensory loss	Motor weakness	Reflex changes
S1	From buttock to back of thigh and leg, lateral aspect of ankle and foot	Lateral aspect of ankle, foot and posterior calf	Plantar flexion of ankle and toes, extension of hip and flexion of knee	Ankle jerk
L5	From buttock to the lateral aspect of leg and dorsum of foot and great toe	Dorsum of foot and great toe. Anterolateral aspect of lower leg	Dorsiflexion of great toe, dorsiflexion of other toes and dorsiflexion in eversion of ankle	Nil
L4	Lateral aspect of the thigh to the medial side of the calf	Medial aspect of calf and shin	Dorsiflexion and inversion of ankle and extension of knee	Knee jerk
L3	Anterior thigh to anterior region of knee	Lower inner aspect of thigh and knee	Flexion, adduction and internal rotation of hip	Knee jerk
L2	Anterior aspect of upper thigh	Upper outer aspect of thigh	Flexion and adduction of hip	Nil

followed by leg pain, but other patterns are possible.

- Back pain alone, intermittent or constant, is usually described as 'aching', related to posture and activity and relieved by rest. It may be felt only in the midline, may spread symmetrically across the back, or may be felt as a sacral or buttock pain. Attacks of mechanical derangement with 'locking' may also occur.
- Sciatic pain alone. Leg pain, usually gradual in onset, either radiates distally from the buttock region or is felt in any part of the dermatome. The distance pain radiates usually depends on the degree of nerve root pressure, but it needs to be differentiated from a peripheral nerve entrapment.
- Simultaneous sciatic and back pain is a less common form of presentation.
- Sudden sciatic pain of such severity that the patient is unable to lie still usually indicates that a large piece of a disc has extruded through the posterior longitudinal ligament.
- Rarely are two ipsilateral nerve roots implicated; or a large posterior prolapse compresses one root on either side of the midline.
- Motor weakness alone without sensory changes may present with a sudden onset of foot drop.
- A rare complication of severe nerve root compression is rupture, or atrophy, of the nerve root. Pain ceases and straight leg raising becomes normal, but motor and sensory signs become more marked.

Natural history

The natural history of disc prolapse has been described in several papers (Saal and Saal, 1989; Saal et al, 1990; Maigne et al, 1992; Bush et al, 1993; Weber, 1994; Komori et al, 1996), and knowledge about the natural history has been increased by the use of CT and MRI (Bozzao et al, 1992; Komori et al, 1996). The history may be one of exacerbations and remissions of pain, with a high chance, approximately 90 per cent, of recovery, especially if pain can be readily relieved. Spontaneous absorption of the prolapsed disc can occur, aided by inflammatory changes that develop around the disc (Ito et al, 1996a; Doita et al, 1996), and especially with a large prolapse (Saal et al, 1990; Maigne et al, 1992).

Management of lumbar disc prolapse

Initial management

A prolapsed intervertebral disc with radiculopathy can be treated very successfully with an aggressive non-operative physical rehabilitation programme (Saal and Saal, 1989). Pain relief is the first requirement, and rest from pain-producing activities is necessary, although how this is best achieved is still debated. Rest in bed may be prescribed (Waddell, 1987b), the rationale being to rest an area of inflammatory oedema around the nerve root and reduce intradiscal pressure, but it should be necessary for a short period only (Deyo et al, 1986; Twomey and Taylor, 1995). There is no evidence that prolonged bedrest or prolonged avoidance of activity reduces the back pain (Twomey and Taylor, 1995) or has any effect on its natural history. Two days of rest is usually considered sufficient (Deyo et al, 1986), as longer periods have not been found to produce any greater improvement. Prolonged bedrest itself constitutes a problem, as it has a deleterious effect on the musculoskeletal system in general, and produces physical deconditioning of muscle with weakness and wasting, which may take some considerable time to recover.

Medication

Simple analgesics should be given in sufficient quantities to ensure pain relief and allow sleep. Non-steroidal anti-inflammatory drugs (NSAIDs) are given in an attempt to control the inflammatory component and also for their analgesic properties (Weber, 1994). Side effects, especially those on the gut and especially in older people (Henry et al, 1996), and their effects on cartilage metabolism (Karppinen et al, 1995), may be limiting factors.

Any method of pain relief without use of drugs, such as TENS or acupuncture, is worth trying, but the results are uncertain (Deyo et al, 1990b, Marchand et al, 1993).

Corticosteroid injections

The painful inflammatory reaction around the nerve root can be eased by an epidural injection (EDI) of corticosteroid. The epidural space lies between the two layers of dura with an outer or periosteal layer, and an inner or dural layer. This space, which is continuous from the foramen magnum to the sacral hiatus, also contains the vertebral venous plexus and fat. The spinal cord usually terminates at about L1 and the dural sac at the S2 level.

Soon after its introduction as a local injection, hydrocortisone was injected extradurally around an inflamed lumbar nerve root. Reports of its use appeared first in the European literature, and in 1961 its successful use in 113 patients was reported (Weinstein et al, 1995). Many reports about its successful use, mainly in uncontrolled papers, have since been published (Watts and Silagy, 1995), and several good reviews have been reported (Kepes and Duncalf, 1985; Bogduk et al, 1994; Koes et al, 1995; Watts and Silagy, 1995; Spaccarelli, 1996). The injection is usually given via the translumbar route, although it can also be given through the sacral canal.

TRANSLUMBAR EDI

The technique is similar to that of an epidural anaesthetic, using a disposable set and scrupulous aseptic technique. The injection must be given only extradurally and must be discontinued should the dura be pierced. The patient lies curled up on the painful side and the injection is given at the involved level. The needle should be felt to lie free in the epidural space, and various techniques, such as the hanging-drop method, have been described to verify its location. An injection of corticosteroid is then given and the patient rests for two days. It may be repeated once or twice more at two- to three-weekly intervals, if necessary.

The major indication is a disc prolapse of recent onset with evidence of nerve root compression, and the best results are obtained with a recent onset of severe leg pain, with or without back pain, and with or without neural symptoms. Other indications, such as back pain alone, rarely produce any benefit.

The injection is never given if there is any nearby skin infection or in people taking anticoagulants. It needs to be given in hospital and old age and pregnancy are not contraindications to its use.

Complications from the injections are rare. The usual problems with corticosteroid injections can occur, including systemic absorption, so diabetes can be exacerbated for a few days. Back pain may be exacerbated for one or two days. Headache may occur in up to 5 per cent of patients, indicating the presence of a dural puncture. It usually settles with rest and rarely requires a dural patch. Serious infective complications are extremely rare.

CONTROLLED TRIALS

Most of the reported trials of EDI have not been controlled (Kepes and Duncalf, 1985; Bogduk et al, 1994; Watts and Silagy, 1995), but 13 properly controlled studies using either the trans-sacral or trans-lumbar routes have been reported. Of these, five (Dilke et al, 1973; Yates, 1978; Mathews et al, 1987; Ridley et al, 1988; Bush and Hillier, 1991) reported favourable results, and eight (Beliveau, 1971; Snoek et al, 1977; Klenerman et al, 1984; Cuckler et al, 1985; Andersen and Mosdal, 1987; Rocco et al, 1989; Serrao et al, 1992; Carette et al, 1997) were unfavourable. However, nearly all of the studies have had their limitations (Spaccarelli, 1996). Two meta-analyses (Rapp et al, 1994; Watts and Silagy, 1995) concluded that corticosteroids are effective in the management of lumbosacral radicular pain. An overall enhanced improvement rate of 14 per cent following the injection, when comparing it to the natural history of the disease, was reported (Rapp et al, 1994). The injection does seem to work best in the short and intermediate term, that is for two weeks to three months after the treatment (Spaccarelli, 1996; Carette et al, 1997).

TRANS-SACRAL APPROACH

The sacrum comprises four fused vertebrae, with a fifth vertebra that remains unfused and ends as two projections or cornua. The opening of the sacral hiatus is normally covered over by a firm, elastic ligament which lies between the two cornua. The hiatus, often at the site of a skin dimple, may be identified between the cornua which are readily palpable on either side.

A solution of 20–30 cc of 0.5 per cent ligno-caine (Xylocaine) without adrenaline is used, to which corticosteroid can be added. The injection is best given in hospital, but can be given in a surgery provided adequate resuscitation facilities are available. The skin is thoroughly sterilized and a 20-gauge needle is inserted at the midline with the patient lying prone and as relaxed as possible, with a pillow under the pelvis. The thumb and finger of the left hand over the cornua help to guide the direction of the needle. There is a sensation of 'giving' as the ligament is pierced, and if the needle is angled slightly down-wards it can then be felt to lie free within the sacral canal. If it impinges on bone, the needle is withdrawn and slightly angled. If it lies outside the canal, the subcutaneous tissue is seen and felt to swell with the injection of fluid (Figure 5.7). Normally the injection is felt to run in without resistance, with repeated aspirations to ensure the absence of any blood or cerebrospinal fluid. A few ccs are injected first, and the patient is observed for about five minutes. The rest of the injection is then given slowly, over at least 10 minutes. The patient is advised that a sensation of warmth, and possibly some exacerbation of pain, may occur, and is asked to report any untoward symptoms such as light-headedness or giddiness. The pulse rate and blood pressure are monitored during and after the injection, and the injection is stopped if any untoward reaction is experienced.

The best results are obtained with a severe degree of sciatic pain of recent origin, with or without neurological signs; the more severe the pain, the greater seems to be the chance of success. It is often a useful method of providing pain relief with either a posterolateral disc protrusion or bilateral leg pain.

The injection is contraindicated with known sensitivity to local anaesthetic or any nearby skin infection.

PRECAUTIONS:
- Strict asepsis is necessary.
- The syringe must be constantly aspirated to ensure that no blood or cerebrospinal fluid is withdrawn. If blood or cerebrospinal fluid is aspirated, the injection is ceased.
- The injection is given slowly.

- Adverse vaso-vagal reactions are anticipated by monitoring the pulse and blood pressure. Facilities for resuscitation need to be at hand.
- The patient stays at rest for approximately 20 minutes after the injection and is then allowed to move about.

The injection may be repeated if necessary two to three weeks later, and may be repeated another two or three times, provided there is some degree of improvement. Pain may be exacerbated after the injection, although rarely for more than one or two days, and in approxi-mately 70 per cent of cases of sciatica there is marked relief of pain and increased mobility so that more active treatment can be instituted.

Manual therapy

The manual therapy techniques best used are lumbar traction and spinal mobilization proce-dures (*see* Chapter 8), both of which are intended to ease pain and increase the range of spinal mobility, and can be continued provided symp-toms are not exacerbated. Other physical methods of treatment such as heat or massage are of no value, and manipulation is contraindicated at this stage (Weber, 1994).

Exercise programmes

Exercise programmes, designed to strengthen muscles, maintain and increase the range of movements and improve endurance, play a central role in management of chronic back disorders (Lahad et al, 1994; Twomey and Taylor, 1995) and help to prevent recurrences (Scheer et al, 1995). Muscle strength decreases and the muscles become more easily fatigued after an attack of disc prolapse with its enforced rest, so that it becomes necessary to prescribe muscle strengthening exercises and stretch tight struc-tures. However, exercise programmes may not play such an important role in the management of an acute attack of low back pain (Dettori et al, 1995; Faas et al, 1995).

Exercises are also needed to correct poor posture (Itoi and Sinaki, 1994; Livingston, 1994) and to help stabilize any segmental instability. However, there is a marked variation in which

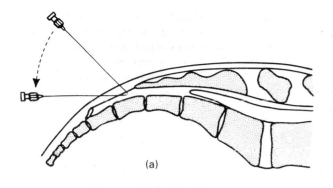

(a)

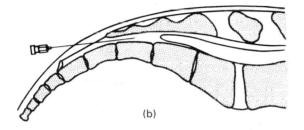

(b)

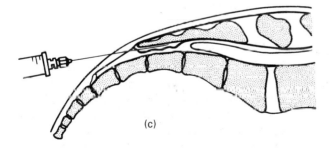

(c)

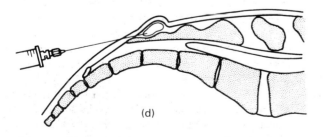

(d)

Figure 5.7 Trans-sacral extradural injection. (a) The needle is first inserted through the sacral hiatus at an angle and then lowered to be directly in line with the sacral canal. (b) The needle lies free within the sacral canal and the injection of fluid runs in freely without any undue pressure. Note the relationship of the dura, which normally ends opposite the second sacral segment. (c) If the needle impinges against bone it is difficult to give the injection. (d) If the needle is placed outside the sacral canal the injection is difficult and a soft-tissue swelling appears over the sacrum

exercises are, or should be, taught (Koes et al, 1991b), and trials have still not confirmed their usefulness (Quebec Task Force, 1987; Koes et al, 1991b; Faas et al, 1995). Patient motivation and compliance are often a problem (Deyo et al, 1990a; Livingstone, 1994). Two months after an active intervention with exercises, most patients had discontinued them, and any initial improvement had gone (Deyo et al, 1990b).

Exercises available are: (1) isometric; (2) extension; (3) flexion; and (4) aerobic exercises (Frymoyer, 1988; Lahad et al, 1994). Each has its rationale; each has its devotees. It may well be that the most important thing is to determine what type of exercise causes the least degree of pain and use that exercise as treatment. The use of modern testing devices such as Cybex (Ito et al, 1996b) provides a means of testing lumbar trunk strength (Robinson et al, 1993), although their role remains controversial and they may not be good predictors of future trouble (Mooney and Andersson, 1994).

In patients with an acute attack of pain, isometric exercises are usually prescribed first (Cady et al, 1979). The rationale for using them is that increasing intra-abdominal and intrathoracic pressures helps to prevent increased intradiscal pressures (Bartelink, 1957; Cresswell et al, 1994). Isometric exercises improve the ability to generate higher levels of voluntarily induced intra-abdominal pressure, and increase the rate of intra-abdominal pressure development during functional situations (Cresswell et al, 1994). They produce minimal joint movement, increase intra-articular pressure to a much lesser extent than do isotonic exercises, and are therefore less likely to provoke pain as other exercises might, especially if they are undertaken too soon or too enthusiastically. However, there is little evidence that they can enhance other forms of muscle function. Isometric exercises are simple to teach and to learn, but they need to be individually tailored, should be performed throughout range, performed as often as possible and regularly supervised by a physiotherapist. Their success, as with other exercise regimens, may well depend upon the ability to convince patients of their long-term benefit.

Spinal flexion exercises are also commonly prescribed. The rationale for their use is that the lordotic curve becomes a major problem, more so on standing, by compressing the posterior structures. Accordingly, the aim of these exercises is to reduce the lumbar lordosis, increase abdominal flexor muscle strength, increase trunk stability, open up the intervertebral foramen and stretch some of the tight posterior structures, including the hamstrings. The increase in muscle strength is designed to create a 'corset of muscles' to support the spine.

McKenzie extension exercises have also been widely advocated, but have a completely opposite rationale (Doneison et al, 1997). The lordosis, by decreasing disc pressure and increasing stability, is now considered to be protective. Extension exercises aim at regaining the lumbar lordosis, reducing stress on the posterior disc and ligaments and moving the nucleus, and with it the patient's symptoms, into a more central position. The centralization of pain means that distal referred pain is moved more proximally toward the lumbar midline. It may be that centralization can predict a more favourable outcome in some patients, although it may just predict those patients who are most likely to improve (Delitto et al, 1993). Although extension exercises are commonly prescribed, many patients do have pain on extension and they find that these exercises exacerbate their pain.

However, the effects of muscle reconditioning and restoration of functional abilities in chronic low back pain patients has not been fully documented in the literature, and trials are difficult to interpret (Quebec Task Force, 1987). Nine clinical trials have been reported comparing flexion with extension exercises (Kendall and Jenkins, 1968; Davies et al, 1979; Zylbergold and Piper, 1981; Buswell, 1982; Ponte et al, 1984; Nwuga and Nwuga, 1985; Elnaggar et al, 1991; Delitto et al, 1993; Dettori et al, 1995), although some other published trials are not valid, in that other treatment modalities were included in the trial (Scheer et al, 1995). Of the nine trials, one (Kendall and Jenkins, 1968) favoured isometric flexion, and three favoured extension (Ponte et al, 1984; Nwuga and Nwuga, 1985; Delitto et al, 1993), although of these, one, Delitto et al (1993) was equivocal. The other five trials showed no difference between flexion and extension exercises. Therefore, there is little evidence in the literature to support a preference for one programme over the other (Elnaggar et al, 1991; Koes et al, 1991b; Livingston, 1994), and it may well be that the most important thing is to perform exercises, rather than what particular method is used.

As pain is relieved, patients should be encouraged to resume normal daily activities, not only to increase spinal mobility and improve disc nutrition, but also for their positive psychological benefits. Aerobic activities such as swimming, walking and cycling can be added and progressed as long as they do not exacerbate symptoms, and stretching (Khalil et al, 1991) or yoga exercises are also added. The intention is to restore as much mobility as possible without the use of forced movements, and the exercise regimes should not cause any exacerbation of pain. Many patients with low back pain feel better after exercise and are able to return to work earlier (Waddell, 1987b; Saal and Saal, 1989). As lumbar function improves with exercise, the level of back pain also declines (Waddell 1987b; Twomey and Taylor, 1995). With a vigorous exercise programme for patients with disc prolapse, 90 per cent of patients had good or excellent outcomes and were able to return to work (Saal and Saal, 1989).

To be effective, an exercise programme requires:

- **Assessment of the patient's isometric, isotonic and isokinetic muscle strength.** This has been aided by the use of isokinetic dynamometers such as Cybex or Kin Com.
- **Individualization.** The programme needs to be prepared and tailored to these individual deficits and requirements.
- **A proper prescription.** Too little exercise may be of no value, too much may be harmful.
- **Specificity.** Specificity of exercises is necessary to obtain the desired training effect.
- **Motivation.** A detailed explanation of the aims of therapy and enthusiasm concerning the results are required to keep patients motivated over the long period before results become apparent.
- **Supervision.** The programme needs to be supervised by a physiotherapist to ensure that the exercises are properly taught and carried out.

- **Correct timing.** Timing is important since starting exercises too soon may aggravate pain and prolong recovery.
- **Progresssion.** The programme needs to be gradually progressed and increased in intensity.
- **Effectiveness.** Exercises should be dynamic and full-range. The programme should produce its desired result without producing any prolonged period of pain or undue fatigue. Should it do so, the programme needs to be revised.

Lumbar supports

Support in a well-fitted corset, with a heat-moulded plastic insert moulded into the lumbar lordosis, is used to help ease pain while allowing the patient to remain mobile (Huston, 1988). Several theories have been proposed, but the exact mechanism by which belts function is not known (Smith et al, 1996). Although a corset cannot completely immobilize the spine, it may help by limiting movement (McGill et al, 1994), especially at the extremes of range. Another proposed mechanism is that it increases intra-abdominal pressure (Bartelink, 1957), and may reduce the load on the lumbosacral disc by up to 25 per cent (Nachemson and Morris, 1964; Walsh and Schwartz, 1990; Lander et al, 1992; Ciriello and Snook, 1995). A corset may allow a better use of body mechanics (de Ruiter, 1990), and so help with lifting, especially if the abdominal or spinal muscles are weak, although this was not confirmed by Smith et al (1996). However, corsets should never be used as the sole method of management. Abdominal and spinal exercises are performed while the supports are worn (Genaidy et al, 1995), and they should be discarded as soon as practical.

Disadvantages of lumbar supports include:

- There may be patient resistance to wearing corsets, unless it can be demonstrated that pain relief will follow
- A placebo effect cannot be overlooked
- Patients may become psychologically dependent upon them
- There is a lack of proof of their benefit (Lahad et al, 1994; Ciriello and Snook, 1995).

Rehabilitation

Patients should be encouraged to return to activity as soon as possible with the use of an active programme (Saal and Saal, 1989). Management in this stage consists of back exercises, postural control and back care. Intensive back exercises are also incorporated into a rehabilitation programme known as 'the back school', in which education, skill and exercise regimes are taught, with the inclusion of basic anatomy, function, posture, proper lifting techniques, and aerobic activities (Lindstrom et al, 1992a,b; Alaranta et al, 1994; Koes et al, 1944; DiFabio, 1995; Hall and Hadler, 1995). It should be supervised by a physical therapist, and a clinical psychologist may assist with behaviour modification therapy and pain management techniques with relaxation and biofeedback (Asfour et al, 1990). Lifting techniques are included for those whose occupation requires them (Professional Development, 1995).

Surgery

There are few absolute indications for surgery and only about 0.25 per cent of patients with back problems will require some form of surgery (Kraemer, 1995). Indications include:

- Cauda equina compression
- A severe degree of pain that increases despite adequate treatment
- Progressive neurological motor deficit.

Surgery should be reserved for those in whom function cannot be satisfactorily improved following a physical rehabilitation programme (Saal and Saal, 1989). The decision regarding whether or not therapy has failed and the type of surgery required, is a difficult one that needs to be considered in light of the natural history with its exacerbation and remission, and the likelihood of recovery over a period of time. In one trial after one year (Weber, 1994), surgery patients did better than did medical ones, but at 10 years the results were identical. The patient's wishes and expectations from surgery plus its cost effectiveness (Hoffman et al, 1993; Shvartzman et al, 1993; Malter et al, 1996) must also be consid-

ered. Operations to relieve back pain alone without sciatica or following an inadequate trial of physical therapy (Errico et al, 1995) are rarely successful. Surgery may need to be considered if symptoms become worse during the initial treatment period, or with no improvement after a minimum of six weeks of treatment, or with recurrent attacks of pain and disability with prolonged loss of time from work.

The type of surgery available and how it relates to the diagnosis also need to be considered. The simplest surgical procedure needed to relieve pain is indicated, and removal of the prolapsed disc material alone is usually sufficient. Open decompressive laminectomy and discectomy has been the standard procedure (Kahanovitz, 1993), and recent changes in techniques have brought about improvements in results (Errico et al, 1995). It is most useful for patients with extruded hard disc fragments (Kraemer, 1995).

Microsurgical discectomy is performed under magnification, and is superior to standard discectomy (Caspar et al, 1991) as it allows a more conservative surgical approach (Williams, 1991) and a smaller incision, better vision, reduced operation time and earlier return to work for the patient. Percutaneous lumbar discectomy has the advantage of being a closed technique, with minimally invasive arthroscopic surgery performed under local anaesthetic. First introduced in 1975 (Hijikata, 1989), it was improved with the use of an automated nucleotome (Onik et al, 1990), which placed a 2-mm probe into the disc to aspirate disc material. Its use increased as disenchantment with the complications following chymopapain injections grew. Its aim is to remove the prolapsed nucleus or to remove it from the centre of the disc, reducing the increased intradiscal pressure (Kambin and Cohen, 1993) and the disc height (Shea et al, 1994). Two prospective controlled trials have demonstrated its success (Onik et al, 1990; Mayer and Brock, 1993), and other trials have reported excellent results (Dullerud et al, 1995; Slotman and Stein, 1996). Complications are rare (Mayer, 1994), as are recurrences (Lowell et al, 1995). Laser discectomy has also been described (Kambin and Cohen, 1993; Ohnmeiss et al, 1994; Sherk et al, 1993).

Spinal arthrodesis

There are three main types of spinal fusion with bony arthrodesis between two or more adjacent vertebrae: an anterior (Faciszewski et al, 1995); a posterior (Lee et al, 1995a); and a posterolateral interbody, which is probably the most commonly used in the lumbar spine. Some problems associated with fusion, its indications, the area to be fused, which type of fusion is preferable, and whether fusion needs be done routinely after laminectomy, remain unsettled. Osteoinductive growth factors may be used to enhance the fusion rates. A major indication for fusion is pain relief in vertebral instability, whether due to degenerative disc disease, spondylolisthesis or trauma. It is most commonly performed for disc disease, but, unfortunately, this is also the least successful indication. The results usually depend on careful case selection rather than operative technology.

Lumbar spondylosis

The term 'spondylosis' causes confusion in that it refers to a well-recognized pathological condition associated with lumbar disc degeneration, but it is also used as a clinical diagnosis. It occurs more commonly in elderly men and may involve all levels of the lower lumbar spine, but especially the lower discs. Its basis is disc degeneration which develops at a more gradual rate, thus allowing reactive changes to take place in the neighbouring structures (Vernon-Roberts and Pirie, 1977; Kirkaldy-Willis et al, 1978), such as vertebral bodies, zygapophyseal joints, intervertebral foramina and spinous processes. As the degenerative changes develop in the annulus, clefts form in the disc and may fill with gas, becoming evident as the vacuum phenomenon on X-ray. These pathological changes are mirrored by radiological changes, which may be graded in degrees of involvement from one to four. The relationship of the X-ray changes to symptoms is, however, inconsistent.

As degenerative changes develop and the disc loses height, the disc space narrows, so that the annulus bulges beyond its normal confines. Osteophytes develop circumferentially around the vertebral margins, most commonly on its

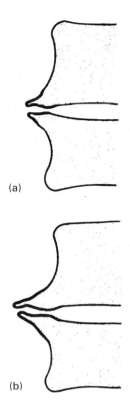

(a)

(b)

Figure 5.8 (a) Early stage of osteophyte formation, which grows outwards around the degenerated disc. (b) Later stage of osteophyte formation

anterolateral borders. They grow outward at first around the cartilaginous mass of the annulus, but may then turn upward or downward and may eventually approximate osteophytes from adjacent vertebrae (Figure 5.8). Anterior and lateral osteophytes are of little clinical consequence, but those protruding posteriorly or posterolaterally may encroach on the neural canal to produce symptoms. Osteophytes tend to develop where pressure changes are greatest and reduce the force per unit area by broadening the area between the disc surface and the vertebral body. They are found more commonly on concavities, such as the concave surface of a scoliotic spine.

Vertebral endplate

The vertebral endplate becomes irregular, and bony sclerosis develops first in the subchondral bone and later spreads to involve a larger area of the vertebral body with pseudocysts and erosions (Francois et al, 1995). Vascular granulation tissue may invade the disc from the vertebral body, so that ultimately it may lead to ankylosis, most commonly in the thoracic spine, with ankylosis of the anterior vertebral margins.

Zygapophyseal joints

Degenerative changes in the disc result in a disturbance of the position and function of the zygapophyseal joints, which become relatively hyperextended. The joints are thus subjected to increasing strains, which result in degenerative changes and capsular thickening. Subsequently, the zygapophyseal joint facets may sublux and impinge against the pedicle of the superior vertebra.

Intervertebral foramen

The diameter of the intervertebral foramen, with its emerging nerve roots, is reduced as a consequence of the diminished disc volume, and of the osteophytic outgrowths on the vertebral bodies and zygapophyseal joints.

The spinous processes

The alteration in the relative position of the vertebral bodies can result in approximation of the spinous processes, evident on X-ray. Ultimately their contiguous borders become sclerotic, with formation of a false joint, known as 'kissing spines', when pain and restricted movement may occur on lumbar extension. How much a problem this represents has been doubted (Beks, 1989).

Clinical symptoms

Patients may complain of back or leg pain, either unilateral or bilateral, with or without neurological symptoms, and stiffness. Pain is typically dull and aching, sited in the lower lumbar midline, and may radiate out to the groin or buttock, but its exact mechanism of production is unknown in any individual case. Pain tends to get worse as the day progresses, but at times it may be more pronounced after a night's rest, and then eases as the patient becomes more mobile. Pain may be exacerbated following overuse or unaccustomed activities by a mechanical derangement with synovitis in the zygapophyseal joints.

Pain in one or both legs may be due to one of three mechanisms:

1. Pain may be referred into the leg.
2. Sciatica may result from nerve root pressure, for which there are three distinct causes. The first is an encroachment on the neural canal by the osteophytes arising from the vertebral and zygapophyseal joints. The second from the disturbance of the normal vertebral relationships that follows disc space narrowing and approximation of the vertebral bodies. The nerve root may be impinged either by the articular facets or by the pedicle of the superior vertebra. Finally, an acute intervertebral disc prolapse may occur, although this is uncommon.
3. Leg pain may be due to a lumbar canal stenosis.

Management

Patients with this condition are usually over the age of 40, may be overweight, and their type of work may aggravate their disorder. They require rest from any known aggravating factors and should avoid activities that involve excessive bending, such as gardening. Support in a corset may help to ease pain and restrict some of their extremes of movement. Passive movement techniques play a major role in management. Lumbar traction and spinal mobilization techniques may be expected to relieve pain and increase mobility. Isometric exercises are used to strengthen abdominal and back muscle groups. Overweight patients must lose weight and should be encouraged to exercise by walking or swimming as much as possible. Anti-inflammatory agents are used for those with evidence of the more severe degenerative zygapophyseal joint changes in an attempt to reduce any associated synovitis.

Surgery is rarely indicated for degenerative changes alone, as they usually involve several discs in older people, and so its role is limited. In patients with sciatica due to lumbar canal stenosis, an operation to decompress the nerve root canal may be indicated.

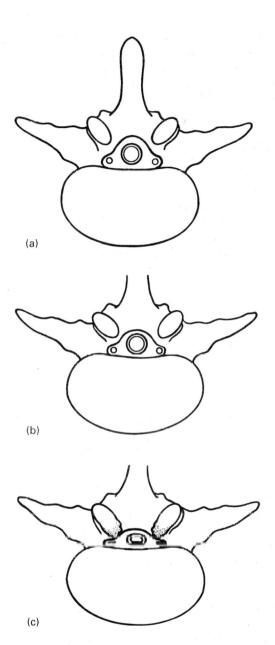

Figure 5.9 The lumbar spinal canal. (a) Normal size and shape. (b) Normal shape but the canal size is diminished. (c) Canal stenosis. The canal size is reduced due to osteophyte formation in the apophyseal joints. The spinal nerves may then be compressed in the para-articular gutter

Lumbar canal stenosis

Stenosis, or narrowing of the lumbar spinal canal is a common cause of back and leg pain in elderly people (Moreland et al, 1989; Deyo et al, 1992b; Turner et al, 1992; Katz et al, 1995a; Stucki et al, 1996). It is characterized by a reduction in the anteroposterior and lateral diameters of the bony spinal canal, and alteration of its shape (Arnoldi et al, 1976). In a normal spinal canal, the neural structures lie within the dural sac between the vertebrae and discs anteriorly and the pedicles and laminae posteriorly, with ample space available for their movement. Spinal stenosis has been described in three anatomic sites: central; in the lateral recess (lateral); or foraminal. Central stenosis involves mechanical compression of the nerve roots in the cauda equina, whereas lateral stenosis involves individual nerve roots outside the dura in the lateral recess. As the size and shape of the canal becomes narrowed (Figure 5.9), and the enclosed nerve roots become compromised, there may be no clear distinction between the two sites (Amundsen et al, 1995).

Lateral canal stenosis (Ciric et al, 1980; Lee et al, 1988; Porter and Ward, 1992; Jonsson and Stromqvist, 1994) results in nerve root compression in the lateral canal. The nerve root, as it descends from the dural sac, passes obliquely around the pedicle. It then runs in a canal formed anteriorly by the disc and vertebral body, posteriorly by the anterior surface of the superior articular facet and superiorly and inferiorly by the pedicles, to emerge through the intervertebral foramen. Its most narrow portion lies between the pedicle and the superior articular facet, where, if degenerative changes with bony hypertrophy occur, the nerve can be easily compressed (Jensen et al, 1994a). The L4 or L5 nerve roots are most commonly involved, and patients present with leg pain, which is usually severe and is more likely to correspond to a dermatomal pattern than is a central stenosis. Symptoms commonly associated with disc prolapse, such as pain made worse by coughing or straining, do not usually occur.

Aetiology

Lumbar canal stenosis may be congenital or acquired. The congenital defect, as for example in achondroplasia, is associated with short pedicles and narrow anteroposterior and transverse diameters of the spinal canal (Hall et al, 1985; Moreland et al, 1989; Kent et al, 1992). The more common acquired condition occurs as a result of degenerative changes in the surrounding bone and soft tissues such as the disc, zygapophyseal joints and ligamentum flavum (Kirkaldy-Willis et al, 1978; Postacchini et al, 1994; Fukuyama et al, 1995). A hard annular bulging with osteophyte formation, together with hypertrophic zygapophyseal joint changes bulging into the spinal canal from its posterolateral angle, produces a typical clover leaf, trefoil shape when viewed from above (Figure 5.10). Some patients may suffer a combination of a developmentally small canal, usually asymptomatic, and degenerative changes, which results in an area of narrowing of the canal. Single or multiple levels may be involved (Frymoyer, 1988). Degenerative spondylolisthesis is also a common cause of both central and lateral stenosis, and may be complicated by the presence of synovial cysts (Jensen et al, 1994a). Rarer causes have been described, including spondylolysis, bone diseases, such as Paget's disease, post-spinal surgery (Louw et al,

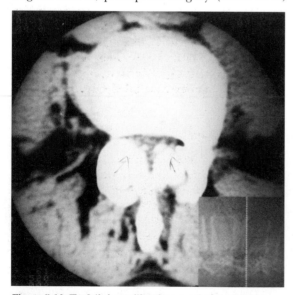

Figure 5.10 Trefoil-shaped lumbar canal stenosis with degeneration in the zygapophyseal joints

1988), neoplasms (Moreland et al, 1989) and isolated disc resorption. Racial differences (Eisenstein, 1977) and familial cases (Varughese and Quartey, 1979; Postacchini, 1985) have been described.

Clinical features

Canal stenosis is usually due to degenerative changes affecting men in their sixties (Dorwart et al, 1983; Hall et al, 1985; Spengler, 1987; Frymoyer, 1988; Lipson, 1989a). Leg pain is always present, although its description may at times be vague. Symptoms are divided into two broad categories: claudicant or neurological. Pain coming on with walking, similar to a vascular claudicant pain, has been termed 'pseudoclaudication'. Pain may be felt in the back, thighs or lower legs, but it is usually poorly localized. Aching pain, or cramps in one or both legs that comes on after walking a certain distance and is relieved by rest or sitting, are most common (Amundsen et al, 1995). When out walking, the patient may have to sit down often on a seat or a fence until the pain eases. Unlike the more rapid disappearance of pain in patients with peripheral vascular disease, pain relief may require a longer period of rest. However, it can be difficult to differentiate them from the history alone, especially should both be present (Dodge et al, 1988). Pain is also made worse when first standing erect or on extension of the spine, gets worse as the day goes on, is relieved by rest and may be relieved on flexion. Pain may involve any part of the limb and may be associated with paraesthesia and/or generalized leg weakness. Sensory impairment in the lower limb is often patchy in distribution. If symptoms tend to be vague or diffuse, they may sometimes be misdiagnosed as psychogenic.

On examination, the patient may present with a wide-based gait, a positive Romberg test and muscle weakness (Turner et al, 1992; Katz et al, 1995a). Other findings may include a typical stooped posture with flexed knees, hips and low back: the so-called simian stance (Simkin, 1982; Kallina, 1985), and patients often have to sleep on the side in a flexed position. Since flexion increases and extension decreases, the anteroposterior spinal canal diameter (Magnaes, 1982; Amundsen et al, 1995; Katz et al, 1995a), altering the back posture may either exacerbate or relieve pain in the back and/or the legs, Pain is absent when the patient is seated. Riding a bicycle to differentiate the pain of lumbar canal stenosis from that of peripheral vascular disease (Dyck and Doyle, 1977), although interesting, is of no great clinical relevance. Tendon reflex and sensory changes are variable, particularly after exercise, and the reflexes should be checked before and after exercising to detect any differences.

Pathophysiology

The exact mechanism of production of symptoms in canal stenosis is uncertain (Moreland et al, 1989; Konno et al, 1995). Normal movements may produce traction on the neural tissues in the spinal canal, but as they can glide and mould within the bony confines, no symptoms are produced (Weisz and Lee, 1983). Symptoms are related to the reduction in spinal canal volume. The anteroposterior diameter of the spinal canal is the most reliable diagnostic parameter (Grabias, 1980; Herno et al, 1994b). It is normally above 15 mm, and less than 11 or 12 mm is definitely abnormal (Eisenstein, 1977; Grabias, 1980; Onel et al, 1993; Herno et al, 1994a). Its minimal cross-sectional area is approximately 77 ± 13 mm (Dommisse, 1975; Schonstrom et al, 1989).

Symptoms could be due to pressure on nerve roots, arteries, veins (Konno et al, 1995) or capillaries (Moreland et al, 1989). Venous pooling can occur in the cauda equina between two levels of low-pressure stenosis (Porter, 1996), and could result in a failure of arterial vasodilatation in the congested roots in response to exercise (Porter, 1996). The nerve roots in the cauda equina derive their blood supply from the radicular arteries (Parke and Watanabe, 1985), which supply only their respective nerve roots and are not distributed to other structures. Actively conducting nerve roots require a large blood supply, which, if reduced, could cause neurological symptoms to develop. Occlusion of a radicular artery and nerve root ischaemia could readily occur in the stenotic spinal canal and be a cause of symptoms (Parke and Watanabe, 1985; Watanabe and Parke, 1986; Porter and Ward, 1992).

Investigations

The diagnosis of lumbar canal stenosis can usually be made on clinical grounds (Deyo et al, 1992a; Katz et al, 1994, 1995; Stucki et al, 1996), with its characteristic history and signs, and is confirmed by radiology. However, symptoms may vary according to their underlying anatomical site (Dauser and Chandler, 1982; Dorwart et al, 1983). Routine spine X-rays are not often helpful (Weisz and Lee, 1983; Amundsen et al, 1995), especially since degenerative changes are so common in this age group (Amundsen et al, 1995). They may, however, lead to a suspicion of the correct diagnosis and help to exclude any alternative diagnosis (Sanderson and Wood, 1993). CT and MR scanning are useful non-invasive techniques which can outline the size and shape of the canal and its contents (Eisenstein, 1983; Simeone and Rothman, 1983; Weisz and Lee, 1983; Bolender et al, 1985; Maravilla et al, 1985; Schonstrom et al, 1985; Kent et al, 1992; Herno et al, 1994a,b), and CT myelography may supply more information (Dublin et al, 1983; Goldberg et al, 1991; Kent et al, 1992; Porter and Ward, 1992). Myelography (Sortland et al, 1977; Uden et al, 1985; Kent et al, 1992) may be needed only as a pre-operative assessment (Herno et al, 1995) to outline the size and shape of the canal. Any alteration to the dural sac, usually an hourglass constriction in the sac at the stenotic level, may be evident (Figure 5.11). EMG changes can be helpful (Yates, 1981; Keim et al, 1985; Tsitsopoulos et al, 1987; Moreland et al, 1989) to indicate degrees of root compression and exclude other diagnoses.

Natural history

The natural history is difficult to determine (Grob et al, 1995) because symptoms may be intermittent (Johnsson et al, 1992, Garfin, 1995), and until recently the initial management strategy was surgical. It was previously believed that surgery was always indicated in most patients, and, especially if only one level were involved, that results would be universally excellent, with success rates of up to 90 per cent reported (Grabias, 1980; Hall et al, 1985; Spengler, 1987; Katz et al, 1991; Johnsson and

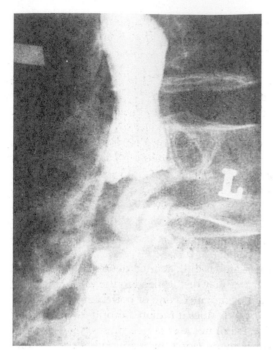

Figure 5.11 An oblique view of a myelogram showing obstruction to the flow of the dye in a patient with canal stenosis and degenerative apophyseal joint changes at L4–L5

Stromqvist, 1994; Grob et al, 1995; Stucki et al, 1996). However, it is now recognized that surgery is neither mandatory nor successful in all cases (Katz et al, 1991, 1995b; Turner et al, 1992; Onel et al, 1993; Postacchini, 1996). Eighty per cent of surgical patients in one report have a good result, but the remaining 20 per cent will develop future deterioration (Postacchini, 1996). In addition, some patients have improved with medical treatment alone, including some in which surgery was contraindicated on medical grounds.

Few controlled prospective trials have been published to compare medical with surgical management (Turner et al, 1992; Onel et al, 1993; Amundsen et al, 1995). A meta-analysis to determine the effects of surgery on pain and disability showed that 64 per cent of patients reported good to excellent results (Turner et al, 1992). However, major defects in reporting were common, and there were wide variations across the studies in the percentage of good outcomes (Turner et al, 1992). A cohort study of 88 patients followed by Katz et al (1995b) for up to 10 years found that 75 per cent were satisfied with their operation. However, one-third had severe back pain, and half were unable to walk two blocks (Katz et al, 1995b). Other problems with surgery became apparent (Katz et al, 1991; Deyo et al, 1992a), including patient satisfaction (Katz et al, 1995b; Stucki et al, 1996), lack of prospective trials (Turner et al, 1992; Onel et al, 1993; Amundsen et al, 1995) and insufficient follow-up. Back pain may remain a problem postoperatively and repeat operations may be needed for other long-term problems (Nakai et al, 1991), such as instability (Hopp and Tsu, 1988; Johnsson et al, 1986, 1989) or restenosis (Herno et al, 1995) due to postoperative bone growth (Chen et al, 1994a).

Management

Medical treatment (Onel et al, 1993; Gregg, 1994; Kana and Weisel, 1994; Garfin, 1995), including weight loss, rest from aggravating activities and suitable analgesia including a TENS machine, a lumbar corset, isometric back exercises and exercises in water should be tried first. Non-steroidal anti-inflammatory agents have little to offer in the way of pain relief and constitute a greater risk in this age group. Extradural injections of corticosteroids may be tried (Ciocon et al, 1994; Stolker et al, 1994), but they are not often successful. Manipulation and traction are contraindicated.

Surgery is indicated in patients with severe pain, major neural deficits, progressive neural damage, lack of medical improvement or if activities or walking distance are limited (Johnsson et al, 1992; Katz et al, 1991), and it is still the treatment of choice for most patients (Hall et al, 1985). Age is no barrier to surgical treatment (Grabias, 1980; Fast et al, 1985; Sanderson and Wood, 1993; Postacchini, 1996). The art of surgery is to provide adequate decompression by removal of sufficient bone, without removing excess bone, which leads to instability. In central stenosis the standard operation has been a total laminectomy (Postacchini et al, 1993), but spinal fusion may be necessary for any resultant instability (Nasca, 1987; Herkowitz and Kurz, 1991; Tuitte et al, 1994; Grob et al, 1995). Multiple laminotomy has been described as being more successful (Young et al, 1988; Nakai, et al, 1991; Postaccini et al, 1993). Decompression and arthrodesis may be necessary for those who have a lumbar canal stenosis due to spondylolisthesis (Herkowitz and Kurz, 1991).

Long-term results may not be as successful as short-term results (Katz et al, 1991; Silvers et al, 1993; Tuitte et al, 1994), and reoperation may become necessary in up to 20 per cent of patients (Johnsson et al, 1989; Katz et al, 1991; Herron and Mangelsdorf, 1991; Caputy and Luessenhop, 1992). Better results may be anticipated with surgery for lateral canal stenosis.

Vertebral instability

Segmental stability in the lumbar spine is dependent upon the surrounding bones, ligaments and muscles, and any degenerative or traumatic disorder that affects any of these structures could result in abnormal segmental movement. The lumbar vertebral instability that results may be a cause of back pain (Nachemson, 1985). However, it is difficult to define, mainly because there are so many conflicting opinions about its existence and diagnostic criteria (Kirkaldy-Willis and Farfan, 1982; Farfan and Gracovetsly, 1984; Stokes and Frymoyer, 1987; Sato and Kikucki, 1993; Sharma et al, 1995; Schlegel et al, 1996). One definition describes it as a clinically symptomatic condition in which, in the absence of a new injury, a physiological load induces abnormally large deformations at the intervertebral joint (Farfan and Gracovetsky, 1984). Its basis is abnormal spinal movement, whether due to an increase in abnormal movement under stress (Kirkaldy-Willis and Farfan, 1982), or abnormal coupling movements (Dupuis et al, 1985). Abnormal rotational or translational movement then leads to rotational or translational instability (Sharma et al, 1995).

It occurs in either sex, usually in the third or fourth decades and usually involves the L4 or, less commonly, the L5 disc (Kirkaldy-Willis and Farfan, 1982). This type of instability usually follows degenerative changes in the disc (Kirkaldy-Willis and Farfan, 1982; Nachemson, 1985; Keller et al, 1990; Mimura et al, 1994) and zygapophyseal joints (Cyron and Hutton, 1980;

Lorenz et al, 1983; Stokes, 1988; Abumi et al, 1990; Pintar et al, 1992; Haher et al, 1994; Patwardthan, 1994; Sharma et al, 1995; Kaigle et al, 1995). It may also occur in patients with spondylolisthesis, following trauma (Cholewicki and McGill, 1996), or postoperatively, such as after decompression of lumbar spinal stenosis (Lee, 1983, Lorenz et al, 1983), all of which should be evident on X-ray. It has also been produced experimentally (Stokes et al, 1989; Kaigle et al, 1995). Loss of muscle function is a common concomitant (Panjabi et al, 1989; Goel et al, 1993; Kaigle et al, 1995).

Clinical findings

Pain, which is dull, aching, deep-seated and often constant, may be localized to the mid-spinal area, or it may radiate to one or both buttocks and legs. Only rarely does it radiate beyond the knees, and evidence of nerve root pressure is usually absent. Pain is made worse by maintaining one posture for a long time, for example standing or sitting, and altering the posture by, for example, lying down or arching the back, may relieve pain. This pattern is typically punctuated by attacks of more severe pain. The spine is vulnerable to any forced or unguarded movements, such as lifting or twisting, which can result in increased strain on surrounding soft tissues, especially the anterior and posterior longitudinal ligaments or the zygapophyseal joints (MacNab, 1971a).

Clinical signs may be difficult to elicit, especially if the overall range of spinal movement be normal, although at times it may be possible to find some loss in the expected range of flexion or extension. The mechanical instability may produce pain on active movement, typically as an arc of pain, which may occur either during flexion or else as the patient straightens up from the flexed position. Tenderness may be found locally over the involved segment of the spine.

Investigations

Although the presence of vertebral instability may be suspected on clinical grounds, the diagnosis needs to be confirmed by X-ray (Mimura et al, 1994; Murata et al, 1994). The significant radiological findings are the demonstration of

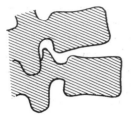

Figure 5.12 Vertebral instability. The upper lumbar vertebra is tilted upwards and backwards on the lower vertebra with overriding of the apophyseal facets

instability in all planes of spinal movement (Dupuis et al, 1985; Frymoyer and Selby, 1985; Nachemson, 1985). In lateral X-rays with the patient in full flexion and extension, abnormal movement with loss of the normal rolling mechanism may be detected. The superior vertebra may move forward on the lower one during flexion, and it may then be associated with a narrowing of the anterior part of the disc. Alternatively, an excessive backward sliding movement of the upper lumbar vertebra may occur on lumbar extension (Figure 5.12).

Other radiological signs have been described, although they have not been fully evaluated. They include:

- The presence of gas within the disc indicates disc degeneration since gas can accumulate following separation of its fibres, but this X-ray sign can be present without any instability.
- A traction spur, which is found approximately 2 mm from the vertebral edge. The outermost fibres of the annulus arise from the anterior margins of the upper vertebral bodies and are inserted into the anterior margin of the lower vertebrae. The abnormal degree of vertebral movement could produce traction on these fibres and accordingly the traction spur develops by growing out horizontally (MacNab, 1971a). (Figure 5.13).

The X-ray changes that have been described may also be present in asymptomatic patients, and so do not necessarily relate to the current symptoms (Sato and Kikuchi, 1993; Murata et al, 1994; Pitkanen and Manninen, 1994; Kaigle et al, 1995). In addition, symptoms may relate to the development of a lateral canal stenosis rather than to the radiological signs of instability (Sato and Kikuchi, 1993).

Management

The patient usually presents with a moderately severe degree of back pain that tends to be constantly present, but may be modified by certain postures. A combination of therapies will be indicated, as the aim of treatment is to control pain, improve posture and attempt to increase the strength and control of the spinal muscles. Exercises to strengthen back and abdominal muscles and correct any postural fault, including hamstring tightness, form the cornerstone of management. Several different trunk and girdle exercise programmes have been used with reported good success (Saal and Saal, 1989), especially if the lumbar multifidus muscle is involved (Wilke et al, 1995). An exercise programme involving the deep abdominal and back muscles to provide joint stabilization has been described in detail by Richardson and Jull (1995).

Pain may be relieved by analgesics and helped by giving advice to the patient about back protection. Such advice includes obtaining extra rest for the back and avoiding postures and movements, particularly prolonged bending and

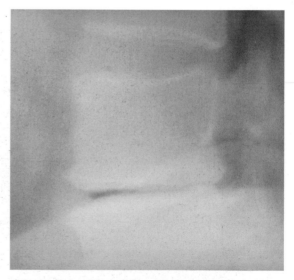

Figure 5.13 L4–L5 instability with gas in the disc and traction spurs

lifting, known to exacerbate pain. Pain may also be relieved with a suitable support, such as a lumbar corset, which has the added advantage of keeping the patient mobile. Lumbar corsets do not need to be worn for any long period. Passive movement techniques, such as spinal mobilization, are used for pain relief, but more forcible manipulative techniques are not indicated. Surgery is a contentious issue in patients with vertebral instability, especially the role of spinal fusion (Frymoyer and Selby, 1985). It does not often need to be considered, but if it is, careful patient selection is required. Fusion is only indicated if pain is severe, prolonged and unresponsive to conservative treatment, with demonstrable radiological evidence of instability.

Isolated disc resorption

In this uncommon condition, severe progressive degenerative changes involve usually only one of the lower intervertebral discs (Jaffray and O'Brien, 1986). The disc is virtually completely resorbed and may develop inflammatory changes (Crock, 1986; Jaffray and O'Brien, 1986), leaving only a rim of annulus (Crock, 1986). Back and leg pain develop, which may be due to altered spinal mechanics, and not to a disc prolapse. Spinal

canal stenosis usually results, with low back, buttock and leg pain. The principal radiological sign is a marked loss of disc space that has developed rapidly, leaving little time for degenerative changes to develop (Figure 5.14). Conservative treatment may settle the symptoms, but surgery for a lateral or central lumbar canal stenosis will often become necessary.

Acute cauda equina syndrome

This acute lesion is an uncommon, most serious, complication of disc degeneration (Choudury and Taylor, 1980; Kostuik, 1993a) that occurs when a mass of nuclear material is suddenly extruded through the posterior longitudinal ligament into the spinal canal. It may follow a sudden flexion strain or a lumbar manipulation (Haldeman and Rubinstein, 1992). The effects of the sudden pressure increase in the cauda equina have been investigated (Glover et al, 1991; Olmarker and Rydevik, 1991). The manifestations include back pain with radiation into one or both buttocks and legs (Floman et al, 1980; Kostuik et al, 1986); sensory and motor neurological defects in the legs, sensory changes in the sacral dermatomes involving scrotal and perianal areas, and alteration or loss of urinary or bowel functions (Lavyne, 1994).

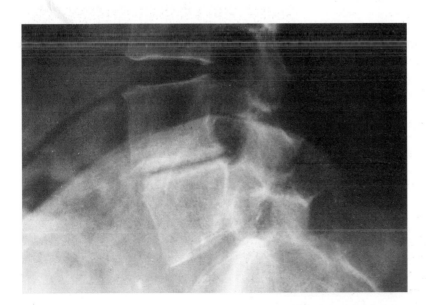

Figure 5.14 Isolated lumbar disc resorption

Early clinical recognition and imaging with MRI, CT or CT-myelography (Kostuik, 1993a; Jensen et al, 1994a) are imperative to allow early surgical decompression to prevent permanent bladder or bowel damage (Kostuik et al, 1986, 1993a).

Juvenile disc syndrome

The pathology and clinical presentation of disc prolapse in adolescents usually differs from that of adults. Most agree that there are sufficient clinical differences to consider it a separate syndrome (Bulos, 1973; Kamel and Rosman, 1984; Ghabrial and Tarrant, 1989), although this is still debated (Ghabrial and Tarrant, 1989). It is more common in boys than girls, although girls may develop it at a younger age than boys. Trauma, either direct trauma to the spine, or indirect trauma following a fall onto the buttocks, appears to play an important role (de Orio and Bianco, 1982). Familial predisposition has been described (Nelson et al, 1972; Zamani and MacEwen, 1982; Clarke and Cleak, 1983; Varlotta et al, 1991).

The patient may complain of varying degrees of pain, but marked spinal stiffness and muscle spasm are the predominant clinical characteristics. Spinal movements, especially flexion, are markedly reduced. A decreased lordosis and a sciatic scoliosis, which become much more pronounced on flexion, may be present.

Neurological symptoms may not be so prominent as in the adult version, but straight leg raising is markedly reduced (Takata and Takahashi, 1994). Hamstring tightness is marked (Takata and Takahashi, 1994), and may also be reflected in a rather peculiar, shuffling gait.

The clinical course is usually prolonged and the diagnosis may often be delayed (Kurihara and Kataoka, 1980; Giroux and Leclercq, 1982; Kamel and Rosman, 1984). Symptoms may persist for up to two years (Bradbury et al, 1996) before resolving, and conservative management does little to influence it. CT or MRI scans (Tertti et al, 1991; Salminen et al, 1993, 1995) are indicated for accurate assessment and to exclude other diagnoses such as a spinal tumour.

Surgery may be indicated in those with severe or persistent root pain or if conservative treatment fails (de Orio and Bianco, 1982; Lorenz and McCullough, 1985; Savini et al, 1991; Silvers et al, 1994; Bradbury et al, 1996). Most series report good initial results, although at follow-up after some years results have been described as disappointing (de Orio et al, 1985; Lorenz and McCullough, 1985). At operation the disc is usually turgescent, diffusely swollen and tightly bulging without necessarily being ruptured (Bulos, 1973), and the posterior portion of the ring apophysis may be traumatically avulsed. Chemonucleolysis using chymopapain has been used with reported good results (Lorenz and McCullough, 1985; Wilson et al, 1992; Bradbury et al, 1996).

6 Mechanical spinal disorders

Zygapophyseal joints

The synovial lumbar zygapophyseal joints can become a source of low back pain and stiffness, with pain commonly referred to the lower limb (Ray, 1991). Difficulties exist, however, in defining its prevalence, how it is to be diagnosed and its management. Opinions range from considering it to be the most common single cause of low back pain, to being an uncommon cause, while some even doubt its existence. The joints were first considered to be a cause of low back pain by Goldthwait in 1911, while Chormley in 1933 was first to use the term 'facet syndrome' (Schwarzer et al, 1995b). Interest in it was relegated to the background after Mixter and Barr's (1934) description of disc protrusion, which soon became regarded as the source of all back pain. It was rediscovered as a source of back pain fortuitously after Rees (1971) claimed to be performing a rhizotomy to the joint, although it was instead a soft-tissue release, and the results he claimed for it were most improbable. Mooney and Robertson (1976) described their facet syndrome, about the same time as Shealy (1975, 1976) described his results with radiofrequency coagulation of the nerve supply to the joints, which has been described in detail by Bogduk (1983). Since then interest in this joint has increased, although its exact role in back pain has remained controversial.

Zygapophyseal joint pain

Zygapophyseal joint pain may be either acute or chronic. Acute pain may follow an injury, often involving spinal hyperextension or hyperflexion (Twomey et al, 1989; Fehlandt and Micheli, 1993). Acute trauma from a motor-vehicle accident may result in severe, but unsuspected, damage (Twomey et al, 1989) with postmortem fractures, undetected on routine X-ray. In the soft tissues, injuries include tearing of the joint capsule, tears in the articular cartilage and separation of the subchondral bone plate (*see* Chapter 16). Acute, non-traumatic attacks of joint pain may also occur. The reasons are not known, and many theories, such as impingement of synovial folds or meniscoid bodies between the joint surfaces, have been advanced to explain their occurrence (Bogduk and Jull, 1985).

Chronic joint pain is more common and may result from long-standing trauma, which may originally have been minor and resulting in degenerative changes in the joint (Lawrence et al, 1966; Lewinnek and Warfield, 1986; Bough et al, 1990) (Figure 6.1). It was previously believed that zygapophyseal joint degeneration occurred only in the presence of, and followed on from, intervertebral disc degeneration (Dunlop et al, 1984; Butler et al, 1990). This is now known not to be the position, and zygapophyseal joint degeneration can develop independently of disc degeneration (Malmivaara et al, 1987; Swanepoel

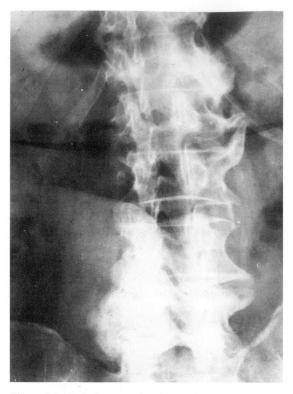

Figure 6.1 Marked zygapophseal joint degeneration at L4 and L5

et al, 1995). Nevertheless, in approximately 80 per cent of cases, zygapophyseal joint changes are associated with disc degeneration, and loss of disc space leads to overriding of the joint facets and abnormal joint movement. The tips of the facet of one joint may then impinge against the pedicle of the superior vertebra (Swanepoel et al, 1995), and be a source of pain.

Articular cartilage in the zygapophyseal joints, as in peripheral joints, is liable to undergo degenerative changes (Eisenstein and Parry, 1987). They are load-bearing joints, with the load varying from 3 to 25 per cent of the axial load (Andersson, 1983; Lorenz et al, 1983; Yang and King, 1984; Kahmann et al, 1990), which becomes higher with standing in prolonged extension or in the presence of degenerative changes in the disc (Yang and King, 1984; Kahmann et al, 1990). Ultimately, degenerative changes develop in the zygapophyseal joints, with erosion and thinning of articular cartilage, and synovitis can result (Swanepoel et al, 1995). The

edges of the articular cartilage are extended as osteophytes and 'wrap-around bumpers', which may be protective (Twomey and Taylor, 1985; Bogduk and Twomey, 1991). Synovitis may be brought on in the degenerated joint especially following overuse activities.

The diagnosis of osteoarthritis in these joints is difficult, as the changes shown on X-ray are of no great help. Degenerative changes seen on CT may not be a source of pain (Revel et al, 1992), although if the changes are severe they are more likely to be painful (Carrera, 1980a,b; Carrera and Williams, 1984; Lewinneck and Warfield, 1986). Other joint conditions, such as synovial cysts, inflammatory diseases, spondylo-arthritis or rheumatoid arthritis, may occur but are not very common.

Provocation tests, mainly using intra-articular hypertonic saline (Hirsch et al, 1963; Mooney and Robertson, 1976; McCall et al, 1979; Marks, 1989) or contrast medium with arthrography (Destouet et al, 1982; Lynch and Taylor, 1986; Moran et al, 1988) have been described, but their specificity is not known (North et al, 1994). Low back pain with ipsilateral pain in the buttocks or referred more distally into the legs was produced with these tests. As in other areas, the distance referred is related to the degree of the under-lying stimulus (Mooney and Robertson, 1976; Mooney, 1987). Normal volunteers were used at first (Hirsch et al, 1963; Mooney and Robertson, 1976; McCall et al, 1979), and subsequently similar results were obtained from patients with low back pain (Marks, 1989). In the earlier study (Hirsch et al, 1963), arthrography was not used to confirm correct needle placement, but it was used in the subsequent studies. The pattern of spinal or referred pain varied in different people and there was a great overlap in any given individual (McCall et al, 1979; Mooney and Robertson, 1976; Bogduk and Twomey, 1991). Stimulating the joint capsule during spinal operations under local anaesthetic (Kuslich et al, 1991) produced a deep, dull, localized low back pain, referred to the buttock, but never to the leg (Kuslich et al, 1991). In operations for lateral canal stenosis, back pain could be produced from the undersurface of the superior articular facet as it impinged upon the posterior surface of the intervertebral disc (Kuslich et al, 1991).

Further evidence was shown to support the notion that pain originated from the intra-articular injections of local anaesthetic, usually bupivacaine, given to produce pain relief (Fairbank et al, 1981; Raymond and Dumas, 1984; Moran et al, 1988). Results were variable and it could hardly be expected that injections of local anaesthetics alone could produce any favourable long-term benefit. However, injections of corticosteroids were also added, but again the results were variable. The reported trials using joint injections are difficult to summarize as they often take varying endpoints, use different injection agents and most are not controlled. The overall results from all tests vary from being very good (Mooney and Robertson, 1976; Carrera, 1980b; Destouet et al, 1982; Carrera and Williams, 1984; Lau et al, 1985; Lynch and Taylor, 1986; Murtagh, 1998; Revel, 1993; Goupille et al, 1993), to moderate (Lippit, 1984; Lewinnck and Warfield, 1986; Helbig and Lee, 1988), and poor

(Raymond and Dumas, 1984; Jackson et al, 1988; Moran et al, 1988; Lillius et al, 1989; Carette et al, 1991; Marks et al, 1992). Three trials have used controls (Fairbank et al, 1981; Lillius et al, 1989; Carette et al, 1991), although the trial by Fairbank et al (1981) used local anaesthetic alone. The other two trials used local anaesthetic and corticosteroids, but their results were not impressive (Table 6.1).

The clinical features associated with zygapophyseal joint dysfunction have been investigated by Schwarzer et al (1992, 1994a,b,c,d,e, 1995b,c) in a series of elegant studies that used double diagnostic blocks for pain relief. Screening was first performed using 2 per cent Xylocaine, as it has a rapid onset and short duration of action. Responders then underwent a separate confirming block with long acting 0.5 per cent bupivarcaine. Double responders were then used to establish the diagnosis and to obviate the problems of a high false positive rate

Table 6.1 Facet joint injections

Name, year	Number of patients	Number of joints	Injection of local anaesthetic	Injection of corticosteroids	Control	Improvement (%)
Carette et al, 1991	49	176	2 cc	20 mg D-med.	Yes	No difference
Carrrera, 1980b	20	20	2–3 cc	10 mg D-med.	No	65
Carrera et al, 1984	143	286	2–4 cc	15 mg D-med.	No	65
Destouet et al, 1982	54	1–4	1 cc	40 mg D-med.	No	54
Fairbank et al, 1981	25	50	0.5% Marcain	None	Yes	56 (acute attacks)
Goupille et al, 1993	206	1–2	None	1 cc	No	76
Helbig and Lee, 1988	99	99	NS	NS	No	82
Jackson et al, 1988	390	2–4	1 cc Marcain	0.5% triam.	No	29
Lau et al, 1985	34	68	1.5% Marcain	20 mg D-med.	No	56
Lewinnek, and Warfield, 1986	20	20	1 cc	20 mg D-med.	No	75
Lillius et al, 1989	28	56	6 cc Marcain	2cc D-med.	Yes	No difference
Lippit, 1984	99	117	11 cc	80 mg D-med.	No	42
Lynch and Taylor, 1986	50	Varied	None	60 mg D-med.	Yes	76
Mooney and Robertson, 1976	100	300	2.5 cc	1 cc D-med.	No	62
Moran et al, 1988	54	143	1-1.5 cc Marcain	None	No	16.7
Murtagh, 1988	100	194	1 cc	6 mg β-methas.	No	94
Raymond and Dumas, 1984	25	50	0.5–1 cc	None	No	16
Revel et al, 1992	40	124	1 cc 2%	2 mg	No	55

β-methas: beta-methasone
D-med: Depo-medrol
Triam: Triamcinolone
NS: not stated

(Schwarzer et al, 1994a) or the use of pain provocative tests alone (Schwarzer 1994d). The diagnosis of zygapophyseal joint pain was confirmed in 15 per cent of 176 patients. No clinical features could distinguish between those who responded and those who did not respond to diagnostic blocks, so they were not able to confirm a diagnosis of a 'facet syndrome' (Schwarzer et al, 1994b). Two models that had previously been used to describe the clinical features of 'the facet syndrome' (Fairbank et al, 1981; Helbig and Lee, 1988) were shown to be unreliable in distinguishing zygapophyseal joint pain from pain of other origins (Schwarzer et al, 1994e). The prevalence rate was higher, 40 per cent, in a study of 63 patients seen in a rheumatological clinic (Schwarzer et al, 1995b).

Pain arising from the disc was determined to be more common than pain arising from the zygapophyseal joint (Schwarzer et al, 1994c), and zygapophyseal joint pain was highly unlikely to occur in patients with symptomatic lumbar intervertebral discs (Schwarzer et al, 1994c). CT was of no value as a diagnostic test for patients with painful lumbar zygapophyseal joints, as its ability to identify such patients was not demonstrated (Schwarzer et al, 1995c).

Clinical findings

The symptoms associated with zygapophyseal joint disorders, pain and stiffness and their localization, are non-specific (Mooney and Robertson, 1976; Raymond and Dumas, 1984), and do not supply a clue to any particular diagnosis or spinal level of involvement (McCall et al, 1979; Lewinnek and Warfield, 1986; Jackson et al, 1988; Schwarzer et al, 1994b). Back pain is usually localized to one side of the midline, and may be referred to the buttock, groin and back of the thigh and leg as far as the knee. It is usually made worse by prolonged sitting, standing or rest, but rarely radiates below the knee. Stiffness is worse in the morning but does not last long. Certain movements involving back extension or hyperextension make the pain worse, whereas others such as flexion may help to relieve it. Zygapophyseal joint pain may be associated with other spinal conditions: synovitis may occur in

patients with lumbar instability or spondylosis, and degenerative joint changes are frequently present in patients with lumbar canal stenosis. Neurological symptoms are absent, unless there is another associated condition, such as lumbar canal stenosis.

Examination

The movements most liable to reproduce pain are extension or extension with lateral flexion, but these tests are non-specific as they can be found in other spinal conditions (Read, 1994). Neurological signs and reflex changes are usually absent. Straight leg raising is usually normal, although it may at times be reduced (Lippit, 1984), but never to a marked degree (Mehta and Wynn Parry, 1994), and presumably occurs due to a reflex hamstring spasm (Mooney and Robertson, 1976; Robertson, 1978). An area of localized tenderness may be palpated to the side of the spine.

Diagnosis

The diagnosis of a zygapophyseal joint disorder is usually made on clinical grounds, even though in most cases it can be little more than an educated guess. Accordingly, it often needs to be made as a diagnosis of exclusion. X-rays are not particularly helpful (Destouet et al, 1982). CT scans can demonstrate joint changes, usually degenerative ones (Carrera, 1980a,b; Hermanus et al, 1983; Carrera and Williams, 1984), but they do not necessarily correlate with the symptoms (Magora and Schwartz, 1976). Arthrography is relatively simple and safe to perform, and it has been of some value as an investigative tool (Carrera, 1980a,b; Dory, 1981; Destouet et al, 1982), but it is too invasive and does not offer sufficient information to be considered a clinical tool (Murphy, 1984). During arthrography the joint is easily ruptured (Maldague et al, 1981; Destouet et al, 1982), which is of some relevance when local anaesthetic is used, as it easily can diffuse out and irritate or anaesthetize surrounding neural tissues. Dual blocks, as described above, appear to be the only certain way to confirm a diagnosis (Bogduk and Schwarzer, 1995).

Management

The mainstay of management is pain relief, mobilization techniques, postural correction and back exercises. In an acute attack of low back pain, rest from the inciting activity may be necessary, although bedrest is rarely indicated and should be discouraged (Deyo et al, 1986). Injections using long-acting local anaesthetic and corticosteroid injections are worth trying (Mooney and Robinson, 1976; Lippit, 1984; Carrera and Williams 1984; Destouet and Murphy, 1984; Lau et al, 1985; Lynch and Taylor, 1986; Lillius et al, 1990), but they require the use of an image intensifier to be certain of correct positioning. Dye may also be injected to ensure proper placement of the needle. The results from the trials that have been reported vary widely. In three trials using controls (Fairbank et al, 1981; Lillius et al, 1989; Carette et al, 1991) results were not impressive. The medial branch of the dorsal ramus can be blocked under radiographic guidance using 0.5 per cent bupivacaine where it crosses in its groove at the base of the pedicle (Mehta and Wynn Parry, 1994).

If simple measures do not suffice, more sophisticated measures to provide prolonged anaesthesia, including radiofrequency denervation, a safe and effective procedure to block the nerve supply to the joint, may become necessary (Mehta and Wynn Parry, 1994). The technique of radiofrequency denervation of the facet joints,

first described by Shealy (1975, 1976), was subsequently refined by Bogduk and Long (1980) to denervate the medial branch of the posterior primary ramus. It is relatively easy, safe and can be effective, but needs to be undertaken in hospital under an image intensifier. It may be more specific than are joint injections (Bogduk and Long, 1980). A large number of case series have been described with high success rates in selected patients (North et al, 1994) (Table 6.2). Surgery (Markwalder and Merat, 1994) is rarely indicated.

Acute lumbago

Since the word 'lumbago' means 'pain in the back', it could be used as a title to describe any type of backache. In its more widely accepted sense, and as it is used here, it denotes an acute lumbar spinal syndrome characterized by a sudden onset of severe persistent pain, marked restriction of lumbar movements, and a sensation of 'locking' in the back. An attack usually occurs after a slight forward flexion movement, such as cleaning the teeth, standing up from a forward flexed position, sneezing, coughing, or bending and lifting a weight with a slight twisting movement (Kanner, 1994). A 'click' may be felt or heard. Pain is made worse by almost any back movement, so that straining, coughing or sneezing can produce intense pain, and even passing

Table 6.2 Radiofrequency denervation results

Name, year	Number of patients	% response
Shealy, 1976	380	80
Burton, 1976	126	42
Lora and Long, 1976	149	6
King and Lagger, 1976	?	27% vs placebo, 0
McCulloch and Organ, 1977	82	50
Ogsbury et al, 1977	37	35
Oudenhoven, 1979	337	83
Ignelzi and Cummings, 1980	41	41
Slujter and Mehta 1981	60	58
Mehta and Ray, 1982	65-	80
Rashbaum, 1983	100+	85
Katz and Savitz, 1986	115	75
Andersen and Mosdal, 1987	47	17
North et al, 1994	82	45

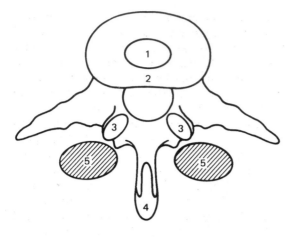

Figure 6.2 Proposed sites in the production of an acute lumbago: (1) the nucleus pulposus; (2) the annulus fibrosus; (3) the apophyseal joints; (4) the spinal ligaments and (5) the muscles

urine can become a problem. The patient, rendered immobile with the back 'stuck' in one position, usually partly flexed, may have to crawl to a bed to lie down immediately, unable to move.

Inspection of the lumbar spine reveals marked bilateral paraspinal muscle spasm, often more prominent on one side than the other. Examination of active movements, especially flexion and extension, is virtually impossible to perform. Laterally flexing the back towards the painful side is also restricted and a scoliosis away from the more painful side is common. Kyphosis, with the patient stuck in forward flexion and unable to straighten up, or a scoliosis towards the painful side, are rare findings.

The severe pain usually eases in a few days, leaving a dull, aching pain, which in a typical attack gradually eases in a week or two and leaves no residual disability. At times, pain may be dramatically relieved after a sudden movement, when the patient may again be conscious of something having clicked in the back. An unexplained feature is that attacks often recurs annually, and then often at about the same time of the year.

Pathogenesis

Acute lumbago is an acute form of mechanical derangement with locking of the intervertebral joint complex. Several theories have been proposed to account for its production, but most have been discarded. They include (Figure 6.2):

- An acute nuclear prolapse of the disc; acute hydrops of the disc; annular tears
- Zygapophyseal joint lesions, include subluxation, synovitis, an impacted synovial fringe or intra-articular structure, such as a meniscoid body
- Ligament tears and a primary muscle lesion.

Acute lumbago is a syndrome in which more than one condition can be the cause of a typical attack. A similar clinical picture also results from a fractured vertebra and, in elderly people, from a pathological fracture due to osteoporosis or secondary tumours. These can be differentiated by the history and X-ray changes. However, in any patient, during an attack, it is usually impossible to diagnose a definite cause, and standard X-rays are normal. It is commonly believed that a disc disorder is responsible, but it is difficult to substantiate this diagnosis during an attack. If a disc prolapse is responsible it can usually be confirmed only after a period of time; either the attack fails to settle over several weeks, or a subsequent attack of acute lumbago is associated with nerve root compression. However, in a sizeable proportion of patients the natural history does not resemble that of disc prolapse and the periodic attacks occur until they finally cease, with no evidence of a disc prolapse ever eventuating.

Management

Acute lumbago usually occurs as a severe attack that renders the patient incapable of movement, so that complete bedrest for a few days in a position of comfort with analgesics, sedation and local heat, such as a hot water bottle, for pain relief is all that the patient can encompass. It is virtually impossible to examine back movements, and manual therapy is also virtually impossible. Gentle, rhythmic manual traction applied to the legs for one to two minutes is all that can be applied. Manipulation is contraindicated if it may exacerbate the condition and it is too difficult to position the patient. As pain eases, other mobilization techniques may be added.

Hypomobility lesions

A hypomobility lesion is a painful, chronic form of a mechanical derangement of the intervertebral joint complex. It is a common condition, and its essential clinical features should include a restriction in the range of accessory intervertebral movements; appropriate testing of these movements will reproduce pain. Pain is often reproduced on testing active or passive spinal movements and if so, a pattern of movement restriction may be built up. X-rays will be normal for the patient's age.

The onset of pain is usually gradual, and it may be related to bending, twisting or some other traumatic event. Pain varies in degree from minor to more severe and is usually described as having a dull, aching quality. It tends to be localized, but may at times be referred more widely into the buttock, abdomen, groin, coccyx or leg. Leg pain is rarely felt below the knee and is never associated with sensory disturbances. At times the distribution of pain may be diffuse and hence the importance of a complete clinical assessment of movement at each lumbar joint for patients with pain of typical or atypical distribution.

Examination

Testing the overall range of the active physiological movements might show some evidence of restriction in movement, although they may at times appear normal. When they are restricted, they should also reproduce the patient's pain. In each area of the spine, the restricted movements tend to fall into certain common patterns. For example, in a patient with unilateral lumbar pain, lateral flexion either towards or away from the painful side may be limited and may reproduce the pain. This is then usually associated with pain either on flexion or on extension, but only very rarely with both. The normal rhythmic pattern of lumbar movement may also be disturbed, best appreciated by standing behind the patient to observe spinal movements. Restricted movement in the intervertebral segment usually results in an alteration in the rhythm of the spinal movements and in their contour.

Should these tests fail to reproduce pain, auxiliary tests (*see* Chapter 4), such as rhythmic over-pressure at the end of the range or the quadrant position, are used to reproduce pain or reveal joint signs at an appropriate level. Other evidence of deranged intervertebral joint mechanics that may be present includes a deformity, such as a scoliosis or loss of the normal lumbar lordosis. In all cases of hypomobility lesions, the normal accessory intervertebral movements, assessed by applying rhythmic pressures against the vertebral bony processes, are lost. The pressures must also reproduce the patient's pain. This may occur at any stage within the limited range, but occurs most often at the limit of the range, and is then often associated with a reflex muscle spasm that produces a characteristic end-feel.

Tenderness may be used as a confirmatory sign, usually felt over the affected joint, either over the supraspinous ligament or more laterally in the paravertebral area. Referred tenderness over the site of referred pain is also common. A thickening of the tissues in and around the relevant interspinous space may be palpable.

Aetiology

Symptoms and signs are related to the loss of the normal intervertebral movements associated with a mechanical derangement of the intervertebral joint. Its aetiology remains unknown, but it seems likely to be related to minor traumatic or degenerative changes in the zygapophyseal joints, and several hypotheses have been presented to explain the syndrome on the basis of such changes. These include degenerative changes in articular cartilage, osteochondral lesions, intra-articular meniscoid structures and adhesions. A form of a post-traumatic lesion can follow manipulation, usually by unqualified practitioners, resulting in a mechanical spinal joint derangement. Patients who have had a previous attack of acute back pain, especially if treated with prolonged rest, may also present with chronic symptoms due to a hypomobility lesion. It may be one cause of back pain in women after a confinement. Hypomobility lesions may be found in any of the spinal intervertebral joints, either in the lower or upper lumbar joints. Lesions may be found at more than one level, when of they are referred to as group lesions.

Lumbar disc degeneration may be associated with a hypomobility lesion at the thoracolumbar junction, with the latter being associated with continuing symptoms.

The importance of a hypomobility lesion could be looked upon in terms of the reduction in function that results from the loss of normal joint range. Most patients with a hypomobility lesion have no specific recognizable underlying pathological lesion, and the exact site of the derangement within the intervertebral joint complex cannot be demonstrated, as no single lesion is responsible for all cases of this joint derangement.

Referred pain

Pain from spinal hypomobility lesions is commonly referred to the back, leg or abdomen, usually to one site, which remains constant.

Sacroiliac pain

The sacroiliac joints can be a source of pain, and their features are described in Chapter 10. Pain and tenderness in the sacroiliac area may also occur with hypomobility lesions of the lower lumbar spine, in which pain is commonly referred to the buttock and over the sacroiliac area. It is then usually misdiagnosed as being due to a sacroiliac joint disorder. Most clinical tests of the sacroiliac joint will also stress the lumbar joints, so that differentiating between the two conditions can be a problem. This may be the reason for the past belief that the sacroiliac joint was responsible for most back problems (*see* Chapter 9). After appropriate treatment is directed to the lumbar joints, most patients with referred pain will respond and so it can be a most satisfying condition to treat.

Coccydynia

With this condition, patients complain of pain in the coccygeal area. Although pain may arise from local trauma, a common cause is a referred pain from hypomobility lesions of the lumbosacral joint. If so, testing of one of these joints must reproduce the pain. Patients are often subjected to many different therapies, including removal of the coccyx, all of which are usually to no avail. Treatment is with manipulative therapy to the lumbar spine.

Abdominal pain

Lumbar spine hypomobility lesions may produce pain that can be felt anywhere within the abdomen and can mimic various intra-abdominal causes of pain. Local abdominal wall tenderness, which is commonly present as a referred tenderness, may also be found. Common sites of involvement include around the iliac fossa or under the costal margin, which may be incorrectly diagnosed as gall bladder disease when the right side is involved. This has lead to claims that manipulation is able to cure some visceral disease.

Management

In hypomobility lesions of the lumbar spine, mobilization and manipulative techniques are the treatment of choice, and should provide relief of pain and restore the restricted range of intervertebral joint movement. With patients who do not respond adequately to mobilization techniques, locally tender areas should be infiltrated with local anaesthetic and corticosteroid, since they may contribute to the perpetuation of the pain. Medication with anti-inflammatory drugs rarely produces any great benefit, but simple analgesics may be used if required. Mobilizing exercises are indicated, especially if the condition has been present for a long time or is recurrent. Prolonged rest and use of supports are contraindicated, as they tend to increase the degree of restriction in the spinal joints.

The hypermobility syndrome

Hypermobility (Figure 6.3) is defined as a range of joint movement in excess of the usually accepted range and it may involve spinal and/or peripheral joints. The range of movement in any joint demonstrates individual variation, as there are inherited differences in the collagen structure of joints and ligaments. In the peripheral joints, the essential feature is that movements can be controlled by muscle activity throughout the

et al, 1990a,b; Grahame 1993; Larsson et al, 1995).

Clinical features

Hypermobility occurs predominately in women and is often familial or racial. It may also be feature in some hereditary connective tissue diseases such as Marfan's syndrome or Ehlers-Danlos syndrome. Hypermobility may be generalized, affecting all joints, or it may involve the spinal joints alone. In the spine, clinical features may include:

- Back pain, either continuous or recurrent
- A generalized increase in spinal mobility and in the range of passive intervertebral movements
- An associated hypermobility of the peripheral joints
- Other investigations, including X-rays, are normal.

Pain in the spine or peripheral joints is presumably due to the joints being more likely to be traumatized during everyday activities. Hypermobility as a cause of back pain was first described as the 'loose back syndrome' (Howes and Isdale, 1971). In their series of 102 patients with back pain (59 men, 43 women), an underlying cause could be diagnosed in virtually all the men. However, in 20 of the women, no definite diagnosis could be made, except that 17 of them had marked hypermobility as the cause of pain. Although the range of physiological movements is increased, a painful reduction in the range of passive intervertebral movement may occasionally be found at one spinal level. Passive movement tests should reveal this relatively hypomobile area, which is also amenable to treatment.

Management

Hypermobile patients with back pain are difficult to manage since pain tends to be recurrent and the underlying hypermobile basis and collagen tissue elasticity is not amenable to therapy. Isometric strengthening and stabilizing exercises form the main basis of management, and at times a support may also be used to relieve pain.

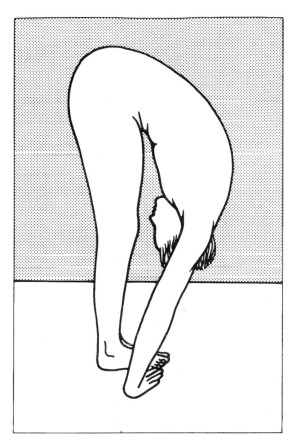

Figure 6.3 Spinal hypermobility

hypermobile range. This differentiates it from joint instability, which has an abnormal range of movement that may also be excessive at times, but which cannot be controlled by voluntary muscular activity. Spinal hypermobility may be confused with two other separate conditions. One is vertebral instability due to disc degeneration. The other occurs with disc degeneration at one spinal level, and the adjacent level may demonstrate a hypermobile range of movement, which may be asymptomatic.

Hypermobility is a fundamental advantage in some sporting pursuits such as gymnastics or ballet. However, for many, often the penalty that has to be paid is the subsequent development of pain in the joints and spine (el-Shahaly and el-Sherif, 1991), while others may develop degenerative joint disease (Bird and Barton, 1993) and some may experience problems with work (Battie

Mobilization techniques are of no benefit unless a painful restriction of intervertebral movement within the hypermobile range can be demonstrated.

Fibrositis/fibromyalgia

Chronic widespread musculoskeletal pain and stiffness is an extremely common symptom (Simons, 1988) that probably involves up to 24 per cent of the American population (Sternbach, 1986). However, in a large percentage of these people, evidence for any underlying recognized pathology is lacking. Many of these patients can be separated into two diagnostic categories: fibrositis (or better, fibromyalgia) and myofascial pain syndromes. Fibromyalgia, which constitutes a large proportion of patients with spinal pain and stiffness (Marder et al, 1991; Wolfe, 1994; Goldenberg, 1995), is a painful non-articular condition predominantly involving muscles (Editorial, 1992). Possibly up to six million Americans suffer from the condition (Wysenbeek et al, 1985), which has a marked morbidity (White et al, 1995), and its prevalence has also been reported to be high in other countries (Bruusgaard et al, 1993, Schochat et al, 1994). Nevertheless, its diagnosis still remains controversial and some deny that it exists at all (Halliday, 1941; Weinberger, 1977; Hadler, 1986; Goldenberg, 1987, 1995; Hassall, 1992; Cohen and Quintner, 1993).

The terminology used to describe this condition has long been a problem. Of the many names given to this clinical condition the most common was 'fibrositis', but this is itself a misnomer since there is no evidence of any underlying inflammatory condition (Bennett, 1981). The term 'fibrositis' was first used by Gower (1904) to describe what he thought were inflammatory changes in the back muscles. This was a popular diagnosis at the time, as it fitted the current medical fad for focal sepsis and ablative surgery. The concept gained further credence when Stockman (1904) described inflammatory changes in muscle biopsies, which were never again confirmed (Collins, 1940). When psychogenic rheumatism became a popular diagnosis, psychological disturbances were also

considered to be its cause (Hudson and Pope, 1989). The term 'fibromyalgia' was first used by Hench (1977), although it might have been chosen because it sounded more scientific (Bennett, 1987). However, it remains the best descriptive title, denoting pain as its major problem in the absence or any underlying inflammatory disorder. Alternative terminology that has been used includes fibromyositis, myofibrositis, non-articular rheumatism and myogelosis, to name but a few. It is a primary condition. The term 'secondary fibromyalgia' has been used, implying that fibromyalgia may be considered to be a part of other rheumatological disorders, such as ankylosing spondylitis or rheumatoid arthritis (Wolfe et al, 1984). This concept is not worthwhile, for once a specific pathological diagnosis has been made, the diagnosis of fibromyalgia becomes redundant.

Since a definite pathological basis is lacking, the idea of fibromyalgia as a disease process has frequently been challenged, and psychological factors have been considered to play a major role in its causation. While there is no doubt that some patients are anxious, tense or depressed (Payne et al, 1982; Ahles et al, 1987), most studies have discounted any major role for psychogenic factors in the causation of fibromyalgia (Wolfe et al, 1984; Clark et al, 1985; Hudson et al, 1985; Goldenberg, 1987; Hales et al, 1987; Yunus et al, 1991; Baumstark et al, 1993). Goldenberg (1987), who described an association with depression, concluded that only a minority of patients was depressed and most patients with fibromyalgia have no psychiatric condition. Recognition of fibromyalgia has increased since the seminal (Schochat et al, 1994) descriptive paper by Smythe and Moldofsky (1977) and the recognition that the central problem is one of pain modulation (Yunus, 1992).

Defining criteria to diagnose the syndrome has been a major problem, and some authors have put forward their own set of criteria (Smythe, 1979; Yunus et al, 1981). The problem of definition is related to the tender points, the widespread areas of hyperalgesia (or tenderness) at specific areas in muscles, their site and number and how many are necessary for diagnosis. Two large series (Yunus et al, 1981; Wolfe and Cathey, 1985), using patients with other rheumatic disorders as controls, determined that a low number of tender points was usually present in patients with other disorders. The number of tender spots needed to diagnose fibromyalgia, out of a potential 14 sites (Smythe, 1979), has been variously given as four (Yunus et al, 1981), seven (Campbell et al, 1983; Wolfe and Cathey, 1985), and 12 (Smythe and Moldofsky, 1977). The American College of Rheumatology (Wolfe et al, 1990) has two major criteria: a history of widespread pain, including axial pain which had to be present for at least three months plus the presence of at least 11 out 18 tender sites on digital palpation. They considered that the presence of another clinical disorder did not exclude the diagnosis. These rigid criteria may be necessary for scientific reporting, but are of no great help in the clinical setting.

Clinical findings

The patient is most often a woman in her forties (Goldenberg, 1987, Wolfe, 1988), with complaints of pain and stiffness involving mainly paraspinal muscle groups, and around the shoulders and hips. Common sites of involvement include the trapezius, the interscapular area and muscle groups related to the iliac crest and buttocks. Pain usually begins insidiously and is usually described as being dull and aching all over. It tends to be worse with prolonged inactivity and may be improved after a period of exercise or heat. The severity of pain may fluctuate, but in most patients it is usually always present to some degree. Pain can be exacerbated by a variety of factors, such as cold, damp, weather changes, stress, noise or bright lights. Associated symptoms include stiffness, which is usually worse in the morning, and fatigue, which is often profound and may be worse in the afternoon. Other problems that have been described include headache, irritable bowel syndrome, lack of concentration, and dysesthesia.

The characteristic findings on examination are localized areas of tenderness in more than one involved muscle group, especially in the spinal and paraspinal areas (Campbell, 1986; Tunks et al, 1988; Wolfe et al, 1990). Practice is needed to develop the correct amount of pressure for accurate testing, as too great a pressure can result in the jump sign, a 'characteristic flinching' (Kraft et al, 1968). However, a marked variation in individual responses may be present: some may have exaggerated tenderness in any area palpated, whereas others may report tenderness with only minimal pressure. The skin over the muscle may be sensitive to rolling.

All ancillary investigations, including X-rays, bone scans using technetium 99M, blood tests and electrodiagnostic tests (Fricton et al, 1985) are always normal. Biopsies of muscle and tender points, and metabolic muscle studies, have been tried, but apart from some minor, non-specific changes, they have been found to be normal (Brendstrup et al, 1957; Awad, 1973; Kalyan-Raman et al, 1984; Bengtsson et al, 1986a,b; Lund et al, 1986; Yunus et al, 1986, 1988; Simms et al, 1994). Endocrine disturbances, especially disorders of the hypothalamo-pituitary-adrenal (HPA) axis, are said to be common (Yunus, 1992; Morand et al, 1996) and may correlate with diurnal variations in stiffness, fatiguability, pain modulation and sleep disturbances (Morand et al, 1996). Other organic diseases should be excluded before the diagnosis is confirmed, and psychogenic symptoms may be difficult to differentiate at times.

Sleep disturbances

Sleep disturbances were first described as playing a role in fibromyalgia by Moldofsky et al (1975). Patients usually have no trouble getting off to sleep or staying sleep, but in the morning they still feel tired and unrefreshed. The non restorative sleep pattern is mirrored in EEG abnormalities, which, during sleep, can be divided into five frequency bands: delta; theta; alpha; sigma; and beta. The abnormal pattern is recorded in the non-rapid eye movement (non-REM) stage IV sleep, which has a slow, one cycle per second, delta rhythm. The abnormality consists of an intrusion of a rapid 8–10 cycles per second alpha rhythm, which correlates with an increase in muscular tenderness and tender points, together with the characteristic fatigue and alterations in mood. The newer computerized techniques that have been used (Drewes et al, 1994, 1995a,b) are also in agreement with this (Smythe, 1995).

Management

Fibromyalgia is a very real condition to those who have it, and a positive diagnosis of its presence can be made in the vast majority of them. The large number of patients who fit its clinical description need to have a diagnostic label, not least for their own satisfaction, and fibromyalgia is the best term to describe their condition. Its natural history usually runs a protracted course, with few remissions, and with persistent pain and fatigue (Felson and Goldenberg, 1986; Goldenberg, 1995). However, it can be a most satisfactory condition to treat and with adequate treatment a remission can be expected in 24 per cent of patients, and pain relief in nearly half (Granges et al, 1994). The patients need be told that there are no simple answers, that treatment can help but is likely to be prolonged, that they will never become a cripple, and that they have to assist with the management. They will often have seen many practitioners, been told that there is nothing wrong or that 'it's all in the mind', or worse that they are suffering from an 'incurable form of arthritis'. Accordingly, there is often a lengthy delay before the correct diagnosis is reached (Goldenberg, 1987).

Fibromyalgia is a problem of pain modulation and there are no easy management solutions. Reassurance and education are essential. Patients need to know that coping with this problem is, to a large extent, up to themselves. When they accept that this is the correct diagnosis, it allows a rational explanation to be given and reassurance that they do not have a progressive crippling or deforming disease. Patient's can very often understand the concept of a muscle being tight or tense and that it can be associated with pain and will take a while to overcome. A simple drawing can help with this, and pamphlets or books may help with patient education. It also helps to have patients' relatives understand the problem.

Medication

Since pain is the problem it would seem logical to offer patients some form on analgesia, but most have already been through most therapeutic options. Non-steroidal anti-inflammatory agents have little to offer, as an inflammatory compo-nent is lacking, and they have the added complication of side effects. Simple analgesics such as paracetamol can be given, but narcotics must be avoided. Antidepressants have been described as being able to relieve pain and tender points (Goldenberg, 1987; Scudds et al, 1989; Yunus, 1992). Tricyclic antidepressants have traditionally been used, and have the advantage that they may help with sleep if they are given at night. Their effect, however, does tend to wear off after some time. Muscle relaxants have also been tried without much effect, and tranquillizers are contraindicated as they have an adverse effect on the sleep pattern. Psychological assessment, especially when combined with attendance at a pain clinic, and other pain-relieving modalities such as TENS, acupuncture, biofeedback, muscle relaxation techniques or meditation may all be needed. Injection with local anaesthetic and corticosteroid into tender points rarely produces any lasting effect.

Aerobic fitness training is one of the mainsprings of management (McCain, 1989; Sherman, 1992). It should begin gradually, as these patients' muscles will be deconditioned because they are likely to have been told in the past that they needed to have extra rest. Stretching and flexibility exercises are best used at first, and aerobic activities (Bennett, 1987), on land or in the water, can then be added. Swimming or walking in warm water is generally best, and may be introduced gradually. Exercises should be individualized as much as possible, supervised and gradually progressed. Heat or ice may help if applied to the muscle prior to exercise. Management in a pain clinic with its multidisciplinary approach, including stress management, relaxation techniques, meditation and biofeedback, is often worth considering.

Myofascial pain syndrome

The basis for the myofascial pain syndrome (MPS) is the trigger point or trigger zone (Simons and Travell, 1983, Simons, 1988). MPS has been described as a condition separate from fibromyalgia, although to many observers the distinctions are arcane. It seems more likely that they are describing the same problem, with one a localized form of the more generalized form (Simons, 1986; Smythe, 1992). Unfortunately, considerable confusion still exists concerning the two conditions (Simons, 1988; Yunus et al, 1988), especially the differentiation between the tender points of fibromyalgia and the trigger points of MPS. The major points of difference that occur with trigger points are:

- Usually only one muscle is involved
- A tender area can be palpated within the muscle
- This can be felt as a taut band
- Palpation of the trigger point produces local pain which may be referred to a more distal site
- A twitch response in the stimulated muscle may be present.

Trigger points, or trigger zones, can be palpated as distinct, firm, taut band-like structures or a feeling of tension within the muscle or its fascia, when rolled with the finger. They can be easily palpated along the long axis, usually best felt with the muscle slightly stretched. A major problem in identifying them is that the patient is usually asked 'Is that tender?' It is preferable, after some practice, to be able to palpate the area and tell the patient 'That is your tender, or painful, area' and have him or her agree that that is correct. The patient should also recognize that the pain that is reproduced is his or her pain and also that the pressure can reproduce his or her area of referred pain. Trigger points can be differentiated from the tender points of fibromyalgia (Smythe, 1992; Wolfe et al, 1992). Pain is more localized than in fibromyalgia, may be acute or chronic, and generalized symptoms such as sleep disorders, morning stiffness and general fatigue are usually absent. Pain may be brought on also by stretching or contracting the muscle, which may have a reduced range of motion and appear shortened. The pain can be abolished, at least temporarily, by injection of local anaesthetic into the trigger zone.

The cause of trigger points remains unknown, although many theories have been described. They may represent a local muscle contraction in an area of high-energy metabolism that has been depleted of its energy supply (Bengtsson et al, 1986b; Lund et al, 1986; Simons, 1988). Many substances, such as substance P, histamine, serotonin, prostaglandins, leukotrienes, kinins, hypertonic saline solutions, potassium and lactic acid have been incriminated as causing a local sensitization of some nerves (Simons, 1988). In some cases they may follow local trauma or overuse, and their prognosis is then usually good. Another localized form may be seen in patients with pain referred from spinal joints around C5–C6 (Smythe, 1986, 1992). A hypomobility lesion at this level very often has a trigger point in muscles around the scapula and usually responds well to spinal mobilization techniques.

Management

Treatment of trigger points forms the basis of treatment of the myofascial pain syndrome (Simons and Travell, 1983; Simons, 1988). Prognosis is much better with this condition than it is with fibromyalgia, and management also differs in several aspects. If only one muscle is involved and the trigger zone is easy to palpate, it usually responds well to local treatment, such as injection of a long acting local anaesthetic, to which a small dose of corticosteroid may be added. The injection is easy to perform and only a small gauge needle is needed. Alternatives include dry needling or deep friction massage, but they are not so comfortable. Muscle stretching is most important and may be combined with mobilization techniques. Heat or ultrasound is of little value in treatment.

7 Vertebral column disorders

The disorders of the vertebral column discussed in this chapter are mainly the rheumatological medical conditions. Surgical conditions such as fracture, fracture-dislocations or structural scoliosis are not included. Rheumatological vertebral disorders may be classified as follows. Inflammatory diseases: spondyloarthritis (ankylosing spondylitis, Reiter's disease, psoriasis, inflammatory bowel disease, reactive arthritis); and rheumatoid arthritis. Metabolic bone diseases: osteoporosis; Paget's disease; osteomalacia; chondrocalcinosis; gout; acromegaly; and ochronosis. Degenerative conditions: diffuse idiopathic skeletal hyperostosis; Scheuermann's disease. Infections and tumours are also discussed.

Inflammatory diseases

Spondyloarthritis

Spondyloarthritis is the best term to classify a closely related group of diseases, which are characterized by an enthesopathy with inflammatory lesions in the spine and synovitis in the peripheral joints. They are linked by inflammatory changes in the sacroiliac joints, and frequent association with skin, mucous membrane, eye, bowel and urinary tract lesions. They demonstrate familial aggregation, related to the presence of the HLA B27 antigen, which is demonstrated by tissue typing. Another related condition is reactive arthritis, in which no infectious agent is found in the joints but an antigen that has been derived from an organism at a distant site may be present. The diseases usually classified under spondyloarthritis include: ankylosing spondylitis; Reiter's disease; psoriatic arthritis; arthritis associated with inflammatory bowel disorders, such as ulcerative colitis and regional enteritis; and reactive arthritis

Ankylosing spondylitis (AS)

The essential diagnostic feature of this disease is the presence of bilateral sacroiliitis, with inflammatory changes usually developing also in the spinal joints. The earliest pathological lesion is characterized by a lymphocytic infiltrate involving primarily the enthesis, a metabolically active area of ligament and tendon insertions into bone and periosteum. Cartilage and subchondral bone are involved in a similar process, and the resulting osteitis and/or chondritis involves mainly central joints of the axial skeleton, such as the sacroiliac joint, symphysis pubis and spinal intervertebral joints. In the spine these changes result in an erosive lesion with the formation of granulation tissue either anteriorly or posteriorly at the upper and lower surfaces of the vertebral body. As it heals the outer fibres of the disc and vertebrae are replaced by a vascular fibrous tissue, which ultimately becomes ossified, leading to bony ankylosis.

The sacroiliac joint changes are described in Chapter 10. Synovitis also develops in the zygapophyseal and peripheral joints, and inflammatory lesions develop in the musculotendinous attachments of the enthesis, especially around the pelvis and heel, with an exuberant periostitis.

Early studies suggested that ankylosing spondylitis was a rare disease, but it is now known to be reasonably common, although the exact prevalence is still debated (Underwood and Dawes, 1995). Early series also reported at least 90 per cent of cases to be men, but these figures have been obtained from radiotherapy departments with predominantly male populations. It is now believed to occur in approximately a 2:1 ratio of males to females. It is quite rare among black races, but it occurs in up to 50 per cent of males in some American Indian tribes in whom HLA B27 is also very common. Its aetiology remains unknown, although gut organisms have been implicated in its pathogenesis (Nissila et al, 1994).

Clinical findings

In most cases the onset is insidious, usually in the late teens or early twenties, and it is uncommon for it to commence at a later age. The disease tends to come in attacks at first, although pain later tends to be more constant. The typical history is one of buttock pain, or pain in the lower back radiating to the buttocks, thighs and groin. Pain tends to be episodic, and often alternates from one buttock to the other. It may radiate down the back of the leg to be confused with true sciatica, but neurological symptoms are absent. Low back stiffness, worse during the early hours of the morning or on awakening, is present, and may be so severe that the patient needs to get up and walk about, as the stiffness tends to improve with activity. The degree of stiffness correlates well with the severity of the inflammatory process. The peripheral joints involved are most commonly proximal joints (shoulders and hips), and lower limb joints such as knees, ankles, heels and feet. Small joints in the wrist and fingers are rarely involved.

Signs

A careful search may be required to detect any early clinical signs, and early diagnosis depends on maintaining a high index of suspicion about the possibility of their presence. Additionally, a diagnosis of a psychogenic illness is often considered in the early stages of the disease when complaints of pain and stiffness are present without any obvious signs. The overall range of lumbar spine movements becomes reduced, often best appreciated as a limitation of lateral flexion. Forward flexion may also be reduced, but, since most of this movement takes place at the hips, this can be missed, as in the early stages the hips may still be able to be fully flexed. Muscle spasm or atrophy (Gordon et al, 1984) is usually evident bilatcrally, giving the spine a straightened, so-called 'ironed-out', appearance. In the later stages of the disease, spinal deformity, especially thoracic kyphosis, is common.

In the early stages, clinical testing of the sacroiliac joints (*see* Chapter 10) is necessary in an attempt to reproduce low back or buttock pain, or produce pain over the sacroiliac joint area. Chest expansion is limited if the costovertebral joints are involved, and is an important and often early sign. Involvement of the cervical spine with pain and stiffness usually occurs late in the course of the disease.

At an early stage, inflammatory changes occur in the enthesis, with involvement of musculo tendinous insertions or tendons, especially around the pelvis and Achilles tendon. Heel pain results from Achilles tendinitis, plantar fasciitis or synovitis of the subtalar joint. Similar changes are found in the symphysis pubis and the manubriosternal joint, with local pain and tenderness. The costovertebral joints are often involved early, resulting in chest pain with restricted respiratory excursion. Temporomandibular joint involvement and dysfunction may also occur.

Other presentations

Ankylosing spondylitis may present first with involvement of the lower limb joints, or less often as a generalized polyarthritis. The hip is commonly involved, but knee, ankle or foot pain

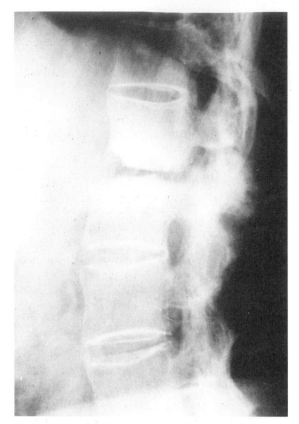

Figure 7.1 Ankylosing spondylitis. Discovertebral involvement in the only unfused spinal segment

usually found at the thoracolumbar junction and is usually associated with a stress fracture in the posterior joints. X-rays show erosive, destructive bone changes with surrounding sclerosis, best demonstrated on CT (Chan et al, 1988) (Figure 7.1). These lesions tend to be found in a mobile segment between ankylosed vertebrae and occur as the result of trauma and not of an inflammatory discitis.

Complications such as neurological disorders (Fox et al, 1993; Ramos et al, 1995), aortic valve or lung disease and amyloidosis are rare.

Confirmatory tests

X-ray evidence of sacroiliitis is necessary to confirm the diagnosis. The radiological changes in the sacroiliac joints should ultimately develop, but since it may at times take several years before they become definite, it may be necessary at times to arrange treatment on the basis of the presumptive diagnosis. Bone scanning may help, but CT or MRI is best to show early changes. These radiological changes are described in detail in Chapter 10.

X-ray changes in the spine during the early stages include a squaring of the vertebrae, as a result of filling in of its normal concavity with periosteal new bone formation and erosion of the vertebral corners. Syndesmophytes are bony bridges formed between the outer fibres of the annulus fibrosus and deep aspect of the anterior longitudinal ligament. They run from the margins of the vertebral bodies in a vertical direction, and can be differentiated from osteophytes, which tend to lie in a horizontal direction (Figure 7.2). Ossification subsequently develops in other areas of the spine such as the spinal ligaments and zygapophyseal joints. The late X-ray picture of 'bamboo spine' is produced by symmetrical paravertebral ossification completely bridging across the disc space. This rigid spine is liable to trauma (Fishman and Magid, 1992), and a fracture may be mistaken for an acute exacerbation of the disease.

Laboratory tests are usually of no special assistance in the diagnosis. There may be mild normochromic anaemia, the erythrocyte sedimentation rate (ESR) is usually moderately elevated and serological tests for rheumatoid

and swelling may be present before spinal involvement. In the upper limbs, the proximal joints are usually involved, but involvement of the small joints of the hand is uncommon.

As a general rule, the spinal disease progresses in an ascending fashion. However, it may present with spinal pain involving the neck, chest or thoracolumbar junction, either in isolation or simultaneously.

It may rarely commence as a generalized systemic illness with weight loss, fever and generalized aches and pains.

Iritis may develop or be the presenting complaint.

Destructive lesions in the disc and vertebral bodies, the so-called Romanus lesion, result from a granulomatous change in the cartilage endplate and the vertebral rim. This spondylodiscitis may occur at any spinal level but is

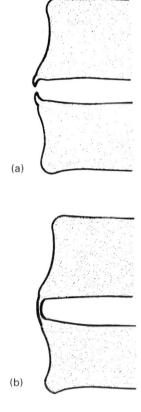

(a)

(b)

Figure 7.2 Syndesmophytes: (a) at an early stage, growing in the outer layers of the annulus; (b) at a more advanced stage

factor are negative. Serum levels of IGA may be elevated (Nissila et al, 1994). The presence of the HLA B27 antigen is usually sought, as it is present in approximately 96 per cent of patients. However, as it is also present in approximately 8 per cent of the normal population, it is of no great value as a diagnostic or screening test, and it is not necessary to make the diagnosis. A positive test may be confirmatory, but a negative test does not exclude the diagnosis. Relatives of AS patients should be advised against having their HLA B27 typed. In the peripheral joints, a bone scan is most useful in depicting early joint involvement. Synovial fluid analysis of involved peripheral joints shows moderately inflamed fluid with predominantly lymphocytic cell infiltration.

Routine measurements

Continued assessment of the patient and the disease is essential. At approximately yearly intervals some basic measurements should be carried out, including:

- Chest expansion, which measures changes in thoracic joints such as the costovertebral joints
- The distance that the tips of the fingers reach from the floor on full forward flexion, to measure both hip and lumbar spine flexion
- When the patient stands upright against a wall the back of the head should touch the wall, easily. With a flexion deformity of the neck, the head is carried forward, and the distance from the back of the head to the wall should be recorded.

Management

The two main problems, control of symptoms and minimizing deformity, need to be assessed and controlled. The symptoms, pain and stiffness, are due to inflammation; the greater the degree of inflammation, the greater the pain and stiffness. Appropriate anti-inflammatory drugs remain the treatment of choice, and they need to be used in sufficient dosage to control inflammation and maintain maximal mobility and activity. Deformity should be prevented by vigorous, organized exercise routines. In the past, management using deep X-ray therapy and immobilization in a plaster cast was disastrous, as symptoms are exacerbated by immobility.

Patient education is most important. The implications and prognosis of the diagnosis are explained, stressing that most patients lead an active life and that the mortality rate from this disease is low. The advantages and limitations of therapy are also explained, and the advantages of remaining as active as possible stressed. Ankylosing spondylitis is a peculiarly flexing disease, and every effort should be made to enable the patient to control his or her posture while sitting or standing and by sleeping on a firm mattress with only a small pillow. Other precautions, including sitting with the back straight and supported to avoid long periods of spinal flexion, are taught. Long periods spent bending and stooping or recumbent in a flexed position are to be avoided (Halm et al, 1995). Patients who become stiff easily while sitting for long periods should get up periodically and walk around.

Medications

The inflammatory changes in the spinal joints usually respond well to anti-inflammatory agents, so much so that they could almost be specific. The smallest dose compatible with clinical improvement is used and may be taken intermittently. Long-term therapy to attempt to control the disease process with sulfasalazine or methotrexate should be considered if simpler methods are not sufficient (Nissila et al, 1994). Injections of local anaesthetic and corticosteroid into synovial effusions in peripheral joints may be of great benefit, but systemic corticosteroids are very rarely indicated.

Physical therapy

Exercises are essential in the management (Hidding et al, 1993; Hidding and Vanderlinden, 1995; Viitanen et al, 1995a,b). They are taught and supervised by a physiotherapist, and may be best performed as a group activity or as a home programme. Postural exercises are also taught, and breathing exercises are needed to maintain mobility in the costovertebral joints. Aerobic activities are undertaken to allow the patient to remain as mobile as possible. Body contact sports will present some difficulty in the young male population, but most other activities, especially swimming, are encouraged. Heat may be of some advantage before an exercise programme is implemented. Traction and manipulation are contraindicated.

Surgery

In the peripheral joints, operations such as synovectomy or joint replacement of the hip and knee may become necessary. Spinal surgery such as osteotomy is only rarely indicated to improve deformity, but it provides worthwhile results in those who would be otherwise condemned to a life spent looking at the ground (Hehne et al, 1990; Jaffray et al, 1992; Halm et al, 1995).

Reiter's disease

Hans Reiter, a German venereologist, described his triad of urethritis, conjunctivitis and arthritis in 1916. Since that time, several other clinical features have been recognized, and the term 'Reiter's disease' is now used to describe their varying combinations. The case that Reiter described followed an attack of dysentery, which may be an initiating factor, but more commonly the disease follows a venereal infection with urethritis. *Chlamydia trachomatis* is the causal agent in most cases and mycoplasma in some. It may also occur in patients with AIDS and may prove resistant to therapy (Keats, 1994). HLA B27 antigen is present in at least 90 per cent of cases.

Clinical features

Most cases occur in young adult males and it is rare in females. Any peripheral joint may be involved, usually in the lower limb, with an often intense and asymmetrical synovitis. Tendon sheath or tendon involvement, such as Achilles tendinitis, is common. Painful heels may also be due to plantar fasciitis, periostitis or erosive changes in the calcaneus. Sacroiliitis, which ultimately occurs in about one-third of patients, may be asymmetric at first and can progress to produce a clinical picture indistinguishable from ankylosing spondylitis. One difference is that the spinal syndesmophytes may be paravertebral: they do not arise at the vertebral margins as do those in ankylosing spondylitis but are separated from the outer margin of the disc.

Management

Rest for the severely inflamed joints is essential, and anti-inflammatory agents are given in a sufficient dosage to control symptoms. Large joints may be aspirated and injected with corticosteroids. Urethritis usually responds to appropriate antibiotics.

Psoriasis

Psoriasis is a very common skin disease, which may be associated with a seronegative inflammatory polyarthritis. Approximately 20 per cent of patients with psoriatic arthritis have spinal involvement, which differs somewhat from ankylosing spondylitis but is similar to Reiter's disease. Sacroiliitis may be asymmetric (Braun et al, 1994) and spinal involvement may be unilateral. Syndesmophytes are paravertebral and develop more randomly than in ankylosing spondylitis. Ankylosis of the neck is relatively common (Jenkinson et al, 1994).

Inflammatory bowel disease

Inflammatory bowel disease, due to granulomatous lesions in ulcerative colitis or Crohn's disease or to infections such as *Yersinia*, may be complicated by sacroiliitis, spondylitis and peripheral arthritis.

Reactive arthritis

In reactive arthritis, the causative organism is usually present on mucosal surfaces, such as the gut, but is not present in the inflamed joints. An antigen from the organism precipitates the inflammatory joint reaction (Inman and Schofield, 1994), usually in HLA B27 predisposed individuals (Hughes and Keats, 1994).

Rheumatoid arthritis

The cervical spine is involved in most cases of rheumatoid arthritis (Clark, 1994; Oda et al 1995), possibly because of its mobility (Casey and Crockard, 1995) and the presence of some 37 synovial joints between the skull and the first thoracic vertebra. The factors that determine its classification include:

● The anatomical site involved
● The underlying inflammatory process in the synovium, bursa or disc
● The destructive changes seen on X-ray (Table 7.1).

Table 7.1 Classification of spinal rheumatoid arthritis

Area	X-ray changes
Upper cervical spine	Erosive changes in: (1) Dens (2) Atlanto-occipital joints (3) Lateral atlanto-axial joints Deformities: (1) Atlanto-axial subluxation, which may be: (i) Anterior: either 'slider' or 'tipper' (ii) Vertical (iii) Lateral (iv) Posterior (2) Collapse of lateral mass of atlas
Lower cervical spine: Discs and vertebral bodies	Disc thinning without osteophytosis, vertebral endplate erosions, vertebral body erosions, osteoporosis and deformities: anterior subluxation of vertebra, and step deformities
Apophyseal joints	Erosive arthritis, blurring of joint space, and fusion
Spinous process	Cortical erosions and thinned out spinous process

The upper cervical spine is the most commonly involved (Lipson, 1989b; Clark, 1994), and results in varying degrees of pain, deformity, instability and neural involvement, including cervical myelopathy (Yonezawa et al, 1995).

Upper cervical spine

ATLANTO-AXIAL JOINT (C1–C2)
In the median atlanto-axial joint, the odontoid process of the axis depends for its stability on the strong transverse ligament that runs between the lateral masses of the atlas. Inflammation in its surrounding bursae (Figure 7.3) produces erosive changes, usually on its posterior aspect, where a synovial bursa lies between the dens and the transverse ligament, leading ultimately to attenuation and loosening of the transverse

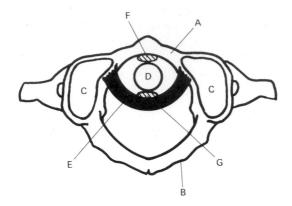

Figure 7.3 The atlas, showing: (A) anterior arch; (B) posterior arch; (C) atlanto-occipital joints; (D) odontoid process; (E) transverse ligament; (F) bursa between odontoid process and anterior arch of atlas; (G) bursa between odontoid process and transverse ligament

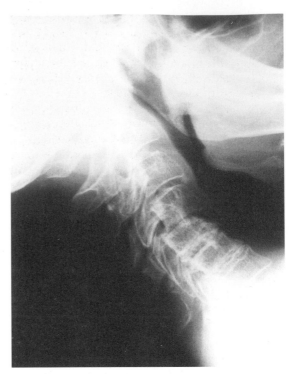

Figure 7.4 RA spine. Subluxation of C4 on C5 and rheumatoid discitis C4–C5, C5–C6 and C6–C7

ligament. The anterior atlanto-axial joint subluxes anteriorly, diagnosed on lateral X-ray by an increased gap above 3 mm between the anterior arch of the atlas and the odontoid process. The body of the atlas can either slide forwards or tip up on the axis. However, measuring the posterior atlanto-odontoid distance is better in order to predict the onset of complications (Boden, 1994). The dens may become completely eroded or it may fracture through its base. A posterior atlanto-axial subluxation is very rare and can occur only if the odontoid process has been severely eroded.

OCCIPITO-ATLANTAL JOINT (O–C1)

Erosive and destructive changes in this joint cause softening and destruction of the lateral mass of the atlas, allowing the occipital condyles to descend onto the axis (Zeidman and Ducker, 1994). The dens can then sublux vertically and may protrude into the foramen magnum. Similar bony destructive changes can occur between the atlas and the base of the skull, altering their relationships and producing a basilar invagination.

Lower cervical spine C3–C7

Discitis is caused by rheumatoid granulation tissue that invades and destroys the intervertebral discs, resulting in spinal ligament laxity and a gradual forward subluxation of one vertebral body on its lower one (Zeidman and Ducker, 1994) (Figure 7.4) Multiple subluxations at C3, C4, and sometimes C5 lead to the classic radiological finding of step-like deformities of the vertebral bodies. Rheumatoid discitis is diagnosed radiologically by a thinning of the disc without any accompanying degenerative changes. Discitis also occurs at the lower cervical levels, but since degenerative changes are also common at this site, radiological interpretation can be difficult.

Erosive changes and osteopenia may be seen in the vertebral bodies. Erosions in the zygapophyseal joints are usually seen at C2–C3, in the neurocentral joints or as cortical erosions of the spinous process, usually at C7. Atrophic changes may lead to a thinning of the spinous process.

Symptoms

Cervical lesions may be asymptomatic for a time or found by chance during X-ray examination.

The main complaint in symptomatic cases is neck pain, which commonly radiates into the head and is usually associated with restriction of neck movement. Other common complaints include vertebrobasilar symptoms (Delamarter and Bohlman, 1994; Zeidman and Ducker, 1994) such as vertigo, and a clicking or clunking sensation in the neck, usually associated with an exacerbation of severe pain. Neurological symptoms are the major complication, although they do not occur as commonly as the X-ray changes might suggest. Sudden head movements can produce pins and needles or numbness in the limbs in shock-like waves, transient blackouts, cord compression or sudden death. Lower motor neurone lesions of the upper limbs may occur with anterior subluxation of the vertebral bodies below C4. In the lower limb, evidence of upper motor neurone lesions may be difficult to evaluate in the presence of arthritic deformities.

Neck X-rays are necessary for diagnosis and assessment (Yonezawa et al, 1995); a lateral view is taken in full flexion and an anteroposterior view is taken through the mouth to view the atlanto-axial joint. MRI, CT or CT-myelography (Pettersson et al, 1988; Dvorak et al, 1989; Larsson et al, 1989; Boden, 1994; Casey and Crockard, 1995) provide definitive views of this area.

Management

The natural history of this disease is most variable (Boden, 1994). The most common complaint is neck and head pain, and relief can usually be obtained with a semi-rigid or rigid collar (Althoff and Goldie, 1980; Kauppi and Anttila, 1995), analgesics and medical management of the rheumatoid disease, so that surgery need rarely be considered.

The presence of neurological lesions requires a greater degree of judgement, and the management of each case needs to be assessed individually. With a lower motor neurone lesion involving the upper limb, a collar may be sufficient to relieve symptoms. Surgery may be indicated with an unstable cervical spine with neurological deficits to prevent irreversible neurological loss (Johnston and Kelly, 1990; Boden, 1994; Grob et al, 1994; Crockard, 1995; Casey and Crockard, 1995; Oda et al, 1995; McRorie et al, 1996). Hospital admission and skeletal traction may be necessary while assessing the severity or progression of symptoms. In the upper spine, stabilization with various types of implants wired in place and cemented with methylmethacrylate or a bone fusion is used (Wertheim and Bohlman, 1987; Zoma et al, 1987; Clark et al, 1989). In the lower cervical spine the choice of operation lies between an anterior or a posterior approach and fusion.

Metabolic bone diseases

Osteoporosis

Osteoporosis may be defined as a reduced bone mass per unit volume (Sambrook, 1996) and results in a reduced bone mineral density. Bone mineral density increases in men and women from childhood to the late teenage years, achieving peak bone mass in both men and women, before it gradually decreases, with losses mainly in trabecular bone, especially about the time of the menopause in women. Bone mineral density in adults is the result of the peak bone mass of early adulthood and the amount of decline since that time. Osteoporosis may result from failure to achieve the average peak bone mass or an accelerated bone loss, or a combination of both. The total amount of bone is reduced, but the bone that is present is histologically normal. The cause of the failure to achieve peak bone mass includes both the postmenopausal and senile forms of the disease. Genetic factors are important, account for up to 80 per cent of the variation in bone mineral density and may be related to the vitamin D receptor gene. Secondary causes of accelerated bone loss include:

- Endocrine disorders: Cushing syndrome; thyrotoxicosis; hypothyroidism; acromegaly; hypogonadism; steroid therapy; and exercise-induced amenorrhoea
- Malignancies, e.g. secondary carcinoma or multiple myeloma
- Medications such as corticosteroids
- Ankylosing spondylitis or rheumatoid arthritis.

Symptoms

Most patients with osteoporosis remain asymptomatic for a long period of time. Pain is usually brought on by a fracture in a vertebra or the femoral neck following the loss of cortical bone in these areas, so that the bone mass becomes insufficient to withstand the normal stresses to which it is subjected. Other common sites of fracture include the wrist, ribs or pelvis. In the spine, the usual complaint is of sudden pain in the thoracic or upper lumbar regions due to a vertebral fracture. Pain may come on spontaneously, follow sudden exertion such as coughing, or sneezing or moving heavy objects, or follow minor trauma. Some may complain of diffuse skeletal pain, whose origin is uncertain, but it may be due to postural alterations in supporting structures. The patient may be conscious of loss of height and the development of a kyphoscoliosis until, ultimately, the lower ribs approximate to the iliac crests. Neural complications due either to cord compression or sciatica are rare.

Investigations

Bone mineral density measurements confirm the diagnosis and severity of osteoporosis, estimate the fracture risk at any one time, determine if treatment is necessary and monitor its effectiveness. It is best measured by dual energy X-ray absorptiometry (DEXA) (Bjarnason et al, 1996) or quantitative computed tomography (QCT). DEXA is simple, accurate, reproducible, fast, with a small radiation dose and it measures the density per area in the spine and hip, expressed in g/cm^2. Fracture risk is estimated by comparing the value obtained against a population of young normal adults. A bone mineral density more than two standard deviations below the mean of the young normal range is defined as osteoporotic. For every one standard deviation that the measurement falls below the mean for young normals, the fracture risk doubles, so that a value three standard deviations below the mean confers approximately eight times the fracture risk. The measurement is then compared with a normal population matched for age, gender and ethnic origin.

Plain X-rays are not sensitive enough for early diagnosis, because of the amount of bone that needs to be lost before the X-ray changes become evident. X-rays are useful to diagnose compression fractures, which occur most commonly at T12, and the incidence decreases with increasing distance from this site. Collapse above the T3 level is rarely due to osteoporosis alone. Biochemical tests are usually normal for primary osteoporosis, but may be more helpful in diagnosing the secondary forms. Markers of bone turnover, such as hydroxyproline, osteocalcin or pyridinoline crosslinks, are research tools that do not add to the clinical assessment.

Prophylaxis

Osteoporosis remains a major health problem (Jones et al, 1994a; Martin, 1995), due to its morbidity, mortality and financial costs (Barrett-Connor, 1995; Randell et al, 1995). At least 60 per cent of women and 30 per cent of men over the age of 60 years will suffer an osteoporotic fracture during their lifetime (Jones et al, 1994b). Prophylaxis, especially in women, consists of recognizing known risk factors and avoiding or modifying where possible (Cummings et al, 1995). These include:

- A family history of osteoporosis (Sambrook et al, 1994)
- Amenorrhoea or premature menopause
- Nulliparity
- Lack of physical exertion or immobility
- Insufficient calcium intake
- Smoking
- Alcohol
- Long-term corticosteroid, thyroxine or anticonvulsant therapy
- Low body weight and an eating disorder.

Management

Long-term management using several modalities to prevent postmenopausal bone loss can be most effective (Ulrich et al, 1996). These modalities include:

Physical activity. Bone mineral density is greater if there is a degree of physical activity (Aloia et al, 1978; Casez et al, 1995; Preisinger et al, 1995). The aim of treatment is to encourage muscle action in stimulating bone development, and exercise may be synergistic with calcium intake. The osteoporotic patient should also be kept as active as possible since osteoporosis will be aggravated by immobilization (Prince et al, 1995). However, a problem in younger women is that an excess of aerobic activity may cause amenorrhoea. Weight-bearing exercises (Ulrich et al, 1996) such as walking and site-specific resistive exercise (Swezey, 1996b) are generally thought to be ideal, but exercises in the water and isometric spinal exercises can also be of benefit (Bouxsein and Marcus, 1994). Exercise can also help to improve posture and may help to avoid falls. However, exercises need to be continued long-term, and so compliance may be a problem.

Calcium intake. Differing opinions as to the efficacy of calcium supplementation have been present for some time (Dawson-Hughes et al, 1990), but it now appears that it has an appreciable protective effect over the long term, especially for the growing skeleton and for postmenopausal women (Reid et al, 1995; Sambrook, 1996). It is possible that those who benefit most may have had a previous low-calcium diet (Elders et al, 1994). In children it has been shown to be of most benefit if given as 1000 mg a day before puberty (Johnston et al, 1992). An adequate calcium intake in women is 800 mg a day before the menopause and 1200 mg a day afterwards (Sambrook, 1996).

Hormone replacement therapy (HRT). Oestrogen has been shown to prevent postmenopausal and post-oophorectomy bone loss. It may be best if it is started immediately after the menopause when bone loss is most rapid, but it also may help with established disease. Its exact mechanism is debated, but is probably due to its action on the oestrogen receptors on osteoblasts. Problems with its use include the risks of endometrial cancer, which may be prevented if progestins are also given, and breast cancer (Colditz et al, 1995), and it needs to be taken over a long period of time. Whether or not a patient should be started on HRT can only be decided only after a full and informed discussion that takes into account several factors, including age and the need for regular screening examinations.

Calcitriol. Calcitrol, a vitamin D analogue, increases the gastrointestinal absorption of calcium and stimulates osteoblastic and osteoclastic activity in the skeleton (Tillyard et al, 1992). It can reduce fracture rates in women with osteoporosis (Chapuy et al, 1992; Tillyard et al, 1992), and can be particularly helpful for patients on corticosteroid therapy (Sambrook et al, 1993). It is used in a dose of 0.25 µg given twice a day. Supplementary calcium or vitamin D must be avoided, and serum levels of calcium and creatinine have to be measured at regular intervals.

Calcitonin. Calcitonin depresses bone resorption and hence it is used as treatment in disorders with a high bone turnover, such as Paget's disease and hypercalcaemia of any cause. Treatment in osteoporosis results in an increase in bone mineral density in the axial skeleton (Civitelli et al, 1988), and it may reduce pain in osteoporotic fracture (Lyritis et al, 1991). It is expensive, is given by injection or an intranasal spray (Overgaard et al, 1992), but resistance may develop.

Bisphosphonates. Bisphosphonates are pyrophosphate analogues which bind to hydroxyapatite crystals and inhibit osteoclast activity so decreasing bone resorption (Fleisch, 1993). It needs to be given in cycles because it can accumulate in the skeleton for a prolonged period (Sambrook, 1995), and so inhibit bone mineralization. Considerable enthusiasm for its use in treating osteoporosis was originally reported (Harris et al, 1993), but was not maintained (Marcus, 1995), as earlier forms of the drug caused disturbances in bone mineralization. New generation agents, such as alendronate or tiludronate, are more potent and have been shown to decrease bone loss and improve the vertebral fracture rate (Liberman et al, 1995; Sambrook, 1995).

Paget's disease

Paget's disease of bone frequently involves the spine, and back pain is a common complaint (Zlatkin et al, 1986). Pathological changes are characterized by an increased bone turnover.

Excessive osteoclastic activity at first with increased bone resorption is followed by osteoblastic overactivity, and the attempt at healing produces excessive and abnormal bone formation. This results in abnormal irregular trabecular surfaces with an increase in vascular and fibrous tissue, and normal compact bone is replaced by a mosaic pattern with widening of the cortex. This bone is physically weaker, and so the normal stresses to which it would be subjected can lead to deformity.

Paget's disease occurs more commonly in men than in women. It is a disease of the elderly (Helliwell, 1995), very rare before the age of 30, occurs in about 3–4 per cent of people over the age of 40, and rises to approximately 5 per cent by the age of 55 (Helliwell, 1995). Its aetiology remains unknown, but genetic factors and a slow virus, a paramyxovirus with inclusion bodies in the osteoclasts, have been implicated. Familial cases are reported, and the disease is most common in western Europeans and is rare in Asians and black Africans.

Its onset is insidious, usually progresses slowly, and most cases remain asymptomatic. It is a focal condition that may be monostotic (in approximately 20 per cent of cases) or polyostotic, with the lumbar spine and pelvis most commonly involved. Pain may be deep, dull, aching, and often worse at night. In only a small percentage of patients is pain severe or intractable. The cause of pain is still debated, but is most likely due to periosteal distortion as the bone enlarges. Pain may also occur because of osteoarthritic changes in joints adjacent to involved bone (Helliwell, 1995). Other musculoskeletal complications include bony deformity, headache from skull involvement or platybasia and basilar invagination, kyphosis, nerve root pain due to bony enlargement, fracture, usually in the femur or tibia, or compression of the spinal cord or cauda equina. Sarcoma, which may develop in less than 1 per cent of monostotic or polyostotic forms, presents with a change in the pain pattern and swelling, and response to treatment is poor.

Diagnosis

Radionuclide bone scans are the most useful imaging technique for early diagnosis. They are highly sensitive, and can be of most help to determine the full extent of the disease in other sites. Typical X-ray changes begin with an area of osteolysis, such as osteoporosis circumscripta in the skull. Subsequent changes, with increased bone density, disordered trabecular pattern and trabecular and cortical thickening, are necessary to confirm the diagnosis, and need to be differentiated from a haemangioma or secondary malignant deposits, especially of the prostate or breast. CT (Zlatkin et al, 1986), MRI or bone biopsy are indicated if there is any doubt about the diagnosis. Serum alkaline phosphatase levels, denoting osteoblastic activity, are higher in this disorder than in most other conditions, and reflect the activity of the disease. An increase in urinary hydroxyproline and markers of bone collagen breakdown, such as deoxypyrridinoline, denote osteoclastic activity. Calcium levels are raised only with immobility.

Management

Asymptomatic X-ray changes or slight elevation of the alkaline phosphatase are not indications for therapy. The main aim of treatment is to relieve pain, but also to maintain mobility and reduce complications such as deformity and nerve compression. Pain can often be relieved by simple analgesics such as paracetemol and nonsteroidals. Specific treatment with three groups of drugs is available. Calcitonin, derived from the parafollicular cells of the thyroid gland, available in human, salmon or pig forms, inhibits bone resorption and slows the rate of bone remodelling. It needs to be given by subcutaneous injection every one or two days for at least six months. Symptoms usually take some four to six weeks to improve, but blood tests take longer to settle. Minor side effects such as flushing, warmth or nausea are common. The development of resistance to its action is a major problem and it has been largely superseded by the bisphosphonates.

The newer forms of bisphosphonates have a marked effect on pain, reduce the bone markers of the disease and are the mainstay of therapy. Cytotoxic therapy with RNA inhibitors such as mithramycin, given by intravenous infusion, is used to inhibit osteoclastic activity. It is indicated if other treatments are not working or if rapid treatment is necessary for serious complications.

Surgery may be indicated for fractures, joint replacement or nerve entrapments.

Osteomalacia

Osteomalacia, and rickets in children, is due to defective calcification of normally produced osteoid tissue with altered structure and weakening of bone. Bone pain and tenderness are common. It results from a disturbed metabolism of calcium or vitamin D, which may result from dietary lack, intestinal malabsorption or renal disease including aluminum ingestion in renal dialysis patients.

X-ray changes showing bone demineralization may be indistinguishable from those of osteoporosis, and softening of bone leads to the appearance of codfish vertebrae and compression fractures. X-ray of the pelvis may reveal pathological fractures, so-called pseudofractures. Blood tests show a low serum calcium and/or phosphate and a raised serum alkaline phosphatase.

Chondrocalcinosis

Chondrocalcinosis is a relatively common condition, characterized by deposition of calcium pyrophosphate dihydrate crystals in cartilage. It occurs most commonly in the large peripheral joints in elderly patients, but may also involve the intervertebral cartilage. In peripheral joints it causes degenerative arthritis and acute attacks of synovitis, pseudogout. Annulus fibrosus calcification leads to degenerative changes with loss of disc space and marked vertebral changes, often asymmetric. One side of a disc may be markedly narrowed whereas the opposite side of the superior disc may be uninvolved. It may be associated with large, often spoon-shaped osteophytes. Acute attacks of spinal pain responding to anti-inflammatory drugs are uncommon.

Investigations to confirm the diagnosis include aspiration of the peripheral joints to find calcium pyrophosphate crystals, and X-ray evidence of cartilage calcification in spine and peripheral joints. Investigations that should be undertaken include tests for serum iron, ferritin and total iron-binding capacity, serum calcium and phosphorous, alkaline phosphatase and fasting blood sugar levels.

Gout

The spine is very rarely involved in gout, as the distal joints of the limbs are the sites of predilection for both acute attacks and tophaceous gout. Despite the rarity of proven cases, the diagnosis is not uncommonly made. The major cause of confusion usually occurs when patients with a degenerative condition are found to be hyperuricaemic, which is insufficient evidence to diagnose gout.

Acromegaly

Acromegaly is caused by a pituitary adenoma producing excess growth hormone that leads to gradual bony enlargement with enlargement of the hands and feet and joint changes due to synovial hypertrophy and cartilage overgrowth. Spinal hypermobility and a dorsal kyphosis are common. The vertebral width is increased due to apposition of periosteal new bone on its anterior border and osteophytosis may lead to bony bridging across the vertebral bodies. The height of the discs is also increased.

Ochronosis

This rare genetic disorder of amino acid metabolism usually occurs in elderly men who present with a stiff and aching spine. Typical X-ray findings are a marked narrowing of the intervertebral discs with relatively little osteophyte formation. Disc calcification is due to hydroxyapatite deposition. Pigmentation is found in the skin and ear, and the urine turns dark on standing, on alkalinization or on adding Clinitest tablets.

Degenerative conditions

Diffuse idiopathic skeletal hyperostosis (DISH)

This common degenerative condition (Resnick et al 1978) was first described as 'senile ankylo-

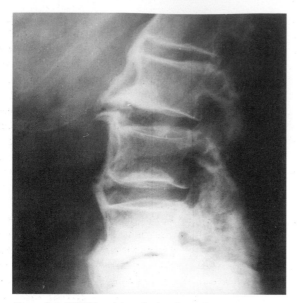

Figure 7.5 DISH involving the lumbar spine

sing hyperostosis of the spine', but its changes are confined neither to the spine nor to older age groups, as it may occur in middle-aged, usually male, patients. The more appropriate terminology is 'diffuse idiopathic skeletal hyperostosis' (DISH) since its pathological changes are found in spinal and extra-spinal structures. It is characterized by an excessive formation of bone at the entheses, and in the spine by prevertebral ossification involving the anterior longitudinal ligament (Figure 7.5), usually on the anterolateral aspect of the vertebrae. Large asymmetric osteophytes and bony bridges are produced across the disc spaces, which remain of normal height (Resnick et al, 1978). The disorder may occur in any area of the spine, but it is most common in the middle and lower thoracic vertebrae, followed by the lumbar and then the cervical spines. The sacroiliac joints remain normal. In the extraspinal sites, excessive bone formation occurs as a 'whiskering' around tendon and ligament entheses, especially in the pelvis, lower limb and heel.

The diagnosis is confirmed on X-ray, where the changes are best seen on the lateral views with exuberant bony masses likened to the flowing of hot wax poured over the anterolateral vertebral surface, which may proceed to complete 'armour-

plated' bony bridging. It may commence first with a ribbon-like prevertebral laying down of calcification (Francois et al, 1995), and a radiolucent line is commonly seen between the vertebral body and its anterior ligament (Sanzhang and Rothschild, 1993). In the thoracic vertebrae, ossification occurs almost exclusively on the right side, presumably because the aortic pulsation preserves the left side from such changes. The vertebral changes occur in the absence of any gross X-ray changes in the disc spaces, zygapophyseal joints or sacroiliac joints, thus differentiating it from spondylosis or ankylosing spondylitis. Thoracic involvement may progress into the upper lumbar and lower cervical spines. Osteoarthritis may develop in weight-bearing joints.

The aetiology of the ossification remains unknown. The HLA B27 antigen is not, but B8 may be, associated. Blood studies such as a full blood count, ESR and biochemical profile are normal. An association with an elevated blood glucose (Resnick et al, 1978) was suggested, but was subsequently disproved (Troillet and Gerster, 1993; Daragon et al, 1995). Differentiation from degenerative disc disease or ankylosing spondylitis is easily made. Similar ossification may occur in hypervitaminosis A, fluorosis and acromegaly, but investigations for them are always negative. Posterior longitudinal ligament ossification is rare, but is more significant since it may encroach on the spinal cord (Francois et al, 1995).

Clinical findings

Although it may be a chance X-ray finding in asymptomatic patients, most patients are conscious of some degree of spinal stiffness, which may occur at any time of the day, although it is usually worse in the morning. Aching pain in the thoracolumbar spine may be the presenting symptom, and is more likely to occur in younger patients who still remain reasonably active. There is little correlation between symptoms and the X-ray findings. As a general rule, stiffness produces little loss of functional capacity, especially when compared to patients with ankylosing spondylitis. Complications, such as a fracture (Hendrix et al, 1994), may follow trivial trauma (Callahan and

[handwritten margin note: occurring in 2nd decade ↑ more commonly]

Aguillera, 1993). Dysphagia may develop in those who have cervical involvement (Jonathan and Baer, 1990). Extraspinal involvement occurs especially around the pelvis, heel and elbow.

Scheuermann's disease

[handwritten margin note: Schmorls nodes r rec. characteristic]

This is a form of osteochondrosis with degenerative changes in the intervertebral disc and cartilage endplate. It is now generally considered to be a growth disorder that involves the discovertebral junction with irregularities in, or absence of, the osteocartilaginous growth zone (Aufdermaur and Spycher, 1986; Francois et al, 1995), leading to irregularities in the transition of cartilage to bone. The cartilage endplate is normally thick, especially at its periphery where it attaches to the annulus fibrosus. If this cartilage is abnormal or weakened, it will allow Schmorl's nodes, a vertical herniation of the nucleus pulposus through the cartilage endplate (Vernon-Roberts, 1994), to protrude into the vertebral body (Ippolito and Ponsetti, 1981). Scheuermann's disease has been considered as an unusually severe expression of Schmorl's nodes, with multiple Schmorl's nodes as a characteristic pathological and radiological feature of this disease. Vertebral growth under the abnormal growth plate becomes impaired, and ossification in the ring aphophysis becomes irregular (Ippolito and Ponsetti, 1981). Abnormality in ossification plus the body weight causes anterior wedging of some of the thoracic vertebrae, allowing the kyphosis to develop (Stoddard and Osborn, 1979). An alternate theory has been proposed (Lowe, 1990), that the kyphosis develops first and the vertebral changes then develop as adaptive changes.

Its aetiology is unknown, although it has been attributed in the past to several different causes, including trauma or overuse at work or sport. The original theory of Scheuermann, that the cause was an aseptic necrosis of the ring apophysis, has long been discounted (Sturm et al, 1993). It was once thought to be an inflammatory disorder, osteochondritis, a mistake that resulted in much unnecessary suffering. Genetic factors may be important (Halal et al, 1978; Lowe, 1990; McKenzie and Sillence, 1992; van Linthoudt and Revel, 1994), and it has been described in identical twins (Bjersand, 1980). It begins in the second decade, more commonly in men. Its exact prevalence is not certain because of the differences in its diagnostic requirements, but it may occur in up to 6 per cent of the juvenile population. The most common site of involvement is the lower thoracic vertebra, usually around T9, and it is extremely rare above T4. In the lumbar spine there is a decreasing incidence from L1, where changes are common, to L5, where they are rare. However, a separate condition may occur in the lumbar spine in boys with back pain, little deformity and typical X-ray changes (Blumenthal et al, 1987; Lowe, 1990).

It is rare for only one vertebra to be involved, and by definition three need to be involved for a diagnosis, whereas in about half of all patients more than five vertebrae are involved. Alterations in vertebral size commonly develop (Scholes et al, 1991). During the pubertal growth spurt, all curves that are greater than 45 degrees will progress (Ponte et al, 1985). The dorsal or lumbar spine may be predisposed to disc degeneration in later life (Stoddard and Osborn, 1979), although this has not been confirmed by Harreby et al (1995).

Clinical features

This common condition (Harreby et al, 1995) may be asymptomatic and so only becomes evident as a chance radiological finding. The usual complaint is of a mild or moderate degree of pain in the thoracic spine, although occasionally pain radiates to the lower lumbar region (Ponte et al, 1985). Pain often follows physical exertion, especially if overuse-type activities are involved. For a patient to present because of deformity alone is not common, and it may be associated with a localized scoliosis. Spinal cord compression or canal stenosis is most rare (Klein et al, 1986; Tallroth and Schlenzka, 1990; Normelli et al, 1991; Bhojraj and Dandawate, 1994). The typical clinical findings include:

- A smooth, rounded dorsal kyphosis that becomes most evident on flexion.
- Loss of spinal mobility. There may be loss of the normal range of flexion and/or extension, and of the passive intervertebral joint range.

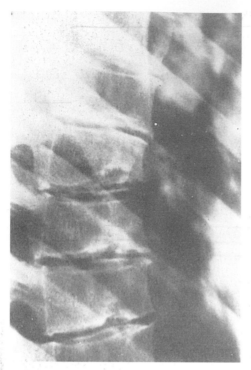

Figure 7.6 The typical radiological features of Scheuermann's disease of the thoracic spine

- Hamstring tightness (Somhegyi and Ratko, 1993).

X-ray changes mirror the pathological changes, and bone scan may help in atypical cases (Mandell et al, 1993). X-rays are necessary to confirm the diagnosis, and at least three of the following changes must be present (Figure 7.6):

- Schmorl's nodes
- Wedging of the vertebral body
- Thoracic kyphosis or a loss of the normal lumbar curve
- Irregular, narrowed intervertebral disc spaces
- Mottling and fragmentation of the ring epiphyses
- Irregularity of the vertebral body surfaces
- Disappearance of the upper and lower outer corners of the vertebral body
- The epiphyses become dense, but the vertebral bodies remain wedged after repair.

Management

The best results are produced if the disease is detected early, before skeletal maturity. When pain is a problem, management consists of:

- Rest from activities that reproduce pain: that includes most sports or work in which bending and lifting are involved.
- Postural correction. Bracing remains the mainstay of management. A Milwaukee brace is used and should be worn for at least six months continuously and then intermittently until pain ceases. Support in a corset alone may be required for lumbar pain. Use of a firm bed and bed-boards in the less severe degrees of deformity is a help.
- Isometric and isotonic exercises, exercises to increase the degree of lumbar lordosis and exercises to stretch the hamstrings and other tight spinal structures are needed. Postural exercises cannot correct an existing deformity but they are used to help prevent an increase in the deformity.
- Manual therapy techniques are contraindicated.
- Surgery is rarely indicated, but it may be necessary for a painful curvature of greater than 65 degrees (Lowe, 1990; Sturm et al, 1993; Ferreira-Alves et al, 1995).

Spinal infections

The most common cause of spinal infection is staphylococcal (Malawski and Lukawski, 1991), and the most common spinal site involved is the lumbar (Malawski and Lukawski, 1991) and lower thoracic spines. The disease may occur at any age, but nowadays is more common in elderly people (Cahill et al, 1991), and its onset may be insidious. A primary source of infection, such as the skin, may be present, and the disease develops due to haematogenous spread through the paravertebral venous system. However, it may also occur from local spread or it may follow spinal operations. As a general rule it involves bone initially (Rothman, 1996), and then spreads early to involve the surrounding disc (Rothman, 1996). The radiological findings are reflected in destruction of the vertebral endplates followed by loss of the disc space (Smith and Blaser, 1991). Spontaneous infectious discitis (Honan et al, 1996) occurs in adults, is rare, and is distinct from infection with postoperative spinal surgery (Honan et al, 1996).

Other causative organisms beside *Staphylococcus* may be involved (Nicholas et al, 1996) including other Gram-positive organisms such as Streptococci or Gram-negative coliform organisms, such as *Escherichia coli* or *Salmonella*. Chronic granulomatous spinal lesions may be caused by tuberculosis, brucellosis or fungal infections. Sacroiliac joint infections are considered in Chapter 10.

Many factors need to be taken into account in assessing a patient with a suspected spinal infection, including age, general health, such as diabetes, drug addiction, immune status, how the infection was acquired and its virulence, recent infections in other sites, including operation or cannulation sites. Investigations in patients with suspected spinal infections include a full blood count, ESR, repeated blood cultures, serum proteins and electrophoresis, an aspiration biopsy of the disc space and specific serum agglutination tests. In staphylococcal infections, the white cell count may be elevated or normal, and the ESR is invariably high, up to 100 mm in one hour. A technetium 99M bone scan should be performed, as it is very sensitive although not overly specific. Radiolabelled white cell scans and gallium scans can be a further help.

X-rays are taken as a routine measure, although they are of little value in the early stages, whereas CT or especially MRI (Post et al, 1991; Smith and Blaser, 1991; Rothman, 1996), which may be gadolinium-enhanced (Donovan et al, 1991), may detect changes at an earlier stage. X-rays ultimately show local destructive changes in the vertebral body with surrounding soft tissue swelling. The disc space becomes progressively narrower, the bony endplate blurred and indistinct, and ultimately the vertebral bodies collapse.

Early diagnosis is essential (Finkenberg, 1993; Rothman, 1996), and definitive treatment will depend upon identifying the causative organism, with repeated blood cultures or repeated local aspiration, which may be performed percuta-

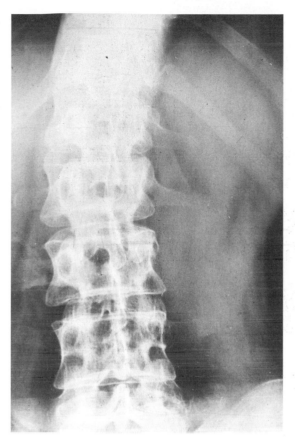

Figure 7.7 Left-sided tumour with scoliosis, soft tissue swelling and loss of the transverse process of L3

neously. Treatment consists of bedrest in hospital with adequate doses of suitable antibiotics, such as flucloxacillin, given intravenously 2 g four times daily combined with probenicid 500 mg twice daily. As healing becomes established over the succeeding months, the patient is mobilized in a spinal brace while antibiotics are continued for at least six months until healing is firm.

Spinal tumours

The spine is a common site for tumours (Figures 7.7 and 7.8), usually due to secondary deposits, and this may become a greater problem with the advancing age of the general population. Pain is usually localized at first to the back, but compression of nerve roots or the spinal cord may also

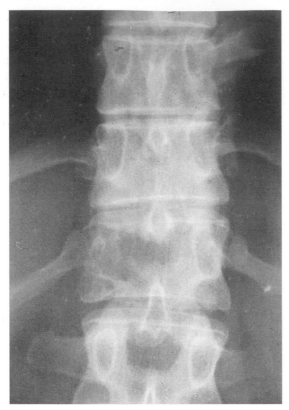

Figure 7.8 Secondary malignancy at T12 with loss of the right pedicle

occur with radiation of pain into the limbs or chest. The presence of a spinal tumour should be suspected clinically in several different situations:

- In a patient known to have had a previous malignancy who now presents with spinal pain
- In a patient over the age of 50 year with back or limb pain without a previous history of a similar problem
- In a patient with exacerbation of spinal pain at night
- In a patient whose symptoms are unremitting or progressively worse
- In a patient who is not responding to conventional therapy (Humphrey and Inman, 1995).

The tumour, either primary or secondary, occurs in the vertebrae more commonly than in the spinal canal. Secondary deposits, much more common than primary tumours, originate most commonly from breast, lung, prostate, kidney and thyroid, may be osteoblastic or osteolytic, and are distributed in bone by closely following the vertebral venous system.

Benign primary bone tumours include haemangioma, aneurysmal bone cyst and osteoid osteoma. Primary malignant bone tumours are rare, although marrow tumours including multiple myeloma or lymphoma are more common.

Spinal tumours are classified as:

- Extradural, such as neuroma, fibroma, lipoma or angioma, which form about 20 per cent of spinal tumours
- Intradural, which may be extramedullary, such as a neuroma, meningioma or sarcoma or intramedullary, such as angioma or glioma
- A neurofibroma (Figure 7.9) may occur singly or multiply as part of Von Recklinghausen's disease. It originates in the spinal nerve root as a smooth or nodular encapsulated growth and is most often intradural but may be extradural or grow outside the spine and produce the so-called 'dumb-bell' tumour

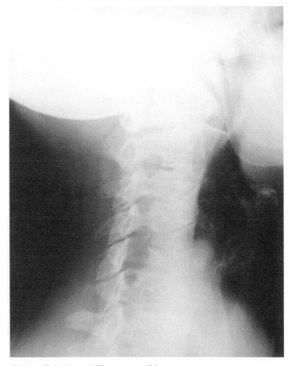

Figure 7.9 Neurofibroma at C5

Investigations for a suspected spinal malignancy include X-rays, full blood count, ESR and a biochemical profile with serum calcium, alkaline phosphatase and prostate-specific antigen levels. The ESR is invariably elevated, especially with multiple myeloma, when serum and urinary EPG and biopsy to show plasma cells are necessary.

X-ray changes occur in the bone without any involvement of the disc, and the vertebral body may collapse with the disc space still intact (An et al, 1995). This is in contrast to spinal infections, including tuberculosis, in which a loss of the disc space is invariable. X-ray changes of bone destruction are a late finding, so bone scanning might be used first to detect any abnormality (Kostuik, 1993b). CT or MRI (Masaryk, 1991; Kostuik, 1993b; An et al, 1995) are then used to confirm the diagnosis. Compression fractures are a common finding and need to be differentiated from other benign disorders. MRI can help here (Rupp et al, 1995) and may be improved with gadolinium enhancement. A bone biopsy (Ghelman et al, 1991) or a bone marrow examination should be performed if the diagnosis remains in doubt.

8 Manual therapy for the lumbar spine

The three manual therapy techniques described for the lumbar spine are mobilization, manipulation and traction.

Mobilization uses repetitive, oscillatory, long-lever, low-velocity, high-amplitude passive movements (Maitland, 1986; Shekelle, 1994). The joint being treated is moved rhythmically within, or at the limit of, its normal range at a speed that the patient can voluntarily resist or prevent. It is usually the first technique used, since complications with it have not been reported, and most cases will improve without any need to consider a full manipulation.

Manipulation is a short-lever, short-duration, small-amplitude, high-velocity passive movement technique. It is used when a joint is moved by the therapist with a sudden movement or thrust, beyond its normal range (Maitland, 1986; Shekelle, 1994). The movement is performed so quickly that the patient is unable to prevent it.

Mechanism of action

The mechanism of action of these techniques is still speculative (LaBan and Taylor, 1992; Lee et al, 1993a), and their use remains empirical. In the peripheral joints, the indications for manual therapy include:

- Replacement of a dislocation or subluxation
- Breaking down or stretching of adhesions
- Reduction of an internal derangement of the joint, such as a loose cartilaginous body
- Hypomobility lesions.

It would be satisfying to be able to translate these examples to the spinal joints, but the evidence that these same mechanisms are at work in the spine is lacking.

Main benefits

- The principal benefit is the restoration of accessory movements, thereby increasing the range of movement in an intervertebral joint segment (Farfan, 1980a).
- Relief of pain. Whatever the underlying lesion producing reduced spinal mobility, it may also result in stimulation of the sinuvertebral nerves and so produce spinal pain. Restoration of spinal mobility will relieve this source of neural irritation.
- Muscles are stretched and muscle spasm may be reduced, which may help circumvent any pain–spasm–pain cycle.
- Disc nutrition, dependent on fluid exchange between the vascular channels in the vertebrae and the disc, is aided by normal joint movement and impeded by loss of normal mobility.
- In the zygapophyseal joints, an internal derangement due to meniscoid bodies

(Bogduk and Jull, 1985) (Figure 8.1), loose cartilaginous bodies, nipped synovial fringes or 'joint lock' have been described.

- In the disc, annular tears or a nuclear prolapse, either bulging into the spinal canal or blocked between vertebral bodies, have been implicated. It would appear extremely unlikely that spinal manipulation can regularly reduce a joint subluxation or reposition a piece of prolapsed disc material (Shekelle et al, 1992).

- Adhesion formation is a popular concept, although it has not been demonstrated around the spinal joints, and it seems highly unlikely that a breakdown of adhesions is a common mechanism. The noise of stretching adhesions as heard, for example, when manipulating a capsulitis of the shoulder is quite different from the crack-like sound on spinal manipulation. If a single manipulation does produce a 'click' with immediate pain relief, it would appear more likely that a loose cartilaginous body within the intervertebral joint complex may have been moved.

- There are psychological benefits. The psychological effects produced by personalized care and the 'laying on of hands' (Farfan, 1980a; Hoehler and Tobis, 1983) implicit in manipulative practice may well be powerful motivating factors.

Precautions

- A careful overall assessment of the patient and his or her musculoskeletal spinal problem is undertaken before any treatment is commenced. A plan is essential. All joints that could be responsible for symptoms must be examined and a treatment plan then devised (Maitland, 1986).

- Contraindications to manual therapy are looked for by history, physical examination and X-ray examination.

- The particular joint at fault is located by clinical testing. If pain is reproduced on passive movement, treatment with suitable passive movements would appear to be a logical extension.

- Extreme gentleness, especially initially, is essential, and is another reason for mobilization techniques to be selected first before manipulation. The depth and strength of treatments should be increased only after reassessing the patient's condition to verify that there is no adverse reaction.

- Mobilization techniques may then be progressed in strength or in their grade of movement.

- Response to the treatment technique is assessed by repeated testing, and considerable practice is needed to recognize the patterns of

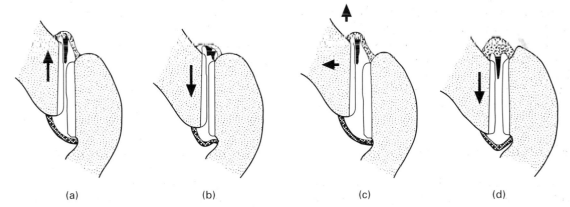

(a)   (b)   (c)   (d)

Figure 8.1 The theory of meniscus extrapment. (a) Upon flexion, the inferior articular process of a zygapophyseal joint moves upwards taking a meniscoid with it. (b) Upon attempted extension, the inferior articular process returns towards its neutral position, but the meniscoid, instead of re-entering the joint cavity, impacts against the edge of the articular cartilage, and buckles forming a space-occupying 'lesion' under the capsule. Pain occurs as a result of capsular tension and extension is inhibited. (c) Manipulation of the joint involving gapping and flexion reduces the impaction and opens the joint to encourage re-entry of the meniscoid into the joint space as shown in (d). Reprinted from *Clinical Anatomy of the Lumbar Spine* by N. Bogduk and L. Twomey with kind permission of Churchill Livingstone.

joint behaviour. A patient with a certain degree of pain and stiffness should improve in an orderly progression after a prescribed level of therapy. Failure to fit into this pattern is an early warning sign to consider an alternate diagnosis.

- It may not be necessary to restore the full range of mobility, as minor increases in the range of movement may suffice if symptoms are improving. The subjective feeling of stiffness does not usually correspond with the objective loss of joint range, as measured by comparing movements to either side.
- Manipulation under general anaesthesia is rarely indicated, and is best avoided since it also prevents any meaningful reassessment of a patient's reaction to a technique. Also, the spine can be much more readily traumatized with the patient unconscious, and it is extremely rare for one manipulation alone to cure a patient's symptoms completely. A spinal joint should never be thrust forcibly in a direction that is protected by muscle spasm. To do so invites trouble. A different direction of movement for the same joint, unprotected by spasm, should be chosen.
- Treatment involving forced flexion of the lumbar spine or manipulation with the patient in a flexed position is extremely dangerous. However, mobilization techniques may be carried out in this direction, particularly if performed in a non-weight bearing position.
- Manipulation using strong manual traction is unnecessary, for it neither improves the results nor renders the techniques any safer.
- Manual therapy is never the sole method of treatment, but should always form part of a total therapeutic management.

Indications

Indications are predicated upon a full clinical assessment of the patient and a review of the diagnosis and treatments available. They may be considered in three groups:

1. Major indications, in which the techniques may be expected to be successful, or at least play a major role, in most cases.

2. Relative indications, in which they may help in some but not in all cases, or other therapies take precedence.
3. Rarely successful conditions, in which they only rarely produce any improvement.

Major indications

The major indication for manual therapy techniques is a painful mechanical derangement of vertebral joint movement in the absence of any neurological lesion, such as:

- A spinal hypomobility lesion with any of its associated pain syndromes
- Lumbar spondylosis. Mobilization techniques usually produce marked improvement in pain, stiffness and function
- A patient with an acute mechanical joint derangement.

Relative indications

- Intervertebral disc prolapse. The role of manipulative techniques in the management of intervertebral disc prolapse remains controversial, and the degree of improvement they can attain is uncertain. Their use may depend largely upon the therapist's experience and expertise. With non-progressive neurological symptoms and signs, such as paraesthesia or an absent ankle jerk, gentler techniques may be used as part of an overall management plan. Gentle mobilization techniques may be of value for patients without severe pain and no neurological deficit. However, disc prolapse with nerve root compression and a neurological deficit should not be treated using these techniques until symptoms are improving. Mobilization techniques may then be added provided clinical improvement is maintained.
- Spondylolisthesis. Patients with either back or leg pain may be helped with mobilization techniques or traction in approximately 60 per cent of cases.
- Hypermobility syndromes with spinal pain usually respond poorly to most forms of therapy, and manual therapy is no exception. However, mobilization is indicated if a hypo-

mobile lesion develops in one spinal segment, and movement reproduces symptoms.

- Pregnancy. The problems with mobilization in pregnant patients with spinal pain relate mainly to the technical problems with adequate posturing of the patient.
- Cervial vertigo (*see* Chapter 15).
- Undiagnosed patients. As a general rule, patients without a firm clinical diagnosis should not be treated with manual methods.

Rarely successful

Patients with pain due to postural disturbances with marked stiffness, or severe degrees of acute lumbago, especially if associated with a marked lumbar kyphosis, are rarely helped by passive movement techniques.

Contraindications

Absolute contraindications include:

- Disease of the vertebral column: the rheumatic and orthopaedic conditions discussed in Chapter 7. They include: trauma, such as fractures, spondylolysis and dislocations; infections; inflammatory disease due to spondyloarthritis or rheumatoid arthritis; metabolic bone disease, such as osteoporosis; tumours, benign or malignant; and developmental anomalies.
- Neurological lesions. Compression of neurological structures within the spinal cord or cauda equina represents an absolute contraindication to any form of manual therapy.
- Vertebral instability.
- Arterial compression. Evidence of vertebral-artery compression is an absolute contraindication.
- Psychogenic causes. Patients whose symptoms are primarily psychogenically determined should never be treated with any of the physical methods of therapy, including manual therapy techniques.
- Patients with bleeding tendencies or who are on anticoagulant therapy.

Technique

For mobilization to be effective, a sense of 'feel' of movement is required, like feeling the meshing of cogs on changing gears. Until this feel has been acquired, treatment by mobilization can never be fully effective. The usual technique employs some two or three oscillations per second. If they are too quick or too slow, it is impossible to gain the proper feel of movement. For a joint to be most effectively moved in any direction it should first be positioned approximately midway between all of its other ranges. An example is found in the metacarpophalangeal joint of the index finger. To achieve maximum distraction with the least effort, a starting position midway between the normal limits of flexion, extension, abduction, adduction and rotation is used. The range of distraction will be limited if the joint is positioned at the limit of any one of these ranges. For lower lumbar mobilization, the lumbar spine is positioned towards flexion; for upper lumbar mobilization, the spine is positioned towards extension.

Mobilization techniques use pressures against some part of the vertebrae. Only the thumbs or the hands should be used to produce movement by transmitting body weight to the vertebrae. If the intrinsic muscles of the hands are used, the technique becomes uncomfortable to the patient and therapist, the hands become tense and the feel of the movement is lost. In all techniques in which direct pressure is applied to the vertebrae, the supporting fingers are positioned with the arms and thumbs over the movement. The correct starting position is important, as it allows the patient to relax and the therapist to work effectively with the minimum of effort and the hands relaxed.

Complications

It is a sound axiom that 'the bad results of manipulation are due to bad manipulators', and considering the many spinal manipulations performed throughout the world each year, the number of recorded complications are extraordinarily few (Shekelle et al, 1992). Most serious complications involve the cervical spine (*see* Chapter 17), and in the lumbar spine, complications should not occur if the necessary precautions are heeded (Haldeman, 1983). Fractures or joint subluxation have been reported, mostly after chiropractic manipulation and often stemming from a failure to recognize the presence of pathology, such as a secondary malignant deposit. Neurological complications that have been described include nerve root compression, rupture of a nerve root cord, compression and cauda equina lesions (Malmivaara and Pohjola, 1982; Dan and Saccasan, 1983; Gallinaro and Cartesegna, 1983; Assendelft et al, 1996).

Controlled trials

Manual methods of treatment can be evaluated only by adequately conducted, controlled, double-blind clinical trials (Koes et al, 1991a), and their acceptance is hindered by the lack of them. There are problems in designing trials, such as assuring that the trial is truly double-blind, since both the doctor and the patient will usually be able to recognize what treatment regimen has been allocated, tailoring the type and degree of manipulative therapy to the patient's clinical problem and comparing one trial with another (LaBan and Taylor, 1992). Some published trials have been heavily criticized on the basis of their patient selection, length of treatment and treatment techniques. Mainly because of these problems, the definitive trial is yet to be done (Twomey and Taylor, 1995).

More recently published trials in the English literature (Coxhead et al, 1981; Hoehler et al, 1981; Farrell and Twomey, 1982; Nwuga, 1982; Godfrey et al, 1984; Gibson et al, 1985; Hadler et al, 1987; Ongley et al, 1987; Kinalski et al, 1989; McDonald and Bell, 1990; Meade et al, 1990; Blomberg et al, 1992; Koes et al, 1992; Powell et al, 1993; Pope et al, 1994; Bradshaw et al, 1995; Triano et al, 1995) are too numerous to review adequately here. However, in general, most trials do show the efficacy of manual methods in a majority of patients in the short term, although at follow-up in all trials at about six months there are no significant differences between the groups. Twenty-five controlled trials were reviewed using meta-analysis (Shekelle et al,

1992), which concluded that manipulation for acute or subacute low back pain produced a 34 per cent improvement in recovery within three weeks from the start of treatment when compared to controls. Several good reviews of the trials have also been published (Ottenbacher and Di Fabio, 1985; Koes et al, 1991a; Di Fabio, 1992; LaBan and Taylor, 1992; Shekelle et al, 1992; Assendelft et al, 1995). The methodological quality, which was low, and the conclusions of 51 reviews, of which 34 reached a positive conclusion, were assessed by Assendelft et al (1995).

The cracking sound

Crack-like sounds coming from the manipulated spinal joints are a well-known, common phenomenon accompanying movement of a joint. The forces exerted during spinal manipulation cause an increase in joint volume with a corresponding fall in fluid partial pressure. Intra-articular gases, drawn out of solution, create a gas bubble (Herzog et al, 1993). Fluid rushes into the area of low pressure, which collapses the gas bubble, and the resultant cavitation process is heard as a crack (Herzog et al, 1993; Brodeur, 1995). Once cavitation has occured, the force–displacement curve changes and the range of motion of the joint increases (Brodeur, 1995). Approximately 20 minutes are required before a joint is again ready to produce a crack, which represents the time taken for the gas to return into solution. Movement at a joint may be produced without any accompanying cracking sound, but if a crack is produced it does indicate that the joint has been moved satisfactorily.

Manipulative techniques

Mobilization

Treatment grades

The degree of movement used during mobilizations is modified according to pain, restriction of movement and muscle spasm. Movements are also graded according to their amplitude and the position within the range that they occupy (Figure 8.2).

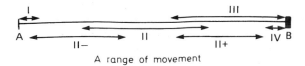

Figure 8.2 Grades of movement. A = Beginning of range of movement; B = end of normal, average range of movement

Grade I is a small-amplitude movement performed at the starting position of the range.

Grade II is a large-amplitude movement that carries well into the range. It can occupy any part of the range but does not reach the limit of the range.

Grade III is also a large-amplitude movement at the limit of the range.

Grade IV is a small-amplitude movement at the end of the range.

Selection of technique

The technique chosen depends on the site of pain, the disturbance in rhythm of spinal movements, and its response to treatment. If pain or restricted movement is unilateral, then unilateral techniques designed to open up or move the same side of the intervertebral joint complex should provide relief. Thus a patient with a right side back pain may be found to have a restriction of lateral flexion to the right. The technique selected aims at opening the right hand side of the intervertebral joint, e.g. by transverse pressures from left to right against the spinous process.

Depth of mobilization

Gentle techniques only are used at first as they are often able to provide a sufficient degree of improvement without any exacerbation of symptoms and signs. Any alteration in the degree of pain, spasm and stiffness, or any change in their position within the range, needs to be constantly assessed both during the treatment session and before the next session. The depth of the mobilization is guided by pain and spasm.

Pain is the most important guide in determining the depth of treatment, and is assessed according to its severity, whether it is localized or referred, and the site within the range of movement at which it is produced. Six factors need to be considered:

1. For patients with severe pain, movements must be small, usually Grade I.
2. With localized spinal pain, mobilization is initially performed in the pain-free range, the movement being carried to the point where pain begins. When pain is felt at the beginning of the range, mobilization must be performed with very small rhythmical movements (Grade I). As the range of pain-free movement increases, mobilization can be performed still further into the range (Grade II).
3. If a mobilizing technique produces distally referred pain, subsequent mobilizing techniques must be performed in the painless range, assessing it immediately after the treatment and again 24 hours later. Provided symptoms or signs have not then been aggravated, the technique may be increased slightly. If referred symptoms become exacerbated, the amplitude of the mobilization and its position in the range must be reduced. Assessment over 24 hours will indicate whether this technique should be continued, although it may be necessary to provoke some degree of pain in order to produce an improvement in movements.
4. When pain, either local or referred, occurs in the last quarter of the range, techniques are more commonly used at the limit of the normal range or until meeting physical resistance, when either a large Grade III or a small grade IV amplitude should be used.
5. With a painful arc in the range of movement, large amplitude Grade II or Grade III mobilization should be performed.
6. In patients with little pain but restricted movement, Grade IV movements are often the only successful treatment. If symptoms are exacerbated, Grade II or gentle Grade III movements are used to relieve local soreness.

Muscle spasm is the other guide to the depth of the mobilization technique to be used. It is a protective mechanism to splint a painful joint and is usually readily apparent on inspection and palpation. Treatment techniques, extremely gentle at first to avoid provoking any sudden, excessive protective muscular reaction, should never be forced beyond this limit. As the patient improves, the depth of mobilization and the range of spasm-free movement should be increased.

Duration and frequency of treatment

Mobilization is usually carried out daily at first. On the first day, mobilization techniques are normally only of short duration, as the examination may have produced sufficient joint movement. The patient should be warned to expect some temporary increase in symptoms, and its degree is assessed the next day. The number of any mobilizations in one session depends on the assessment of the degree of the symptoms. With moderate degrees, three or four mobilizations of a joint, lasting approximately 30–60 seconds each, are given. If symptoms are minimal, six mobilization treatments are given. If reaction is not excessive, treatment can be progressed in subsequent sessions.

Assessment of techniques

The initial technique must be used gently without provoking any pain. Symptoms and signs are then reassessed, the range of movements and pain being compared to those previously present. If the clinical findings are unaltered, the same technique may be repeated more firmly and the patient reassessed. If there is still no improvement, an alternative technique is selected. If symptoms have been exacerbated, that particular technique is discarded. A good guide to the success of treatment is whether the joint range that is subsequently retained is at least 50 per cent of the increase gained during treatment.

Reaction to treatment

Mobilization techniques should result in an improvement of symptoms over a few days. Some degree of soreness may be experienced for a time after treatment using strong techniques, but this should have eased before the next treatment.

Many mobilization techniques for the lumbar spine have been described and only the five most commonly used will be described here: rotation; posteroanterior central pressure; posteroanterior unilateral vertebral pressure; transverse pressure; and longitudinal movement. The indications for these techniques are summarized in Table 8.1.

Table 8.1 Indications for lumbar spine mobilization techniques

Technique	Main indications
Rotation	This is usually the first technique indicated and is especially useful in patients with unilateral pain
Posteroanterior central vertebral pressure	Patients with midline pain or with some radiation to either side; spondylosis
Posteroanterior unilateral vertebral pressure	Unilateral pain particularly arising from the middle or upper lumbar spine
Transverse vertebral pressure	Unilateral pain especially arising from the upper lumbar spine
Straight leg raising	Pain and restricted movement in the pain-sensitive elements in the vertebral canal and foramen
Longitudinal movement:	
Using two legs	Bilateral pain arising from lower lumbar region
Using one leg	Unilateral pain arising from lower lumbar region
Lumbar traction	If symptoms are of gradual onset; if pain is not aggravated by active movements; spondylosis

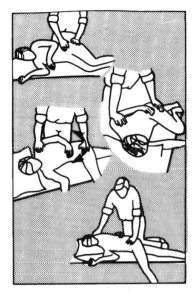

Figure 8.3 Mobilization of the lumbar spine: rotation

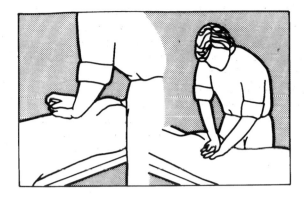

Figure 8.4 Mobilization of the lumbar spine: posteroanterior central vertebral pressure

Rotation

This is the most common and effective mobilization technique for the lumbar spine. Indications include unilateral back or leg pain, or central back pain with a restriction of movement to one side only.

The patient lies on his or her side with the head on a pillow. The localization of this movement to one area in the lumbar spine is obtained by the degree of rotation. This is attained by appropriate positioning of the patient's thorax and pelvis and then positioning the lumbar spine towards either flexion or extension by flexion or extension of the hip (Figure 8.3).

An oscillatory movement is produced by the therapist's left hand rotating the patient's pelvis while the right hand stabilizes the thorax. For the upper lumbar spine, rotation is used with the spine in minimal extension; for the lower lumbar spine, rotation is used with the spine towards flexion; and for the lower lumbar spine, rotation is used with the spine towards flexion.

Posteroanterior central vertebral pressure

Indications include midline lumbar pain with some radiation out to both sides, as in mechan-

ical derangement of a lumbar joint or lumbar spondylosis.

The patient lies prone with the arms by the side and the head turned to one side. The therapist stands on the left side and places the pisiform area of his or her left hand over the spinous process, reinforcing it with pressure from the right hand.

An oscillating movement is obtained by the therapist rocking his or her upper trunk up and down, pressure being transmitted through shoulder and arms (Figure 8.4).

Posteroanterior unilateral vertebral pressure

Indications include hypomobility lesions involving the upper or middle lumbar spine associated with localized back pain and muscle spasm.

The patient lies prone, arms to the side and the head turned to one side. The therapist stands on the side to be treated with thumbs placed lateral to the spinous process at the appropriate level (Figure 8.5).

By positioning the shoulders directly over the hands, pressure can be transmitted by movement of the trunk to the thumbs so that the thumbs themselves do not need to move.

Transverse vertebral pressure

Indications include unilateral lumbar pain, especially in the upper lumbar spine.

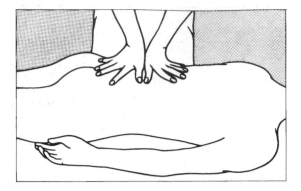

Figure 8.5 Mobilization: posteroanterior unilateral vertebral pressure

The patient lies prone with the arms by the side and the head turned to one side while the therapist stands to the right side with thumbs against the right side of the vertebra to be mobilized (Figure 8.6).

Oscillatory pressure is applied through the thumbs against the spinous process. Greater range of movement is produced in the upper spine than in the lower spine.

Longitudinal movement

This is a useful and gentle technique in which a rhythmic longitudinal movement is applied to one or both legs. It is used especially on patients with sudden severe pain, either in the lower lumbar midline or radiating to one side, who may not be able to be positioned for any alternative mobilization technique.

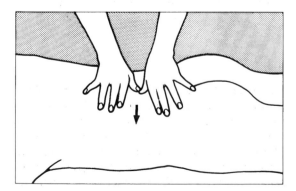

Figure 8.6 Mobilization: transverse vertebral pressure

Manipulation

Manipulation techniques are classified as being either: non-specific, i.e. applied to an area of the spine; or specific, in which movement is localized to one intervertebral segment only.

Non-specific techniques

These are an extension of the mobilization techniques described above but with a rapid thrust now applied at the limit of the normal range. The two most important techniques are rotation and posteroanterior pressure.

ROTATION

The therapist stands on the right side of the couch with the patient supine. The therapist's left hand steadies the patient's left shoulder and his or her right hand positions the left hip and knee into flexion at a right angle. The patient's pelvis is rotated to the right by pulling the left knee across the body and down towards the floor (Figure 8.7). The therapist next grasps the posterolateral aspect of the patient's upper calf with the right hand and applies counter-pressure against the shoulder with his or her left hand. By positioning the patient's underneath leg, the lumbar spine may be placed into a position of either flexion or extension.

With the patient suitably positioned, an oscillatory rotational movement is supplied by each hand, and then a sudden downward and rotary thrust is added to the leg while maintaining strong counter-pressure to the shoulder. It is essential that this movement should produce a

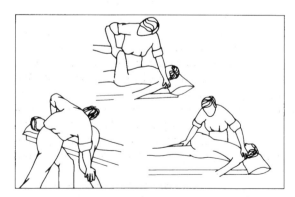

Figure 8.7 Manipulation of the lumbar spine: rotation

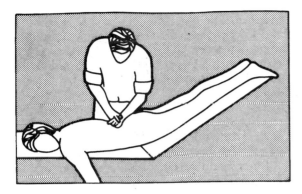

Figure 8.8 Manipulation of the lumbar spine: posteroanterior vertebral pressure

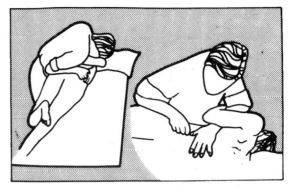

Figure 8.9 Manipulation: rotation of intervertebral joints

rotation of the pelvis and spine and not just an adduction of the leg.

POSTEROANTERIOR PRESSURE

With the patient lying prone, the therapist uses the pisiform bone of his or her right hand to stretch the intervertebral joint to its limit.

By suddenly increasing the pressure on the hands, a movement of very small range is produced. To increase its effectiveness, the patient's trunk or legs may be supported in a position of extension (Figure 8.8).

Specific techniques

LUMBAR ROTATION

The therapist stands facing the patient, who lies on the right side with the left knee and hip flexed. The patient's lower right leg is then moved into sufficient flexion to position the appropriate lumbar intervertebral joint midway between its range of flexion and extension. The patient's thorax is then rotated by pulling on the right arm with the left forearm against the patient's shoulder and the right upper forearm behind the patient's left hip. The therapist's left thumb presses downwards against the left side of the spinous process of the upper vertebra of the joint to be manipulated. At the same time, his or her right middle finger pulls upwards against the spinous process of the lower vertebra (Figure 8.9).

The patient is rocked back and forth with the therapist's forearms until the maximum rotary

stretch is applied. At the same time, the pressure against the spinous processes is increased until the joint is felt to be tight. The manipulation is performed by an increased push through both forearms while suddenly increasing the pressure against the spinous processes.

Lumbar traction

Traction is a very useful form of treatment (Pal et al, 1986), although its exact mechanism of action is uncertain. It is usually considered to produce spinal elongation (Pellicchia, 1994; van der Heijden et al, 1995). More likely, it is one particular form of mobilization technique, now applied in a longitudinal direction along the long axis of the spine by a harness and a machine of some description of which some 10 types have been described (Pellecchia, 1994). It may be constant or intermittent, standing or lying, straight or flexed, at home, in hospital or in the rooms. A friction-free couch is not essential, but it is of great advantage and many varieties of it are available.

Method

The patient first stands while a belt is firmly fixed around the thorax, and then lies down while a second belt is applied around the pelvis. Clothing must not be caught under either of these belts. The patient then lies either prone or supine on the traction couch. If supine, the hips and knees may both be flexed. For maximal effect, the intervertebral joint being treated should be positioned midway between its position of flexion and extension. The belts are then attached by straps to fixed points beyond the ends of the couch and tightened to remove any looseness from the harness.

The site and degree of the patient's pain is first determined. Traction is then applied from the head end, the foot end, or from both ends. If a roll-top traction couch is not being used, friction is eliminated between the patient and the couch by alternately raising or lowering the patient's thorax and pelvis. A maximum of 13 kg should first be used for a period not exceeding 10 minutes and pain reassessed after 10 seconds. A careful watch is kept for any back symptoms, even if induced by movement or coughing. If low back pain is induced, the duration and pressure of this first treatment is reduced.

Progress

This depends on:

- If severe symptoms are completely relieved, the strength of traction should be reduced by at least half, and its duration should not exceed five minutes, to prevent any exacerbation of symptoms.
- If symptoms are only slightly relieved by 13 kg traction, the strength may be increased to approximately 20 kg for 10 minutes. However, if 20 kg then completely relieves symptoms, the strength should be reduced to below 18 kg.
- If symptoms remain unchanged, traction should be increased to 20 kg and sustained for 10 minutes.
- If symptoms are exacerbated, traction should be reduced and its duration limited to five minutes.

Traction is slowly released, while the patient gently tilts the pelvis from side to side. If pain is then experienced, traction should be held until the pain disappears. After the traction is removed, the patient should rest a few minutes before standing, especially after the first treatment, and warned that it is normal for the back to feel strange for approximately two hours.

Progession

On the day following the first treatment, symptoms and signs are reassessed to determine whether traction should be repeated, and if so, how it is to be graduated. Signs may be assessed immediately after the first traction, but flexion is often more limited at that time. One way to gauge its success is whether at subsequent treatments the weight known to produce pain can be increased without producing any discomfort.

If symptoms are exacerbated during the first treatment but remain unchanged after reducing the strength, traction must be discontinued. If, however, symptoms and signs do not deteriorate, traction can be reinstituted and an assessment made of the strength that can be applied without increasing the symptoms. It is a good sign if a greater strength can be applied.

When symptoms are relieved on the first day, progression is guided mainly by the severity of any temporary exacerbation after treatment. During the first three or four treatments, improvement will probably be small but noticeable, and treatment should be increased in time, not strength. If no exacerbation follows treatment, the weight can be gradually increased. Otherwise strength and time can be increased together. The usual strength used is between 30 and 45 kg, but, if the rate of progress is slow at the lower strength, traction up to 65 kg may be necessary. In general, the length of treatment need not exceed 15 minutes, since longer periods do not produce any further progress. Strength should not be the controlling guide to treatment and is referred to only when traction has been set. The scale measurement is valuable mainly as a record.

Intermittent variable traction can be used for the lumbar spine; as in other areas of the vertebral column, its duration, strength and indications are similar to those for other forms of traction.

Precautions

No soreness should be felt following the lower strengths of traction, although there may be some discomfort from the harness. After the traction has been applied, the patient should attempt alternate flattening and arching of the

Table 8.2 Selection sequence of techniques for the lumbar region

Unilateral symptoms	Bilateral symptoms
Rotation or posteroanterior central vertebral pressure	Posteroanterior central vertebral pressure
	Rotation
For upper lumbar region:	For upper lumbar region:
Transverse vertebral pressure	Transverse vertebral pressure
Traction	Traction
For lower lumbar region:	For lower lumbar region:
Traction	Traction
Longitudinal movement	Longitudinal movement

lumbar spine and coughing to test for any back discomfort. The first session of traction is used in the form of a trial run to avoid the embarrassing, although harmless, situation where a patient has difficulty regaining his or her feet after excessive traction.

Indications

- Nerve root pressure due to intervertebral disc prolapse
- Non-traumatic symptoms of gradual onset, either localized to the lumbar area or referred into the leg
- Lumbar spondylosis usually responds to gentle or intermittent variable traction

- Back pain without any obvious loss of normal range of active lumbar movement usually responds better to traction than to manipulation
- When no further progress can be obtained by use of mobilization techniques
- It may be necessary to precede traction with a manipulation, particularly if the intervertebral joint is stiff. If traction does not result in any further progress, it is best to revert to mobilization techniques.

Contraindications

Traction is contraindicated in hypermobility syndromes of the spine or sacroiliac joints, and in patients with ligament injuries.

9 The spine in sport

Back pain is a very common symptom among athletes (Sward, 1992; Harreby et al, 1995), just as it is in the general population. This could well be related to the high physiological loads that are placed on the spine in most athletic pursuits or during athletes' intense training loads (Milgrom et al, 1993). Prophylaxis is important, and guidelines to ensure proper musculoskeletal development need to be instituted at an early age in an attempt to prevent future problems. Good coaching, ergonomic education, and safe training programmes may be prerequisites (Harreby et al, 1995; Burton et al, 1966a).

The pathological basis of spinal disorders in sports people is, as might be expected, the same as that which will be found in the rest of the population, and has been described in previous chapters. Accordingly, mechanical back (Figure

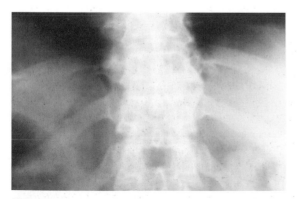

Figure 9.1 T10 degenerative changes in a top golfer

9.1) and zygapophyseal joint problems, intervertebral disc degeneration with prolapse, juvenile disc syndrome and sacroiliac disorders are common causes of back and leg pain in most sportsmen or women. Pain from these conditions may be referred widely, and pain referred into the hamstring area may present as what is taken to be a recurring hamstring problem.

Spondyloarthritis usually presents in young men in their early twenties, and so it may commonly occur in sportsmen and the diagnosis is often delayed. Quite commonly, pain is related to an injury, even a relatively minor one, and so patients may present first to a sports clinic. Another common presentation is with swelling of one or both knees. Hypermobility is a common finding in sports people, as it is an advantage, even a necessity, for ballet dancers and gymnasts.

The injuries that involve the spine may be due to direct, indirect or overuse injuries, and some injuries may commonly occur as the result of specific activities (Sward et al, 1990a; Tertti et al, 1990; Hainline, 1995; O'Brien, 1996). Special problems that may be found in individual sports include lumbar vertebral compression fractures or neck fractures in rugby (Silver, 1984; O'Brien, 1996). Traumatic disc rupture is a rare event, but it may occur with flexion, axial rotation and high-impact loading in football and skiing (Adams and Hutton, 1982; White and Panjabi; 1990, Haher et al, 1993). Fractures of the transverse process of L2 or L3 may occur as a direct injury, but more commonly they are the result of an indirect trauma, when a sudden severe contraction of the psoas muscle pulls the transverse process off its vertebra. Muscle tears, although a commonly made diagnosis, are relatively rare.

A growing adolescent back has special problems that may require attention (Dommisse, 1990; Sward et al, 1990a; Harvey and Tanner, 1991; Micheli and Wood, 1995; Morita et al, 1995; Burton et al, 1996), and symptoms are often related to the growth spurt (Harvey and Tanner, 1991). Disc degeneration can also commence at an early age (Elliott et al, 1993). An acute injury to the vertebral endplate and apophysis may occur at this age (Sward et al, 1990b; Tertti et al, 1990). Such injuries occur anywhere from the midthoracic to the midlumbar regions and may involve one or two discs. In many sports, the most common overuse injury is a spondylolysis, and young sports people presenting with unilateral low back pain related to activity should be considered as having a spondylolysis until proved otherwise. Scheuermann's disease is a common problem at this age (*see* Chapter 7), and it may first present with pain brought on from any sporting activity (Horne et al, 1987). Other causes of low back pain, such as infections, osteoid osteoma or tumours, might still present in young athletes and require urgent investigation.

Clinical examination of the spine in sports people is conducted along the routine lines described in Chapter 4. Special attention needs to be given to any tightness of the hamstrings and lumbodorsal fascia; leg length; muscle strength testing; weakness of abdominal muscles; spinal deformity; scoliosis or kyphosis; and hip joint contractures, all of which may be predisposing factors to spinal pain. Investigations need be carried out according to the proposed diagnosis. X-rays, except in cases of trauma, rarely offer much assistance. In a review of routine X-rays for the initial evaluation of low back pain, less than 2 per cent showed any significant findings (Curd and Thorne, 1989).

Spondylolysis

Spondylolysis is the most common overuse sporting injury of the lower back. This stress fracture of the pars interarticularis of the lumbar spine is characterized by a defect in the pars without any forward vertebral displacement. The pars is a narrow strip of bone that lies between the superior and inferior articular processes. It consists of two layers of dense cortical bone, one running in an anterolateral direction and the other posteromedial. They are joined by thick, bony trabeculae, so arranged because of the need to transmit compressive loads (Cyron et al, 1976). The pars progressively increases in thickness from the first lumbar to the fifth lumbar vertebra, as increasing stress is placed upon it (Cyron and Hutton, 1978). The force required to produce a fracture also increases from the first to the fifth vertebra (Cyron et al, 1976).

Spondylolysis was previously considered to be a congenital defect (Nordstrom et al 1994; Newell, 1995), but the ossification centres in the vertebral body and neural arch do not correspond to the site of the defect. It is not present at birth (Fredrickson et al, 1984; Nordstrom et al, 1994), nor in fetal skeletons (Willis, 1931). It is related to the bipedal gait, does not occur in primates (Ciullo and Jackson, 1985) and is quite rare in children before ambulation (Rosenberg et al, 1981). It usually develops during the first decade of life (Nordstrom et al, 1994), and there is an increasing incidence with age (Fredrickson et al, 1984) up until the age of about 20, after which the incidence remains steady (Nordstrom et al, 1994).

Spondylolysis is now recognized as being a stress fracture of the pars interarticularis (Hutton and Cyron, 1978; Newell, 1995), which differs from other stress fractures in the limbs in that it has a hereditary predisposition, an earlier age of onset, a lack of periosteal reaction, and the defect may persist on X-rays (Wiltse et al, 1975). The fifth lumbar vertebra, where the mobile lumbar spine meets the fixed pelvis, is the most common site of involvement. The incidence decreases as one proceeds cephalad, although at times more than one spinal level may be involved. Spondylolysis may be bilateral or unilateral (Morita et al, 1995), and bilateral spondylolysis may be associated with an isthmic spondylolisthesis. Unilateral spondylolysis occurs more commonly in sporting people, and it is usually found on the side opposite to the side most involved in an activity. Thus, in right-arm fast bowlers, it occurs in the left pars interarticularis, and similarly it occurs in the right pars in left-arm fast bowlers. This may be related to a greater degree of lumbar rotation and/or extension that is necessary on that one side. After a spinal fusion, a pars fracture may develop in the vertebra above the fused segment. An acute pars fracture may occur, but it is rare (Cope, 1988), and may follow a major traumatic event such as in parachute jumping or a fall from a roof.

Genetic or racial tendencies may play a role in the causation of spondylolysis (Wiltse et al, 1975; Green et al, 1994). It is more common in males than in females (Fredrickson, et al, 1984), there is some evidence for an increased familial incidence (Green et al, 1994; Miyake et al, 1996), and pars defects have been described in identical twins. It is reported to occur in approximately 5 per cent of the American and European population (Green et al, 1994). In one series of 500 children, the incidence was found to be 4.4 per cent at the age of 6 years, and it increased to 6 per cent at maturity (Fredrickson et al, 1984). However, marked racial differences occur, with black races having the lowest reported incidence, approximately 2 per cent (Roche and Rowe, 1952), while it can occur in approximately 50 per cent of Eskimos (Stewart, 1953). A lumbar lordosis or some inherent weakness in the pars (Porter and Park 1982, Foster et al, 1989), including hypoplasia of the neural arch and other congenital spinal defects, especially spina bifida occulta, may be present (Roche and Rowe, 1952; Wiltse et al, 1975; Miyake et al, 1996).

Clinical findings

Spondylolysis often remains asymptomatic (Fredrickson et al, 1984; Saraste, 1987; Stinson, 1993; Nordstrom et al, 1994), and so remains clinically unrecognized. The patient will usually present following activity (Hardcastle et al, 1992; Green et al, 1994) with pain in the lower lumbar region, often localized to one side of the spine. Pain may be referred to the buttock or leg, especially after a long-continued activity in which back movements are involved. The mechanism of pain production is not certain (Eisenstein et al, 1994; Nordstrom et al, 1994; Schneiderman, et al,

1995), although it is probably due to stretching of local neural elements in the pars defect (Nordstrom et al, 1994; Schneiderman et al, 1995). Spondylolysis does not usually cause nerve root pressure. However, if it fails to heal, a pseudarthrosis with hypertrophic changes forms around the pars defect, which can entrap the nerve root as it runs under its pedicle. Nerve root pressure can also occur with disc degeneration (Hardcastle et al, 1992; Stinson, 1993) or with vertebral instability, either of which may be present concurrently.

Physical examination may fail to reveal any specific diagnostic features. The patient first stands and indicates with one finger the site of pain, often localized to one side of the spine. An increased lordosis (Kraus, 1976) and hamstring spasm may be present. Standing on one leg and extending the spine is a most useful test for reproducing pain (Figure 9.2). Pain may also be reproduced on extension and rotation of the lumbar spine, or in the quadrant position. Tenderness is localized over the affected site.

The diagnosis is best confirmed using technetium 99M bone scans (Pennell et al, 1985;

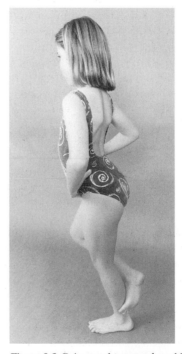

Figure 9.2 Pain may be reproduced by standing on one leg with the back in extension

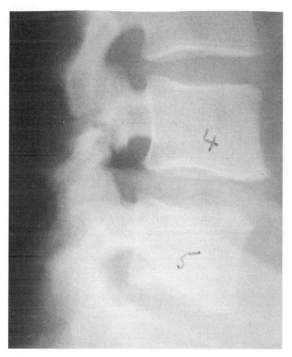

Figure 9.3 Spondylosis at L4 is evident in a lateral view

Bellah et al, 1991; Pettine et al, 1993) to reveal a localized hot spot in the pars, and it is usually positive before any radiological change becomes evident. X-rays are, however, necessary to confirm the diagnosis (Hellstrom et al, 1990) and to exclude other, rarer, diagnoses, such as a stress fracture in the surrounding bone structures (Ireland and Micheli, 1987; Weatherley et al, 1991; Fehlandt and Micheli, 1993). X-rays may appear normal at first, and can also be difficult to interpret (Porter and Park, 1982). The defect may at times be evident on the standard X-ray views (Figure 9.3), but oblique views are usually necessary to demonstrate it (Figure 9.4). They are best obtained with the X-ray angulated with a 20-degree tilt towards the head. In the oblique view in normal subjects, the pars has been likened to a Scottie dog, with the ear represented by one superior articular process, the face by the transverse process, the eye by one pedicle seen end on, and the foreleg by the inferior articular process. The body of the dog is formed by the lamina, and its tail and hindleg by the opposite articular process (Figure 9.4). In X-rays of spondylolysis, the defect in the pars is seen in the dog's neck and resembles a collar placed around the neck.

CT (Grogan et al, 1982), which is best used with a reverse gantry (Hardcastle et al, 1992) and SPECT scanning (Raby and Mathews, 1993; Read, 1994; Lusins et al, 1994), are also most useful to confirm the diagnosis. CT shows more detail about the defect, such as fragmentation or other changes in the bone. MRI may not add much more to the diagnosis, although it has been described as showing earlier changes (Yamane et al, 1993) and may demonstrate any concomitant disc degeneration that is present (Saraste, 1987; Hardcastle et al, 1992), which is more likely to occur with a spondylolisthesis than with a spondylolysis. Other bony changes that may be present are usually seen clearly on CT. They include a stress reaction at the same intervertebral level, with sclerosis, thickening and enlargement of the bone of the contralateral pedicle (Wilkinson and Hall, 1974; Sherman et al, 1977; Hardcastle et al, 1992; Miniaci and Johnson, 1993; Elliott et al, 1995), and the pars may appear elongated (Morita et al, 1995). The pars elongation is also due to overuse, in which repeated stresses lead to microfractures, so that as they heal, the pars become elongated. It was once considered that it may be a factor in causing spondylolysis but it is now recognized as being a consequence of the stress (Morita et al, 1995). In children and adolescents with spondylolysis, growth of the zygapophyseal joints and laminae may become retarded (Eisenstein, 1978; Grobler et al, 1993; Miyake et al, 1996).

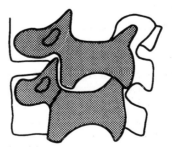

Figure 9.4 An oblique X-ray of the lumbar spine, which has the appearance of a Scottie dog. In the lower segment, a spondylolysis through the pars interarticularis appears as a collar around the dog's neck

Pathogenesis

The pars is a remarkably strong, but not rigid, structure (Lamy et al, 1975), that is capable of deformation (Green et al, 1994). This region of the lumbar spine is subjected to the highest mechanical stresses (Dietrich and Kurowski, 1985), as it acts as a pivot between the vertebral body and posterior zygapophyseal joints and is capable of deformation (Green et al, 1994). Humankind's erect stance and lumbar lordosis may accentuate the stress placed upon this area. When a child first begins to stand and walk, the combination of a lumbar lordosis and a relative restriction in hip extension could produce such stress on the pars interarticularis, with the result that a stress reaction or fracture may develop.

Experimental studies in isolated cadaver vertebrae using mechanical loading of the spine have been undertaken to determine which spinal movements are most likely to produce spondylolysis (Dietrich and Kurowski, 1985; Stokes, 1988). Several experimental mechanisms have been proposed, but activities that produce alternative flexion and extension movements, which then cause large stress reversals in the pars, seem to be the most likely mechanism (Green et al, 1994). Other investigations that have produced a stress fracture include the role of compression, shear or torsion (Green et al, 1994), torsion (Troup, 1976), flexion (Lamy et al, 1975; Farfan et al, 1976), and forces applied posteriorly to the inferior articular processes (Cyron et al, 1976; Cyron and Hutton, 1978). There is no consensus among them as to which of these experimental mechanisms are the most relevant to the human condition (Green et al, 1994). However, they all conclude that a stress fracture is most likely to be produced, and not an acute traumatic one.

Spondylolysis is a common sporting overuse injury, and sports that involve lumbar extension, but especially extension and rotation, are recognized for their propensity to cause it. The prevalence varies in individual sports, but 20 per cent, a four-fold increase in prevalence compared to that of the general population, is a commonly used figure. Sports that spondlyolysis develops in, and in which extension and rotation have been reported, include: gymnasts (Jackson et al, 1976; Ciullo and Jackson, 1985; Micheli, 1985; Walsh et al, 1985), wrestlers (Rossi, 1978; Granhed and Morelli, 1988), divers (Rossi and Dragoni, 1990), athletes (Hoshina, 1980; Rossi and Dragoni, 1990; Sward et al, 1990a), ballet dancers (Micheli, 1983; Fehlandt and Micheli, 1993), pole vaulters (Gainor et al, 1983), football players (Ferguson et al, 1974; Wiltse et al, 1975; Semon and Spengler, 1981; McCarroll, et al, 1986) and water skiers (Horne et al, 1987). In weightlifters, the spine is axially loaded, and spondylolysis is present in at least 22 per cent of them (Kotani et al, 1971; Ichikawa et al, 1982, Granhed and Morelli, 1988).

Spondylolysis also occurs in throwing sports such as javelin, baseball pitchers and fast bowlers in cricket. In fast bowlers it is an extremely common overuse injury, reaching almost epidemic proportions (Foster et al, 1989), with a prevalence of 55 per cent in one study (Hardcastle et al, 1992). It occurs mainly in the young, enthusiastic, developing fast bowlers, placing a large load on the pars (Reilly and Chana, 1994), so that few top level fast bowlers have escaped having at least one spondylolytic fracture during their career. A detailed literature has been produced, illustrating many of the underlying biomechanical features associated with its production (Elliott and Foster, 1984; Foster et al, 1989; Bell, 1992; Elliott et al, 1992, 1995; Annear et al, 1994; Bartlett et al, 1996). The action of fast bowling involves a run-up at a fast speed (Elliott and Foster, 1984), followed by two large impacts, one as the back foot is planted, then by another as the front foot is planted. Sudden hyperextension, rotation and lateral flexion of the lumbar spine then takes place, before the follow-through follows with flexion of the spine. A fully side-on or a fully front-on bowling action can help to avoid the development of a spondylosis. However, an action that is midway between these two involves either a rotation, or more particularly a counter-rotation, of the shoulder and lumbar spine, and so increases the likelihood of developing a spondylolysis (Hardcastle, 1993, Elliott et al, 1995). The safest action is one in which the hips and shoulders are aligned as much as possible, so as to minimize the degree of counter-rotation. Other mechanical causative factors to consider besides overuse include the height of the arm at delivery and the degree of extension of the front foot (Elliott et al, 1995). The same mechanisms that cause spondylolysis can also be a factor in causing an increased lumbar or thoracolumbar disc degeneration (Hardcastle et al, 1992, Bartlett et al, 1996).

Management

This fracture can usually heal if it is detected and treated early (Eisenstein, 1978; Pettine et al, 1993; Daniel et al, 1995; Merbs, 1995, Morita et al, 1995), and preventive programmes are instituted to prevent recurrences. When spondylolysis becomes symptomatic, pain relief is the immediate therapeutic need. This requires rest from all aggravating activities, together with the use of suitable analgesics. The player and coach must realize that it will not be possible to continue to play or train through pain, due to the risk of developing more serious damage. A lumbar brace or support (Micheli, 1985; Daniel et al, 1995) is worn to relieve pain and restrict extension and bracing and electrical stimulation have been described (Pettine et al, 1993). Isometric exercises are necessary and can be performed while the brace is being worn.

As pain settles, the aim is for the patient to become as active as possible within the limits of pain. Aerobic activities such as swimming and walking are usually ideal at this stage, and can be introduced after warm-up exercises and stretching routines have been performed. Running cannot be undertaken until pain has resolved, and it may need to be modified should pain return. Back exercises are essential (Foster and Fulton, 1991), and weights and pulley exercises can be introduced slowly, as strength and flexibility need to be increased for all muscle groups. Activities can then become more sport specific as the patient is eased back into full activity.

Surgery is not usually often indicated (Kip et al, 1994), although it may be considered if after six months of conservative therapy there is still some doubt about healing or if a pseudarthrosis is present. The choice of surgery then lies between using a Buck screw, the Morscher hookscrew, or Scott wiring (Johnson and Thompson, 1992; Hardcastle, 1993; Dreyzin and Esses, 1994). Somewhat similar results are reported for each method.

Aftercare and prophylaxis

Warm-up procedures and stretching are carried out before any training or playing, and general aerobic fitness training is maintained. A corrective exercise programme is instituted off-season, with emphasis on specific functional back activities. Return to full playing activity should be gradual and consultation between the player, coach and medical adviser should be undertaken to assess any problems or improvements with style and the sporting action. A major problem is that it is often the most talented youngster who has the greatest workload, and every effort should be directed towards recognizing overuse as well as poor techniques and poor preparation. Restricting the number of balls bowled in a training session or in a game, especially by junior bowlers, has become a necessity.

Spondylolisthesis

Spondylolisthesis is the forward displacement of one vertebral body on its lower neighbour. It was first described 200 years ago by obstetricians, who recognized that, in its severest form, it could lead to an obstructed birth. The slip may be measured in millimetres, but more commonly it is divided into four degrees by measuring the distance that the slipped vertebra travels forward on its lower counterpart. A first-degree slip is a displacement of one quarter of the anteroposterior vertebral body diameter, and a fourth-degree slip is a full diameter displacement (Figure 9.5). Any vertebra may be involved, but most commonly it is the fourth or the fifth lumbar.

The anatomical structure of the lumbosacral spine plays a major role in its production. While the body is in a standing position, there is a constant downward and forward thrust on the lower lumbar vertebrae, especially at the lumbosacral junction, where a 30-degree slope is present. Accordingly, body weight helps to predispose to spondylolisthesis, especially in the presence of any mechanical weakness. The potential slip is normally counteracted by a bony hook, which consists mainly of the inferior facet that hooks into the superior facet of the vertebra below. This hook has to become deficient for a

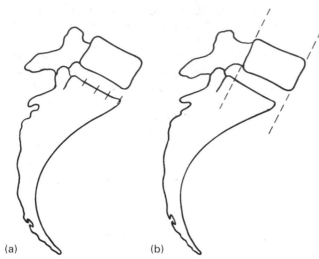

(a)   (b)

Figure 9.5 (a) Normally, the posterior margin of L5 is continuous with a line drawn from the posterior margin of the upper sacrum. The upper border of the sacrum is shown divided up into four equal segments. (b) Grade 1 spondylolisthesis. The body of L5 slips anteriorly as far as the first division on the sacrum

forward slip to occur, and the upper vertebral body with its pedicles and inferior articular facets slips forward, away from the lower vertebra with its laminae and superior articular facets, which remain in their original position. This accounts for the palpable gap that may be present above the affected level on clinical examination.

Spondylolytic or isthmic spondylolisthesis

Isthmic spondylolisthesis is most commonly due to a bilateral spondylolysis as the result of bilateral stress fractures of the pars. The pars fracture separates the articular facets allowing the body to slip forward. Other subtypes may also occur, including an elongated but intact pars, or rarely due to an acute fracture. The orientation of the zygapophyseal joints remain in their normal relationships, in contrast to the dysplastic type, although congenital anomalies, such as hypoplasia of the posterior neural arch, may occur in about one-third of cases (Wiltse and Rothman, 1989). It is the most common form of spondylolisthesis in young adolescents, and most commonly involves males at the L5 level (Newman, 1976; Fredrickson et al, 1984). The greatest degree of slippage occurs at L5 between the ages of 9 and 14 years (Ciullo and Jackson, 1985), and after the age of 15 it rarely increases in degree, although at the L4 level it may become more progressive and symptomatic (Saraste, 1987; Grobler et al, 1994).

The usual presentation is with back or back and leg pain, and the severity of symptoms may relate to the degree of the slip. As the body of L5 slips forward, a shear stress is created on the adjacent disc, which may result in degenerative changes in the disc. The role of trauma in spondylolisthesis is complicated by several factors. Patients with a previously asymptomatic spondylolisthesis may develop symptoms after an injury (Bell et al, 1988), or, in patients with a known spondylolisthesis, it may increase the degree of the existing slip. In patients with a spondylolysis, trauma may precipitate a spondylolisthesis.

The other types of spondylolisthesis: congenital; traumatic; degenerative; and pathological (Wiltse et al, 1976), need to be differentiated.

Dysplastic spondylolisthesis

This type of spondylolisthesis occurs as a slip of L5 on S1, usually associated with an elongation of the pars. Congenital abnormalities, such as inadequate development of the upper sacral facets, spina bifida occulta or evidence of a congenital dysplasia in the neural arches, are commonly present. A familial history is common, and hereditary factors have been described (Shahriaree et al, 1979; Wynne-Davies and Scott, 1979), while up to 50 per cent of the first-degree relatives of index cases may also be affected (Wynne-Davies and Scott, 1979). The zygapophyseal joints are dysplastic and become incompetent, unable to resist shear forces, and so they cannot prevent the facets of L5 slipping forward. It occurs in about one-third of the symptomatic children and adolescents with spondylolisthesis (Hensinger, 1989; Ishikawa et al, 1994). It is twice as common in girls as in boys, and symptoms usually become evident in the early teens during the growth spurt and with increased activity. It may present with evidence of neurological defects and may develop into a grade 4 spondylolisthesis.

Patients may present with back pain, abnormal gait and marked hamstring tightness. Neurological symptoms can develop after the slip reaches about 30 per cent (Wynne-Davies and Scott, 1979), although cauda equina compression is unlikely. A radiological reassessment should be carried out periodically to assess progress in young people who have this problem.

Degenerative spondylolisthesis

This type of spondylolisthesis occurs most commonly as a slip of L4 on L5 (Grobler et al, 1993; Nugent and Kostuik, 1993). It is found much more commonly in women than in men (Rosenberg, 1975; Nugent and Kostuik, 1993), in black women (Rosenberg, 1975; Grobler et al, 1993), and in people with an increased lumbar lordosis. It occurs in elderly people, and it is not at all common below the age of 50 years (Herkowitz, 1995). It may occur also in patients with a primary generalized osteoarthritis (Grobler et al, 1993), with Heberden's nodes in the terminal interphalangeal joints of the fingers and degenerative changes in the zygapophyseal joints (Grobler et al, 1993). The slip is usually a grade 1 or 2, and it may at times be progressive (Matsunaga et al, 1990). Anatomical considerations are important in its development. The fourth lumbar vertebra is more mobile than the fifth lumbar, which tends to be wedged between the iliac bones, and the ilio-lumbar ligament gives more stability at the L5 level (Rosenberg, 1975; Luk and Leong, 1986; Grobler et al, 1994). The more mobile L4–L5 intervertebral joint at the apex of the lumbar curve is usually subjected to greater stress, with consequent degenerative changes in the disc and zygapophyseal joints (Rosenberg, 1975; Farfan, 1980a; Jensen et al, 1994a) with loss of their structural supports

(Herkowitz, 1995). A sagittal orientation of the zygapophyseal joints may contribute to it (Grobler et al, 1993).

Back pain may be due to the degenerative disc changes, and the severity of pain correlates with the degree of dynamic instability present (Friberg, 1991). Pain may also occur if a lumbar canal stenosis (Herkowitz and Kurz, 1991), or often a lateral canal stenosis, is present, when CT or MRI will be necessary for diagnosis. Sciatica may also result from the development of an intraspinal synovial cyst (Kiely, 1993; Maheshwaran et al, 1995).

Traumatic spondylolisthesis

This is rare, is due to a severe degree of trauma, and may be associated with a fracture in other parts of the neural arch.

Pathological spondylolisthesis

This is also rare. It can result from a local or generalized bone disease, including Paget's disease, tumours and infections, leading to failure of the integrity of the bony hook of the neural arch.

Clinical findings

Back and/or leg pain may be related to the effect of the spondylolisthesis on spinal mechanics. The effects vary with the degree of the slip, so that with a minimal degree of slip the effect on surrounding tissues may also be minimal. When progression is gradual, a buttress of bone may form at the anterior border of the first sacral segment, so reducing the tendency to slip. However, with increasing degrees of spondylolisthesis, the soft tissues may be stretched and traumatized. The hamstring and back extensor muscles tend to be tight, presumably in an attempt to stabilize the pelvis. A scoliosis is not uncommonly present.

Back pain may be due to vertebral instability, or to recurrent attacks of synovitis in the posterior joints. Back and leg pain are most commonly due to L5 nerve root pressure, may be unilateral or bilateral, and may arise from:

- A pseudarthrosis at the site of the neural arch defect with an hypertrophied mass of fibrous tissue, which at operation can be picked up by a pair of forceps and 'rattled' around, giving it its name of a 'rattler'. It may protrude into the intervertebral foramen and can compress the nerve root at the same level (Shiraishi and Crock, 1995).
- Disc degeneration may develop (Szypryt et al, 1989; Grobler et al, 1994), most commonly at the next level above the spondylolisthesis (Elster and Jensen, 1985).
- Spinal canal stenosis or lateral recess stenosis may occur in up to 25 per cent of patients (Elster and Jensen, 1985).

Diagnosis

The diagnosis of spondylolisthesis may be suspected on clinical grounds from a history of low back pain that is made worse by standing and eased by sitting. On inspection, an increased lumbar lordosis and bilateral extensor muscle spasm may be present. Examination may reveal a gap or dimple at one level and a step-like protuberance due to the spinous process of the lower level. The spinal movement most commonly altered is extension, which becomes painfully limited, and other movements may be of full range with pain experienced at the limit of the range. Hamstring spasm is common. Passive intervertebral pressures applied to the spinous process over the affected level may also reproduce pain.

X-rays are necessary to confirm the diagnosis, assess the degree of the slip and evaluate any instability (Wood et al, 1994). MRI may be a help in assessment (Ikata et al, 1996), and the status of the discs above and below the level of the spondylolisthesis may also need to be assessed with CT or MRI (Hardcastle et al, 1992).

Management

Spondylolisthesis may be asymptomatic and require no active treatment (Rosenberg, 1975; Fredrickson et al, 1984). In symptomatic patients, treatment is designed to relieve symptoms, attempt to stabilize the spinal defect and reduce

the degree of lumbar lordosis. It has a benign natural history in most young and adult patients (Frennered, 1994), and conservative treatment is usually sufficient to control symptoms (Frennered, 1994). Management depends on the severity of pain. If it is not a major problem, rest from activities known to exacerbate pain and the use of a corset or brace may produce sufficient pain relief (Willner, 1985; Bell et al, 1988). If pain is severe, rest, with or without traction, local heat, analgesics and pain-relieving modalities may be required.

Treatment with passive movement techniques can be helpful, especially with lumbar traction and mobilization techniques that use lumbar rotation. These are always applied gently at first, but may be gradually increased in strength, provided improvement is maintained. Forceful movements are always contraindicated. As symptoms improve, exercises are given with a view to improving the patient's posture, together with isometric exercises to the abdominal and extensor muscles to increase the muscular control of the lumbar spine. The patient is instructed in the techniques of back care, as in Chapter 4, including avoidance of occupational and postural strains, care with lifting, and a long-term exercise programme with weight reduction if necessary. Reassessment of the degree of the slip should be carried out periodically, especially in young children.

Surgery may be indicated with a prolonged history of back pain or sciatica that has not responded to routine medical management; spinal canal stenosis or rapid progression to a grade 3 or 4 slip. However, the type of surgery required (decompression, fusion or internal fixation) remains debated (Ricciardi et al, 1995). In spondylolitic spondylolisthesis, surgical excision of the hypertrophied mass of fibrous tissue at the site of the defect may be indicated (Shiraishi and Crock, 1995), and good results have been described (McGuire and Amundson, 1993; Ricciardi et al, 1995; Shiraishi and Crock, 1995). In patients with spinal canal stenosis, decompression with or without fusion may be necessary. Whether decompression alone will lead to further instability, necessitating a spinal fusion, remains a problem.

10 The sacroiliac joint

The sacroiliac joint is a synovial joint formed between the medial surface of the ilium and the lateral aspect of the upper sacral vertebrae. It is divided into a dorsal, ligament portion and an inferior, ventral synovial portion, with an S shape in both vertical and anteroposterior directions. The sacrum has the appearance of a double wedge as it lies between the two iliac bones with its upper portion, or base, wider than the lower apex and tapering anteriorly to posteriorly. The articular surface of the sacrum is shaped like a letter L lying on its side, so that its upper, more vertical, limb is shorter than its lower, more horizontal, limb (Figure 10.1). The joint surfaces are lined by articular cartilage on its sacral aspect and with thinner fibrocartilage on its iliac side (Walker, 1986; Bernard and Cassidy, 1991). The articular surfaces are slightly irregular, roughened and interlocked with ridges and depressions (Bowen and Cassidy, 1981; Vleeming et al, 1990a,b; Daum, 1995). A depression at the junction of the upper and middle thirds of the sacrum corresponds to a prominent protuberance on the ilium, so helping to provide stability (Vleeming et al, 1990a,b). The joint is surrounded by a capsule lined by synovial membrane. It participates in the transmission of weight-bearing forces from the trunk to the lower limbs, and it plays a role in energy absorption (Wilder et al, 1980; Alderink, 1991).

The pelvis is made up of three bones and constitutes a bony ring containing two posterior sacroiliac joints and one anterior median joint, the symphysis pubis (Gamble et al, 1986), in an inherently stable arrangement (Alderink, 1991). Anterior and posterior sacroiliac ligaments connect the sacrum and ilium. The posterior ligament is thick and strong, whereas the anterior ligament is thinner and weaker. An interosseous ligament joins roughened tuberosities on the sacrum and ilium dorsal to the joint surface. On weight-bearing, the upper sacrum is driven forwards and downwards into the pelvis, as a shear force is developed (DonTigny, 1985, Daum, 1995). Three other accessory ligaments: iliolumbar; sacrospinous; and sacrotuberous

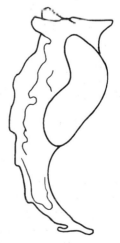

Figure 10.1 The sacroiliac joint. The articular surface of the sacrum is shaped like a letter L lying on its side

(Vleeming et al, 1989; Smidt et al, 1995), are strong, help in stabilization of the joint and prevent any backward movement of the lower sacrum (Miller et al, 1987; Vleeming et al, 1989; Daum, 1995). Surrounding muscles, which neither span nor control this joint (Walker, 1992), are invested in a strong aponeurosis, which may be placed under tension when the muscles contract and so may become a source of pain (McGill, 1987; Walker, 1992). Age changes in the joint may ultimately result in obliteration of the joint space by fibrous bands, which may develop into bony ankylosis (Resnick et al, 1975; Stewart, 1984; Walker, 1986, 1992; Bernard and Cassidy, 1991; Smidt et al, 1995). The joints have a complex innervation (Dietrichs, 1991, Fortin et al, 1994a), mostly by the L2–S2 nerves (Bernard and Cassidy, 1991; Dreyfuss et al, 1994a; Fortin et al, 1994a; Daum, 1995).

Movements

Over the years, considerable speculation and controversy have arisen about whether the sacroiliac joints move, and, if so, what is their significance. It is now agreed that the range of movements that is present is important, even though it is normally only a few millimetres (Grieve, 1976; Alderink, 1991). Movement also takes place in relatively young subjects and there are no gender differences (Smidt et al, 1995). Movement takes place simultaneously in all of the three linked pelvic joints (Kapandji, 1983), and ligament laxity about these joints is enhanced during pregnancy and labour under the control of the hormone relaxin (MacLennan, 1991; Walker, 1992).

A variety of methods, analytic and empirical, have been used both in living subjects and in cadavers to describe and quantify the movements.

A simple rotatory movement around one axis, nutation, (Kapandji, 1983) or around three axes (King, 1992) was used to describe them, but had to be discounted since the axes of rotation are much more complex and will vary according to individual and asymmetric movements (Wilder et al, 1980; King, 1992). The exact biomechanical axes, which can vary according to the complex movements in the trunk and hip, remain unknown (King, 1992), Owing to inherent difficulties in finding appropriate tests, confirming the various hypotheses about sacroiliac movement has not been possible.

Among the methods described are X-ray stereoradiography and roentgen stereophotogrammetry (Frigerio et al, 1974; Egund et al, 1978; Lavignolle et al, 1983; Grieve, 1983; Bakland and Hansen, 1984; Walheim and Selvik, 1984; Miller et al, 1987; Pierrynowski et al, 1988; Scholten et al, 1988; Sturesson et al, 1989; Brunner et al, 1991; Vleeming et al, 1992; Jacob and Kissling, 1995; Smidt et al, 1995) with markers placed under the skin on the sacrum and iliac bones. These papers mostly agree that the range of movement is small, with a range of angular rotation of approximately 4 degrees and a translation of approximately 3 mm. Lower figures have also been reported (Jacob and Kissling, 1995), as well as higher ones which range from 9 (Smidt et al, 1995) to 26 degrees (Frigerio et al, 1974), although the latter paper had only one subject and major faults in its technology (Sherlock, 1981). Three-dimensional X-ray stereophotogrammetry, using two X-ray beams and plates placed orthogonally to each other, has been used to obtain objective evidence of the quality and quantity of sacroiliac joint movement in cadavers and living subjects (King, 1992) with varying results (Egund et al, 1978; Lavignolle et al, 1983; Sturesson et al, 1989; Jacob and Kissling, 1995; Smidt et al, 1995) (Table 10.1).

Table 10.1 Three-dimensional X-ray stereophotogrammetry

Name, year	Number and status	Rotation (degrees)	Translation (mm)
Egund et al, 1978	4 symptomatic patients	2	Approx. 2
Lavingolle et al, 1983	5 athletic young adults	10–12	6
Sturesson et al, 1989	25 symptomatic patients	1–3	—
Jacob and Kissling, 1995	24, age 20–50 years	1.7	0.7
Smidt et al, 1995	32 young, normal	9	—

Although a unifying model of sacroiliac function still has not been found, perhaps the best model is supplied by Lavignolle et al (1983), who used X-ray stereophotogrammetry at first to describe movements in cadavers, and then to study five athletic adults. The subjects were placed supine, with the trunk immobilized and the hip movements arranged to simulate running and walking, so that the right hip was actively flexed and the left actively extended. In this model, the right ilium rotated posteriorly with hip flexion, and the left iliium rotated anteriorly relative to the sacrum. The innominate bone rotated around axes that changed according to these movements and the axes did not lie in the conventional coronal or sagittal planes (Lavignolle et al, 1983). Six degrees of freedom were described, and the axes described did not correspond to any of the previously described models. It was concluded that knowledge of the function of the joint was incomplete and that all the old models should be abandoned (Lavignolle et al, 1983).

Sacroiliac pain

Sacroiliac joint pain has been a controversial subject for many years (Greenman and Tait, 1988; Nachemson, 1992; Schwarzer et al, 1995d). There is no doubt that inflammatory sacroiliitis causes pain, and its features are well described. Patients often have a history of alternating buttock pain, usually worse at night, associated with back stiffness and unrelated to posture. Other causes of pain in this area include secondary malignant deposits or metabolic bone diseases.

However, the problem has been if, or how often, do mechanical joint disorders cause pain? For many years, until the description of intervertebral disc prolapse (Mixter and Barr, 1934), a diagnosis of sacroiliac joint sprain was commonly considered to be a major cause of low back pain. Further confusion also arose because referred pain and tenderness from the lower lumbar spine is commonly felt in the sacroiliac area. This pain and tenderness can be reproduced by injections of hypertonic saline into ligaments around the lumbosacral joint.

That pain does arise from the sacroiliac joint itself has now been determined in several series. On clinical grounds, pain was considered to have arisen from these joints in 22.5 per cent of one large series of 1293 patients (Bernard and Kirkaldy-Willis, 1987). Using double diagnostic joint blocks, Schwarzer et al (1995d) found that pain may arise from this joint in probably up to 30 per cent of patients with low back pain. This confirmed the figure by Fortin et al (1994a,b), who used provocation tests in normal volunteers and in patients with low back pain. Using double blocks, Maigne et al (1996) considered that in 18.5 per cent of patients with low back pain, it was of sacroiliac origin.

The mechanical type of sacroiliac joint pain is normally described as a dull ache felt in the buttock (Fortin et al, 1994,b), rarely radiating below the knee, and sometimes referred to the groin (Schwarzer et al, 1995d), the posterior aspect of the thigh or the lower abdomen. In patients with a mechanical sacroiliac joint lesion, pain is unilateral and can be exacerbated by movements that stress the sacroiliac joint. Pain may also be referred to the iliac fossa, where it is usually associated with a localized area of deep tenderness over the iliacus muscle, Baer's point, which is often confused with tenderness due to an intra-abdominal lesion. It is also commonly felt anteriorly over the pubic symphysis or the origin of the adductor tendon. Patients may at times report a dull, heavy feeling in the leg, but characteristically neurological symptoms, such as paraesthesia, are absent. Low back pain in pregnancy is a common problem, and pain often arises from the sacroiliac joint (Berg et al, 1988; Broadhurst, 1989b; Ostgaard et al, 1991, 1993, 1994; Hainline, 1994, 1995; Orvieto, et al, 1994).

Sacroiliac joint examination

This should commence with a general examination focusing especially on the spine and lower limbs, followed by sacroiliac joint inspection, assessment and palpation.

Inspection

The overall posture is inspected first: patients with unilateral sacroiliac disorders tend to stand or sit with the body weight supported on the opposite side. Any asymmetry of the skin creases or gluteal folds is looked for. The pelvic level is then assessed and the leg length measured (*see* Chapter 4) (Cibulka and Koldehoff, 1986), since any differences in leg length can produce rotation of the innominate bone (Cummings and Crowell, 1988; DonTigny, 1990).

The bony prominences of the pelvis, and the relative positions of the posterior superior iliac spine (PSIS) and anterior superior iliac spine (ASIS), are assessed. Although they may provide a clue to diagnosis, the diagnosis can never be made on the basis of bony asymmetry alone. The patient first stands while the examiner crouches behind and places the hands at the top of the iliac crests with one thumb on each PSIS. Then, while kneeling in front of the patient, the examiner's hands are placed along the iliac crests with the thumbs on the ASIS. The relative positions of each PSIS are then reassessed with the patient sitting down. These tests are used in an attempt to assess any innominate rotation, although these anatomical landmarks are a poor criterion for sacroiliac joint dysfunction, and there is poor inter-tester reliability between them (Potter and Rothstein, 1985; Herzog et al, 1989).

If the patient is then asked to bend forwards, the position of the spines may become reversed, so that the spine that previously lay at a lower level is now higher than its opposite number. In unilateral mechanical sacroiliac disorders, these prominences may be found to lie at different levels, usually with the PSIS on the painful side found to be at a lower level than the other.

Two screening tests have been derived from these observations, although they also are not reliable (Dreyfuss et al, 1994a). In the standing flexion test, the patient bends forward with the knees straight and the PSIS movement is observed on each side. With sacroiliac joint restriction, the PSIS moves higher in a cranial direction on that side. The test is then repeated in the seated flexion test, in which PSIS movement is usually not so marked, but with joint restriction it again moves higher on that side.

Sacroiliac joint tests

These tests attempt to stress the joint by using a series of passive movements. The essential point, however, is not the assessment of movement, but the provocation of pain, so that to be considered positive the test must reproduce the patient's pain. The numerous tests devised to test the joints attest to their inadequacy. Since they also stress other potential pain-producing structures in this region, such as the hip or lumbar spine, false positives and false negatives are not uncommon (Potter and Rothstein, 1985; Beal, 1989; McCombe et al, 1989; Gemmell and Jacobson, 1990; van Duersen et al, 1990; Dreyfuss et al, 1994a; Laslett and Williams, 1994). Also, no single clinical test is sufficiently sensitive to differentiate between the different tissues that could be stressed (Maigne et al, 1996). In the absence of any gold standard to evaluate the test, it is best if several of them are always incorporated into the examination (Cibulka et al, 1988; Dreyfuss et al, 1994a).

The first three tests are performed with the patient lying face downwards. The remaining six tests are performed with the patient lying supine.

1. With the patient lying prone, a rhythmic oscillatory pressure is applied to the apex of the sacrum with the heel of the hand, with the arm being kept fully extended. This springing movement produces a shearing movement across the sacroiliac joints, although it also produces movement also in the lumbosacral joint (Figure 10.2a).

2. The sacroiliac joint may be stressed by stabilizing the ilium with one hand and then moving the sacrum in a cephalad direction with the other hand (Figure 10.2b).

3. This test may then be repeated by stabilizing the ischial tuberosity with one hand and moving the sacrum caudally with the other (Figure 10.2c).

4. The patient lies supine and pressure is applied by the examiner's hand against each anterior superior iliac spine, as though trying to spread them apart (Figure 10.2d).

5. The patient lies in the same position as in 4 and the iliac crests are compressed, as though they are being squeezed together (Figure 10.2e).

6. The patient lies supine with the hips and knees flexed to 90 degrees. The adductors of

the hip are isometrically contracted by the patient attempting to squeeze the examiner's hand placed between the knees (Figure 10.2f).

7. The patient lies in the same position as in 6 and the attempt to spread the knees apart is fully resisted, producing an isometric contraction of the hip abductors (Figure 10.2g).

8. The patient lies on the back at the edge of the couch and the examiner takes the leg and hip backward into full extension (Figure 10.2h).

9. The FADE test (**F**lexion, **AD**duction, **E**xtension of the hip) is a most useful test as it applies a posterior shearing stress to the sacroiliac joint. The patient lies supine and the hip is taken first into flexion and is adducted across the body. One hand is placed under the buttock, and the other around the knee. Pressure is applied along the shaft of the femur to compress it. (Figure 10.2i).

Palpation

It is customary to palpate these joints for the presence of any tenderness, but the synovial portion of the joint lies deep to the overlying ilium, where it is inaccessible to direct palpation. Tenderness in this area usually represents a referred area of tenderness from disorders of the lower lumbar spine.

Disorders of the sacroiliac joint

These may be classified as: inflammatory; mechanical (hypomobility or hypermobility lesions); osteitis condensans ilii; the piriformis syndrome; infective; and osteoarthritis.

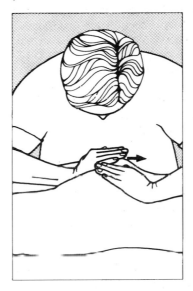

Figure 10.2 (b)

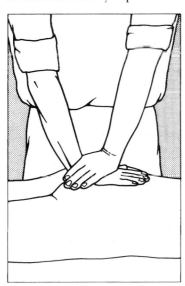

Figure 10.2 (a)

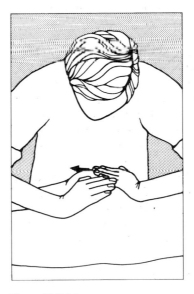

Figure 10.2 (c)

Inflammatory diseases

Inflammatory disease of the sacroiliac joint (*see* Chapter 7) is most commonly associated with the seronegative group of spondyloarthritis (Khan, 1992), and may be due to: ankylosing spondylitis; Reiter's disease; psoriatic arthritis; arthritis associated with inflammatory bowel disease, such as ulcerative colitis or Crohn's disease.

The diagnosis, or at least suspicion, of sacro-iliitis is first made on clinical grounds but confirmatory tests are then necessary, and X-ray remains the procedure of choice. Technical problems may arise in obtaining satisfactory views of the sacroiliac joint (Fewins et al, 1990), and careful positioning of the patient is necessary to obtain an adequate view of the entire length of the joint (Rothschild et al, 1994). X-ray changes,

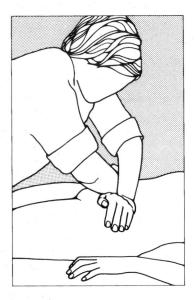

Figure 10.2 (d)

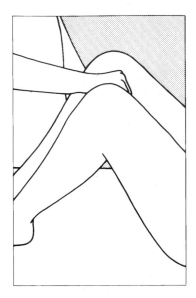

Figure 10.2 (f)

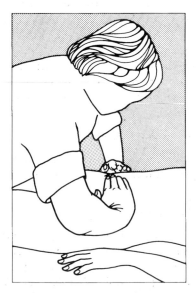

Figure 10.2 (e)

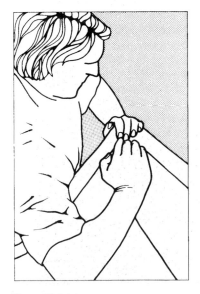

Figure 10.2 (g)

especially in the early stages, may also be difficult to interpret accurately (Rothschild et al, 1994), as sometimes these may take up to several years to develop (Mau et al, 1988). Since they are necessary to confirm the diagnosis (Vogler et al, 1984,

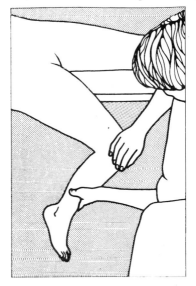

Figure 10.2 (h)

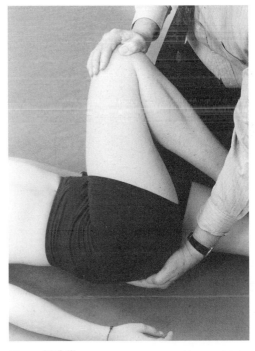

Figure 10.2 (i)

Braun et al, 1994), it remains a presumptive one until the appropriate radiological changes become evident.

If there is doubt about the diagnosis, other modalities including technetium 99M bone scans (Vesterskold et al, 1994), CT or MRI (Vogler et al, 1984; Ahlstrom et al, 1990; Fewins et al, 1990; Aliabadi and Nikpoor, 1991; Murphey et al, 1991; Battafarano et al, 1993; Edelmann and Warach 1993; Braun et al, 1994; Daly et al, 1994; Hanly et al, 1994; Rothschild et al, 1994; Bollow et al, 1995; Wittram et al, 1996) are indicated, as they provide a better appreciation of the presence and extent of any inflammatory changes.

The early radiological changes of sacroiliitis appear in the lower half of the joint and involve especially its iliac side, since this has the thinner cartilaginous surface. Osteopenia with bone demineralization around the joint margins leads to a loss of the subchondral bone, which normally appears as a white line of increased density in the joint X-ray. The joint loses its normally well-defined contours as its margin becomes blurred, and in some areas an apparently increased widening develops, while in other areas it becomes narrowed and irregular. The irregularity is further increased by the appearance of erosions along the joint margins, with areas of bone condensation or sclerosis adjacent to the joint margin producing a mottled or 'moth-eaten' appearance. The joint cartilage is lost, and in the process of repair, fibrous bands bridge the joint to lead to a fibrous ankylosis, which subsequently becomes a bony ankylosis. The late stages of this disorder are characterized by complete bone fusion across the joint and ossification in the surrounding ligaments supporting the joint.

Mechanical sacroiliac lesions

Mechanical lesions may be due to either hypomobility or hypermobility of the sacroiliac joint.

Hypomobility lesions

These lesions are a cause of lower back pain, and have received more attention in the recent literature where they are also termed 'sacroiliac joint dysfunction' (DonTigny, 1985; Dreyfuss et al, 1994a; Fortin et al, 1994a; Daum, 1995; Maigne et al, 1996). Their importance may lie not so much in how common they might be, but that, if recognized, they should be amenable to treatment. They usually occur in young people, and may be associated with activities in which movements place a rotational stress on the sacroiliac joint. They occur especially as a result of athletic pursuits (Chisin et al, 1984; Lindsay et al, 1993) such as golfing, tennis or ballet dancing, but may also follow pregnancy, childbirth or trauma (Daly et al, 1991). Pain, as described above, is usually felt in one buttock, but it may radiate much more widely. Examination may reveal associated structural faults, such as an asymmetric development of the pelvis (Lewit, 1985) or unequal leg length (Lewit, 1985; Cummings and Crowell, 1988). The natural history is unknown (Bernard and Cassidy, 1991; Daum 1995) as there are no satisfactory ancillary tests such as X-ray, bone scan or blood studies that are able to confirm the diagnosis (Davis and Lentle, 1978; Sturesson et al, 1989; Dreyfuss et al, 1994a). Diagnosis depends clinically on the sacroiliac tests, outlined above, with the aim of reproducing the pain. However, diagnostic sacroiliac joint blocks (Schawartzer et al, 1995d), which are not difficult to perform, but do need to be performed under fluoroscopic control, are the only certain way of confirming the diagnosis.

Treatment with passive movement techniques is usually eminently successful (Cibulka, 1992). Injection of the sacroiliac joint with a long-acting anaesthetic plus a corticosteroid, using a direct posterior approach into the most inferior aspect of the joint, is a relatively easy technique to perform using an image intensifier (Hendrix et al, 1982; Maugars et al, 1992). A heel lift is supplied if necessary, and an exercise programme, especially involving strengthening the pelvic floor muscles is instituted (DonTigny, 1985; Daum, 1995).

Hypermobility lesions

Hypermobility lesions of the sacroiliac joint are not common (Jacob and Kissling, 1995), although they may occur in one of two situations. The first is secondary to instability of the symphysis pubis and osteitis pubis, which occurs predominantly as a common overuse condition in some athletes (Corrigan and Maitland, 1994) (Figure 10.3). This may be complicated by hypermobility of one or both sacroiliac joints and may also be associated with an osteitis condensans ilii. The second occurs in young women, usually during or soon after pregnancy. The patient presents with sacroiliac and pelvic pain made worse by standing, walking or turning over in bed.

Treatment of hypermobility is extremely difficult and consists of rest: from any known aggravating activities; analgesics; pelvic floor exercises; swimming; anti-inflammatory agents; and the newer form of sacroiliac belt, which may help to provide pain relief. Manual therapy techniques might exacerbate the symptoms, and surgery is rarely indicated (Daum, 1995).

Osteitis condensans ilii (OCI)

This benign condition is characterized by condensation of bone, usually on the iliac side of the sacroiliac joint (Olivieri et al, 1990). Diagnosis is made on X-ray, which shows a dense triangular sclerosis on the lower portion of the iliac bone. It occurs mostly in young adults, more commonly in females. First described in women after childbirth, when complaints of pain in the back or sacroiliac area are common, it was then

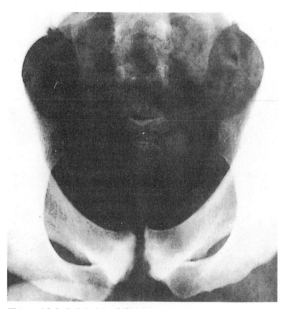

Figure 10.3 Pelvic instability

considered to be only a coincidental radiological finding, unrelated to any symptoms. However, it is now recognized that the underlying cause is a hypermobility of the sacroiliac joint. OCI is produced as a stress reaction, and the bony reaction results in thickening of the surrounding bone around the sacroiliac joint (Dihlmann, 1991).

The radiological picture of OCI is characterized by a well-defined area of bone sclerosis with increased density along the inner, lower border of the ilium adjacent to the sacroiliac joint. The X-ray findings should not be confused with sacroiliitis (Withrington et al, 1985), for, in this condition, the sacroiliac joint itself is normal, as the joint space and articular surfaces are not involved. OCI may be bilateral, and is then usually symmetric, or it may uncommonly occur on the sacral surface of the joint (Olivieri et al, 1994). The X-ray changes may be confirmed by CT and MRI (Olivieri et al, 1990; Clarke et al, 1994). The HLA B27 antigen is absent.

Osteitis condensans ilii has a variable course, as pain derives from the sacroiliac instability and can be prolonged, although ultimately, spontaneous resolution, either partial or complete, may occur (Bellamy et al, 1983). Treatment consists of reassurance, analgesics and correction of any pelvic instability. A sacroiliac belt, if properly applied, may be quite a help in relieving pain.

The piriformis syndrome

This condition is due to an entrapment neuropathy of the sciatic nerve in the piriformis muscle (Broadhurst, 1990; Rich and McKeag, 1992). The symptoms may be similar to those due to lumbar intervertebral disc prolapse, but without back pain. The pyriformis muscle runs from the anterior sacrum to be inserted into the upper surface of the greater trochanter of the femur. The sciatic nerve usually runs under its lower surface, but, in approximately 10 per cent of people, it will run through the muscle where it can be entrapped. It usually occurs as an overuse condition in active people, especially as a result of activities involving twisting, but it may also follow direct trauma.

Pain is usually located deep in the buttock (Broadhurst, 1990). There may be difficulty

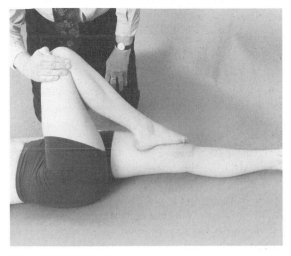

Figure 10.4 Pyriformis test

walking up stairs or on an incline, and pain may be made worse by sitting, when standing up from sitting or at night. Pain is best reproduced with the patient supine, the hip flexed, adducted and internally rotated and hip abduction is then resisted (Figure 10.4). External rotation may also be painful and weak, especially if the hip is abducted simultaneously (Rich and McKeag, 1992; Hainline, 1995). Other clinical tests have been described, and may also be positive (Beatty, 1994). Diagnostic aids include MRI to delineate the muscle and nerve (Jankiewicz et al, 1991) and nerve conduction studies (Fishman and Zybert, 1992).

Treatment is difficult. It relies mainly on correcting any underlying biomechanical faults (Barton, 1991) and appropriate stretching of the muscle. Local anaesthetic and corticosteroid injections are usually worth trying (Barton, 1991; Sayson et al, 1994). A heel raise may be necessary. Surgery has been described (Solheim et al, 1981; Cameron and Noftal, 1988; Vandertop and Bosma, 1991), but all other possible causes need to be excluded first.

Infections

Infections of the sacroiliac joint are rare. They usually only involve one joint (Abbott and Carty, 1993; Bohay and Gray, 1993; McGaughey, 1994;

Osman and Govender, 1995), but the diagnosis is often delayed or is mistaken for other causes (Abbott and Carty, 1993; Carlson and Jones, 1994). Pyogenic infections involve either the bone or the joint itself, may occur due to haematogenous spread, by direct spread or following surgery, and are most commonly caused by staphylococcal infections. Infections also occur in intravenous drug addicts due to a variety of organisms, and are often unusual ones such as fungi.

The patient usually has an elevated temperature, ESR and white cell count. Clinical signs are easily missed in the early stages of the disease, but the tests described above are usually positive, and the gluteal muscles on one side appear wasted.

Blood samples are taken for culture and sensitivity, and are repeated if necessary. Needle biopsy, either closed or open, is essential to confirm the diagnosis and to identify the causative organism and its sensitivity (Hendrix et al, 1982; Maugars et al, 1992). X-rays are usually normal in the early stages, and so are of no help in diagnosis. A bone scan is probably the best early test (Abbott and Carty, 1993; Bohay and Gray, 1993; McGaughey 1994), and if it is positive, a CT or MRI scan is of most benefit (Haliloglu et al, 1994). Ultimately, X-rays will show erosive, destructive joint changes.

Osteoarthritis

Changes due to osteoarthritis may occur in the articular cartilage of these synovial joints (Resnick et al, 1975), and develop with increasing age, although they are usually asymptomatic. Osteoarthritis may be unilateral or bilateral. Degenerative changes first involve, and are more severe in, the middle third of the joint (Brunner et al, 1991) and usually on its iliac surface (Bowen and Cassidy, 1981; Bellamy et al, 1983), where the cartilage is thinner than on the sacral surface. The changes in cartilage are similar to those in peripheral joints. Degenerative changes are increasingly more common with advancing age, and may occur secondary to disorders in which movement of the joint is decreased. This occurs in people who are immobilized, or in patients with hip joint disease. With unilateral hip disease, degenerative changes usually occur in the

contralateral sacroiliac joint. Degenerative changes occur in patients with DISH, who develop pararticular osteophytes, although the joint surfaces are maintained.

These changes are reflected in the X-ray appearances as loss or irregularity of the joint space, subchondral sclerosis and osteophyte formation. Cystic and erosive changes are rarely seen. Osteophytes may form on the inferior surfaces of the joint, more commonly in women (Stewart, 1984), and are easily recognized on X-ray. They may also appear on the superoanterior joint aspect, more commonly in men (Stewart, 1984), and appear on X-ray as dense bony deposits (Valojerdy et al, 1989). They may give the appearance of bony ankylosis of the joint, but this is most rare in osteoarthritis (Resnick et al, 1975).

Passive movement techniques

The three commonly used mobilization techniques for the sacroiliac joint are: posteroanterior pressure; backward rotation of the iliac crest; and forward rotation of the iliac crest. The best technique to use first is generally the one that reproduces the patient's pain.

Posteroanterior pressure

The patient lies prone with the arms by the sides. The therapist stands by the patient's left side, places his or her left hand over the sacrum, reinforcing it with the right hand, with the shoulders positioned over the hands.

Posteroanterior pressures are applied using small oscillations to the dorsal surface of the sacrum. The direction may be inclined cephalad, caudad, towards the right or the left side, or any combination of these, and may be complemented by an equal and opposite pressure over the adjacent ilium.

Backward rotation of the iliac crest

The patient lies on his or her right side and the therapist, standing in front, places the left hand over the anterior superior iliac spine with the heel of the right hand against the posterior

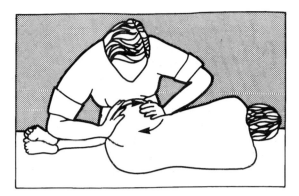

Figure 10.5 Backward rotation of the iliac crest

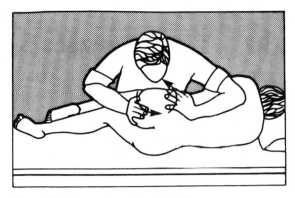

Figure 10.6 Forward rotation of the iliac crest

surface of the left ischial tuberosity. By leaning over the patient, both the therapist's forearms are pointed in opposite but parallel directions (Figure 10.5).

The therapist holds the patient's pelvis firmly between his or her hands and rocks his or her body so that the ischial tuberosity moves posteroanteriorly and the anterior superior iliac spine moves anteroposteriorly, producing a backwards rotation of the iliac crest.

Forward rotation of the iliac crest

This is similar to that described for the previous technique, except that the left hand is placed on the posterior surface of the iliac crest and the heel of the right hand under the ischial tuberosity, reaching as far anteriorly as possible.

Holding the pelvis firmly between his or her hands, the therapist moves the anterior superior iliac spine posteroanteriorly and the ischial tuberosity anteroposteriorly by a swinging movement of his or her trunk (Figure 10.6).

Manipulation of the sacroiliac joint

The technique for manipulation of the sacroiliac joint also involves rotation of the lumbar spine (Figure 10.7) and is the same procedure as a rotational manipulation of the lumbar spine (*see* Chapter 8).

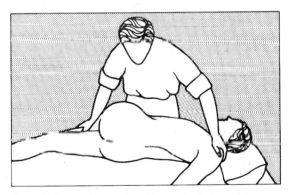

Figure 10.7 Lumbar rotation for manipulation of the sacroiliac joint

11 The cervical spine

The cervical spine provides great flexibility with motion around three axes (Heller, 1992), together with protection for the neural and vascular tissues contained within it as they pass to and from the skull. It protects the spinal cord while balancing a skull weighing approximately 6 kg on its upper joints (Bland and Boushey, 1990). The size and volume of the spinal canal display marked individual variations (Bland and Boushey, 1990; Kamiyama et al, 1994). During physiological movements of the cervical spine, the nervous tissues contained within the spinal canal need to adapt so that no significant stress is placed upon them (Panjabi and White, 1989). The spinal cord is lengthened during flexion and it is shortened on extension.

Thirty-seven joints are to be found in the relatively small area of the cervical spine, which may for convenience be divided into upper, C1 and C2, and lower, C3–C7, areas. The upper cervical spine comprises the atlas (C1) and the axis (C2), which have distinctive structures that are well adapted to their specialized function of providing mobility at the cranio-vertebral junction (Kramer et al, 1991).

C1

The atlas, which supports the skull, is shaped like a ring, with an anterior and a posterior arch. The anterior arch articulates on its posterior aspect with the odontoid process of the axis. The atlas lacks a vertebral body but has two lateral masses, each of which bears a superior and an inferior articular facet. The superior articular process, concave from side to side and from back to front, articulates with the occipital condyle to form the occipito-atlantal joint. Its medial to lateral concave inferior articular process articulates with a convex articular process on the upper surface of the axis to form the lateral atlanto-axial joint (Figure 11.1). Its transverse process is relatively long and is easily palpated just below the mastoid process. The small posterior tubercle is difficult to feel, although it may be possible with deep palpation.

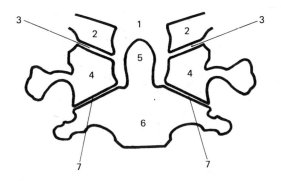

Figure 11.1 The C1–C2 region: (1) foramen magnum; (2) occipital condyles; (3) atlanto-occipital joint; (4) lateral mass of C1; (5) odontoid process; (6) body of C2; (7) lateral atlanto-axial joint

C2

The anterior body of the axis carries a central portion, the odontoid process or dens, which articulates with the posterior aspect of the anterior arch of the atlas to form the median anterior atlanto-axial joint. The dens forms the fulcrum around which C1 rotates, and articulates behind with the stout transverse ligament. On each lateral aspect is a convex articular process, which articulate with the lateral mass of the atlas to form the lateral atlanto-axial joints. Two strong alar ligaments pass upwards and laterally from the dens to the medial aspect of the occipital condyle.

The posterior arch of the axis is formed by two pedicles and two laminae. The inferior articular process arises from the inferior surface of the pedicle and articulates with the superior articular process of C3.

C3–C7

The mobile intervertebral segment, from C3 to C7, comprises an anterior cartilaginous joint and the two posterior zygapophyseal joints (Figures 11.2 and 11.3). In the lower cervical spine, the flattened zygapophyseal joint facets are so placed that the facet on the superior process faces

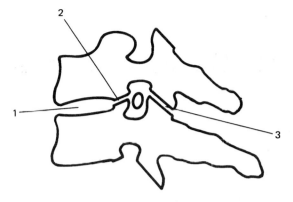

Figure 11.3 The lateral view of the cervical spine. The mobile intervertebral segment comprises the disc (1) and neurocentral joint (2) in front and the apophyseal joint (3) behind

upwards and backwards while the facet on the inferior articular process downwards and forwards at an angle of about 45 degrees. They are richly endowed with proprioceptive and nociceptor fibres.

The anterior joint is modified by the presence of the neurocentral joints, also known as the joints of Luschka, uncovertebral, or lateral interbody joints, which abut across the posterior margin of the vertebral body. For many years it has been debated whether they represent true synovial joints or are pseudarthroses. It seems that they are not true synovial joints that would contain hyaline cartilage and synovium, and are not present at birth (Bland and Boushey, 1990; Connell and Wiesel, 1992). They are formed from spaces in the posterolateral region of the intervertebral disc that develop, at about the age of 20 years, as the result of movement and weight-bearing (Kokobun et al, 1996). They aid in providing vertebral stability, and degenerative changes may develop as part of the process of spondylosis, in which their osteophytic outgrowths may subsequently encroach upon the nearby transverse foramen, through which runs the vertebral artery.

Cervical movements

The type and range of movements in the upper cervical spine vary to a large extent, since the

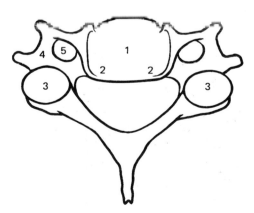

Figure 11.2 Cervical vertebra viewed from above. The mobile intervertebral segment comprises the disc (1) and neurocentral joints (2) in front and two apophyseal joints (3) behind. The transverse process (4) also contains a foramen (5), through which the vertebral artery passes

vertebrae do not move in a simple manner about a single axis. Movements in one axis can result in simultaneous movement in another axis and translation in a third. The usual figures given here or in the literature serve only as guide, and the range will also vary with age and build (Dvorak et al, 1992).

Atlanto-occipital joint

The main physiological movement at the atlanto-occipital joints is flexion–extension, which produces a nodding movement of the head as the occiput tilts backwards and forwards on the concave surface of the upper facets of the atlas. On flexion of the head, the occipital condyles glide backwards on the concave facets of the atlas, and the reverse movement takes place with extension.

A few degrees of range of lateral flexion and rotation are possible in this joint. As the occiput glides over the superior articular process of the lateral mass of the atlas, movement is coupled with a small degree of simultaneous movement into lateral flexion and rotation. Rotation here is coupled with lateral flexion to the opposite side.

Atlanto-axial joints, Cl–C2

The atlanto-axial joints are comprised of two lateral joints and a central joint which is formed between the anterior arch of the atlas and the odontoid process of the axis. Two active movements take place at these joints: rotation and flexion–extension.

The principle movement is rotation, which takes place by pivoting of the atlas around the immobile odontoid. At least 50 per cent of total neck rotation takes place at this joint (Penning and Wilmlink, 1987). As the atlas rotates, so do the atlanto-occipital joints and the head. Rotation is limited by the alar ligaments that run from the odontoid to the occiput, and is accompanied by movement in the lateral axial joints, in that one moves forwards and the other backwards.

Flexion–extension also occurs in this joint, and it has a range of approximately 10 degrees. On flexion, the posterior arch of the atlas tips and slides forwards on the axis and approximates it

on extension. The anterior arch of the atlas moves anteriorly up to 3 mm, and any movement beyond that is abnormal. The lateral atlanto-axial joints are unusual in that both surfaces are convex, so that the movement involves both a rolling and a sliding movement of the two articular facets.

Active lateral flexion does not occur in the atlanto-axial joints, but there is a small range of passive accessory movement that is necessary for movement.

Lower cervical joints, C3–C7

Intervertebral discs are present between C3 and C7. The greatest range of motion takes place at C5–C6 (Holmes et al, 1994), which is also the site of maximal disc degenerative changes.

During flexion, the upper vertebral body tilts and slides anteriorly over the lower body and, as in the lumbar spine, is accompanied by an appropriate movement in the zygapophyseal joint. Similarly, during extension, the upper vertebral body tilts and slides posteriorly, accompanied by a movement in the zygapophyseal joint.

Lateral flexion and rotation in the lower cervical vertebrae are combined movements, because the oblique orientation of their zygapophyseal joints does not allow one to take place without the other. After only a few degrees of lateral flexion, the joints come into apposition and so force the vertebrae into rotation towards the same side. Conversely, after a few degrees of rotation, apposition in the zygapophyseal joints forces the vertebrae into lateral flexion towards the same side. Approximately 7 per cent of rotation takes place at each individual cervical joint.

Summary

1. Flexion–extension occurs at the 0–C1, C1–C2 and lower cervical joints with a total range of approximately 105 degrees, made up of approximately 45 degrees of flexion and 60 degrees of extension. At 0–C1 the range is approximately 35 degrees; at C1–C 2 the range is approximately 10 degrees.
2. Lateral flexion occurs at the 0–C1 and the

lower cervical joints. The range is approximately 45 degrees to either side, of which 4–8 degrees occurs in the 0–C1 joint. A small range of passive lateral flexion occurs in the C1–C2 joints.

3. Rotation occurs mainly at the C1–C2 and lower cervical joints. The total range is approximately 80 degrees to either side, of which over half occurs in the upper cervical spine (Crisco et al, 1991). At 0–C1 there is a very small range of 3–4 degrees; at C1–C2 the range of rotation is from 35–47 degrees.

12 Cervical pain

Cervical pain is a common symptom in the adult population (Bovim et al, 1994; Leak et al, 1994), as 50 per cent could experience an episode of pain during their lifetime (Barry and Jenner, 1995). At any given time, up to 12 per cent of the adult population has some discomfort in the neck with or without arm pain (Wilson, 1991). In a long-term follow-up of 205 patients with neck pain over a 15-year period, one-third had persistent moderate to severe pain and their outcome was both clinically and radiologically difficult to predict (Gore et al, 1987). Reliable epidemiological studies concerning the prevalence of cervical pain have been sparse (Bovim et al, 1994), and compared to the lumbar spine, little attention in the literature has been paid to discussing its aetiology or natural history. A major problem with discussion about the cervical spine is that it has been looked upon simply as a smaller version of the lumbar spine, even though there are structural, biomechanical and pathological differences (Bogduk, 1994). Pain is the major presenting complaint, but it is often poorly localized, and signs may lack sensitivity and specificity or may be difficult to demonstrate (Leak et al, 1994), while X-rays and CT scans play little role in determining most of its underlying causes.

Symptoms and signs in the neck range in severity from minor to severe, and treatment needs to be adjusted accordingly. Minor complaints such as grating or creaking sensations in the neck may only require reassurance. The vast majority of patients with cervical pain and stiffness will respond to a suitably arranged therapeutic regime and surgery needs to be considered in only a very small percentage of cases. Spondylosis (Swezey, 1996a) and hypomobility lesions are found more commonly in the neck than in the lumbar spine, and usually respond well to mobilization techniques.

Potential sources of neck pain include that it may: arise from non-vertebral structures, including the thyroid, larynx, chest or diaphragm; arise from rheumatological disorders (*see* Chapter 7); or be musculoskeletal in origin. Pain can arise from any of the musculoskeletal structures in the neck (Wilson, 1991), but mostly it will arise from the vertebral column and may be divided into those involving either the upper cervical spine or the lower cervical spine.

Vertebrogenic disorders in the neck

Upper cervical spine

Pain may arise from: the atlanto-occipital (0–C1) joint; the lateral median atlanto-axial (C1–C2) joints; and the zygapophyseal joints (C2–C3). Innervation of the atlanto-occipital and the atlanto-axial joints is derived from the ventral rami of C1 and C2, respectively (Dreyfuss et al, 1994b,c).

Atlanto-occipital joints

Dreyfuss et al (1994b) used provocative injections into the atlanto-occipital joints under fluoroscopic control to determine their pain patterns. Pain was described as being deep, aching, suboccipital and referred widely towards the vertex of the head. Pain from this joint was more severe and was referred more widely than was pain from the atlanto-axial joint.

Lateral atlanto-axial joints

Pain arising from the lateral atlanto-axial joints has been described in cases of unilateral osteoarthritis involving the joints (Ehni and Benner, 1984, Busch and Wilson, 1989; Star et al 1992; Dreyfuss et al, 1994b,c). It is more localized and less intense than atlanto-occipital pain, felt laterally and posteriorly at the C1–C2 segmental level. This distribution was confirmed subsequently by Ehni and Benner (1984) using local anaesthetic to abolish the pain, and by Dreyfuss et al (1994a,b), who used provocative injections into the joint.

Median atlanto-odontoid joint

This joint may also be a source of pain due to degenerative changes (Zapletal et al, 1995), but these are uncommon and difficult to detect clinically or on routine X-rays (Zapletal et al, 1995).

Zygapophyseal joints

C2–C3 zygapophyseal joint pain has been described (Trevor-Jones 1964; Bogduk and Marsland, 1988). Dwyer et al, in two papers (Dwyer et al, 1990; Aprill et al, 1990), used joint provocation in normal, asymptomatic subjects and in symptomatic patients with degenerative changes to describe the referral patterns that arose from C2–C3 (Figure 12.1). Pain is referred laterally and also up to the occipital area of the skull (Dwyer et al, 1990).

Lower cervical spine

Earlier studies to investigate soft tissue pain were performed using provocative tests, such as saline

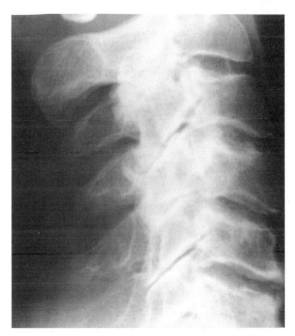

Figure 12.1 Zygapophyseal joint degeneration C2–C3, C3–C4, C5–C6

injections into the deep structures, to produce posterior neck and head pain (Campbell and Parsons, 1944; Feinstein et al, 1954).

The cervical disc including the posterior annulus is innervated, as in the lumbar disc (*see* Chapter 1), by the sinuvertebral nerves (Bogduk et al, 1988a), and can be a source of neck and referred pain (Cloward, 1958, 1959; Hodgkinson, 1979; Kikuchi and MacNab, 1981; Schellhas et al, 1996). In the cervical vertebral canal, the nerves supply the disc at their own level and at other levels, then take an essentially upwards course to supply the disc above and penetrate into the depths of the annulus fibrosus (Bogduk et al, 1988a). Provocation and analgesic discography were used to investigate the role of the disc in patients with post-traumatic neck pain (Bogduk and Aprill, 1993), and it was concluded that disc pain alone was responsible for the pain in 20 per cent of the patients. Cervical discography was compared to MRI in another trial (Schellhas et al, 1996) to assess the role of discogenic pain.

The zygapophyseal joints in the lower cervical spine, which are orientated differently from those in the rest of the spine, can also be a source of pain (Dwyer et al, 1990). Each cervical zygapophyseal joint is innervated by the medial branches of the cervical dorsal rami that run above and below it (Bogduk, 1982). The dorsal rami arise from their spinal nerve and pass over the root of the transverse process. Their medial branch runs posteriorly around their articular pillars, and ascending and descending branches supply the zygapophyseal joints above and below.

Zygapophyseal joint pain may be referred to the head or towards the shoulder (Dory, 1983; Wedel and Wilson, 1985; Dussault and Nicolet, 1985; Bodguk and Marsland, 1988; Aprill et al, 1990; Dwyer et al, 1990). It was assessed by Bogduk and Marsland (1988) on the premise that complete pain relief identifies that joint as the source of pain. This was achieved under fluoroscopic control using joint blocks with up to 1 cc of local anaesthetic injected into the joint or by injecting the medial branch of the dorsal ramus (Barnsley et al, 1993a,b; Barnsley and Bogduk, 1993; Lord et al, 1995a). Since single blocks have a high false positive rate (Barnsley et al, 1993b), the joint should be injected at two levels on two separate occasions with two different local anaesthetics, lignocaine and bupivacaine, using a double-blind, controlled technique (Barnsley et al, 1993a). Criteria for a positive test were complete pain relief on both occasions, and that the relative durations of the two local anaesthetics could be correctly discriminated.

Alternatively, these joints can be blocked by the use of percutaneous radiofrequency ablation (Lord et al, 1995a), which is safe but technically demanding, and has its limitations (Bogduk et al, 1988b), including a high failure rate, and so it is not recommended (Lord et al, 1995a).

Dwyer et al (1990) used provocative injections on normal volunteers to derive maps describing the segmental pain referral patterns. They were then used to treat a group of neck pain patients using zygapophyseal joint blocks (Aprill et al, 1990). The prevalence of intervertebral disc pain and zygapophyseal joint pain in the same cervical segment was assessed using discography and joint blocks (Bogduk and Aprill, 1993). A symptomatic disc and a symptomatic zygapophyseal joint were identified in the same segment in 41 per cent of patients, discs alone in 20 per cent, and zygapophyseal joints were symptomatic but the discs were asymptomatic in 23 per cent. They concluded that an anterior cervical fusion should not be undertaken on the basis of a positive discogram alone, as that does not exclude zygapophyseal joint pain (Bogduk and Aprill, 1993). This is further discussed in Chapter 6.

Neck pain

This is usually described as a deep, dull, aching pain, usually not particularly severe, but often constantly present and made worse by sudden movements or most physical activities involving the neck. Pain is felt diffusely in the neck, interscapular region or shoulder and is commonly associated with stiffness. Pain may also be referred distally into the arms, but its site does not always indicate the spinal level of the disc degeneration. A previous history of acute attacks of pain is often present. Minor attacks of pain or stiffness felt in the same distribution may have occurred, and been labelled previously as fibromyalgia.

Shoulder pain

Pain in the shoulder can be referred from the neck, and if so it may present in three separate clinical situations:

1. Pain may radiate from the neck above the scapula into the shoulder. Clinical examination then shows that shoulder movements are painless but that neck movements are painfully restricted and may reproduce the shoulder pain.
2. The patient may present with shoulder pain alone, without neck pain. Shoulder movements are normal but the pain should then be reproduced on neck movements.
3. There is another, less common, clinical setting in which shoulder movements are painful but neck movements are either clinically normal or only slightly painful. This is usually taken as being due to shoulder, and not neck, pathology. However, some may improve with neck treatment alone, usually traction and mobilization techniques to C4–5, C5–6. If improvement does occur, it

will be within one or two treatments, so repeated neck treatments are unnecessary.

Arm pain

Pain in the arm may be either:

- Referred pain from the neck. This usually radiates into the extensor aspect of the upper arm, although at times it may be felt anywhere in the limb, associated with sensations of heat or cold or other non-segmental dysthaesia.
- Due to nerve root pressure. The C6 or C7 nerve root is most commonly involved, but a disc prolapse is uncommon and it is more likely to be due to degenerative changes in the zygapophyseal joints. It usually follows minor degrees of trauma or overuse, and is commonly precipitated by activities with head extension or excessive use of an arm, for example, after painting a ceiling.

Scapular pain

Pain, usually described as dull and aching or occasionally throbbing like a toothache, occurs either in the interscapular region or over the upper scapular border. It may occur with or without neck pain on the same side. Both the sixth and seventh cervical nerve roots supply fibres to a wide distribution in the neck and chest muscles. A lesion that produces irritation of these nerves may cause pain felt widely over the trunk or chest. Another common clinical finding is the presence of localized areas of tender, readily palpable, thickened areas of fibromyalgia. Their origin is uncertain, although it is presumed that they represent localized areas of muscle spasm due to mechanical derangement of the intervertebral joint with referred pain and tenderness. They usually disappear after mobilization of the appropriate spinal segment.

Anterior chest pain

Chest pain may be referred from the cervical spinal joints and has been described by the not very appropriate term as 'cervical angina' (Booth and Rothman, 1976). It may be substernal, felt in the anterior chest wall or be bilateral. Its character, site, severity and radiation can vary markedly and may be related to exertion, posture or breathing.

The essential diagnostic feature is that pain will be reproduced on spinal movements, or that local joint signs are found at an appropriate spinal level. The effect of several mobilization treatments in easing or abolishing pain also tends to confirm the diagnosis. Diagnosis is more difficult in elderly people, when changes in the coronary arteries and in the spine are common and may be present together. X-ray changes of cervical spine degeneration are so common as to be of no value in confirming the diagnosis.

13 Examination of the cervical spine

- Inspection. Observe posture, body build, gait, and head movements
- Active movements. Test flexion, extension, lateral flexion and rotation. Observe the range, reproduction of pain, and rhythm
- Auxiliary tests: overpressure; repeated movements; sustained pressure; the quadrant positions; upper limb tension tests; vertebral artery testing
- Passive movements. Test the passive range of flexion, extension, lateral flexion and rotation at each joint. Test the accessory movements at upper and lower cervical spine
- Palpation
- Neurological testing of upper and lower limbs
- General medical examination.

Inspection

Posture is observed, as it may provide a clue to the diagnosis. A common postural abnormality, associated with prolonged static working positions, is characterized by a protracted chin, increased cervical lordosis, and rounded shoulders with the head poked forward. Patients with acute torticollis hold the head laterally flexed and rotated to one side, usually away from the painful side. With cervical nerve root pressure, a hand may be held under the elbow of the affected limb to relieve tension, otherwise relief may be attained by placing the hand on the head.

Standing with the head poked forward tends to throw the C7 spinous process into prominence and it may be associated with an overlying fat pad, or dowager's hump.

Active movements

Active movements are best tested with the patient seated, as this stabilizes the trunk. The patient is asked whether any symptoms are experienced in this position, and if so, to indicate their site. The patient then moves the neck into full flexion, followed by extension, lateral flexion to each side and then rotation to each side. These movements are observed while first standing in front of, and then beside, the patient, and noting:

- The range of movement. The normal range is usually measured in degrees, and varies with age and build
- Whether or not the movements reproduce any symptoms
- Disturbances of rhythm and the presence or absence of any deformity.

If no pain is present at rest, the patient is asked to move the head in the direction to be tested until pain is felt. If pain is present at rest, the head is moved until pain begins to increase and the range is noted. Provided the pain is not too severe, the head is then moved further into the range and any difference in its severity, site, distribution and area of referral is reported. The movement is stopped before the pain becomes too severe. If pain is not a problem the patient continues to move the head to the limit of the available range, reporting any alteration in symptoms.

Active movements should be repeated while standing in front of, and then to the side of, the patient, while observing the patient's rhythm and any local restriction in movement. A typical pattern of movement restriction in a cervical hypomobility lesion is a painful limitation of extension, usually associated with a restriction of lateral flexion and rotation towards the painful side.

Flexion

The examiner stands in front of the seated patient, who is asked to bend the head forwards, while noting whether the head or neck tends to deviate to either side. Then the examiner looks down on the muscular contour of the neck from the occiput to C7, noting any difference in the degree of prominence on either side of the spinous processes. One side becomes higher than the other with a rotational deformity.

Then the examiner stands alongside the patient and asks him or her to flex the head forwards, noting whether the cervical spine is unrolling evenly from the head downwards. With pain or muscle spasm in the lower cervical spine, flexion occurs mainly in the upper cervical and upper thoracic areas.

over pressures for upper & lower Cx spine.

Extension

Extension should first be assessed with the examiner standing in front of the patient to observe whether the head deviates to one side or the other. The relationship between the deformity and the symptoms are assessed by manually countering the deviation and then comparing the new range, and whether it reproduces pain, with the previous one. Extension should also be observed from the side to determine if it occurs mainly in the upper cervical area. If so, the head is held extended at its limit and pressure applied to move the lower cervical spine also into extension. If it is the site of pain, the movement is restricted and pain is reproduced or exacerbated.

OP for upper & lower Cx

Lateral flexion

This movement is observed with the examiner standing in front of the patient and watching the contour of the side of the neck from the mastoid process to the C7 level. The presence of any restriction of movement may be visible (Figure 13.1), and, if so, overpressure is applied to stretch the segment to determine whether it reproduces symptoms.

OP for upper & lower Cx

Rotation

Rotation should also be observed with the examiner standing in front of the patient and noting whether the head tends to tilt forwards or backwards during the movement. By countering this abnormal rotation, symptoms may be related to the deformity.

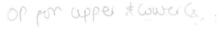
OP for upper & lower Cx

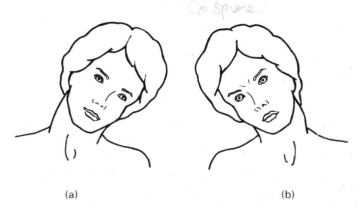

(a)   (b)

Figure 13.1 (a) Lateral flexion to the left is normal and is accompanied by a smooth curve in the right side of the neck. (b) Lateral flexion to the right is abnormal and is accompanied by a loss of the normal curve on the left side of the upper neck. This limitation is often easier to observe on repeated neck movements

Auxiliary tests

If symptoms still could be arising from the neck, further rests need to be assessed. These are: overpressure; repeated movements; sustained pressure; the quadrant position; and the upper limb tension test.

Overpressure

Overpressure is applied at the end of the painless range with small oscillatory movements and determining its end-feel.

Repeated movements

If pain is not provoked at the usual testing speed, the movements are repeated and at an increasing speed.

Sustained pressure

This test is used, especially in patients with arm pain, to demonstrate the cervical origin of the pain. The neck is moved into extension, rotation and then lateral flexion towards the painful side. The head is moved either to the limit of range or where pain is experienced and gentle pressure is then applied and gradually increased for 10 seconds to determine if arm pain is reproduced. Occasionally, pain is first felt as this movement is released or just after its release. Compression is then applied to the head, with the neck held in slight extension and slight lateral flexion towards the painful side. It is slowly applied and progressed only in the absence of pain.

Active NvB

The quadrant position

The quadrant position is a most useful test for either the lower or upper cervical spine that is used to place the joints under maximum stress.

The lower cervical quadrant position

For patients with left-sided pain, the neck is tilted back until the lower cervical spine is fully extended and it is then laterally flexed to the left. While held in this position, rotation to the left side is added (Figure 13.2a).

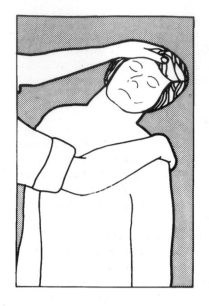

(a)

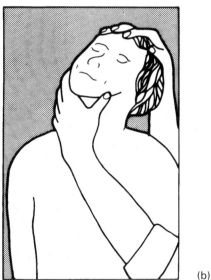

(b)

Figure 13.2 Cervical quadrant position: (a) lower; (b) upper

The upper cervical quadrant position

Standing to the left side of the patient, the examiner guides the head into extension. Pressure is applied to localize the movement to the upper cervical joints by grasping the patient's chin in the left hand, the forehead in the right hand, and the trunk is stabilized by the examiner's arm from behind. The head is then held in extension and rotated to the left with oscillatory movements to the limit of its range. The head, fully rotated, is then laterally flexed, using an oscillatory movement (Figure 13.2b).

Upper limb tension tests

These tests are similar to those for the lumbar spine in that they apply tension in order to test movement of the cervical nerve roots or their root sleeves in the neural canal (Elvey, 1986; Pullos, 1986; Kenneally et al, 1988). The role of these movements has been confirmed in a cadaver study (Selvaratnam et al, 1994). Clinically, a stepwise increase in tension is applied (Quinter, 1989) to the neuromeningeal structures in the neck by altering the positions of the limbs (Maitland, 1986). A number of tests have been described that are valuable for the diagnosis of previously undiagnosed neck and/or arm pain. The tests are sensitive but not overly specific, as they do not provide evidence about any specific underlying pathology, and several different tissues may be involved in the tests. Nevertheless, it has been shown that they can discriminate between referred and local causes of upper limb pain (Selvaratnam et al, 1994). They can also be used as a starting point for some treatment techniques. To test for shoulder pain, the patient lies supine and the arm is placed in a position behind the coronal plane. The shoulder is depressed and abducted in a slight degree of extension (see Figure 13.3). The shoulder is externally rotated (Figure 13.4), and forearm is supinated, the elbow is extended and the wrist and fingers are extended (Figure 13.5) The head is then turned to the painful side (Figure 13.6) and to the non-painful side (Figure 13.7). Then neck is flexed and laterally flexed to either side. Straight leg raising of both legs may be added (Figure 13.8).

Vertebral artery testing

Testing the vertebral arteries should always be part of a general neck examination. In all patients with neck pain, but especially if there are also complaints of giddiness, an attempt must be made to assess the relationship between neck

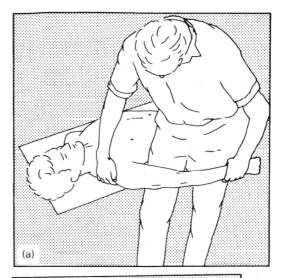

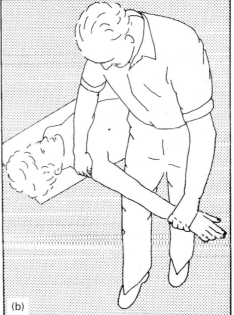

Figure 13.3 (a) Abduction arm in test for shoulder pain. (b) Abducted until symptoms change

movements and whether any giddiness is produced (*see* Chapter 16). This is done first by direct questioning and then by testing neck movements. Dizziness or pain may be experienced at any stage during the test, or with a sustained position or upon its release. The test must be abandoned if any symptoms are produced.

These tests are descibed in full in Chapter 16.

Passive movements

The two passive movements of the intervertebral joint complex are tested: the passive range at each individual joint, and then, the accessory movements. The passive range at each individual joint is tested by moving the head and neck into flexion, extension, lateral flexion and then rota-

tion, while feeling for movement between the adjacent bony processes of the spinous processes and the articular pillars.

Upper cervical spine

Atlanto-occipital joint

This may be tested in: lateral flexion; rotation; and flexion–extension.

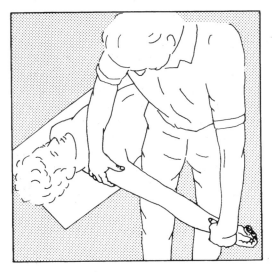

Figure 13.4 Release of abduction tension followed by external rotation

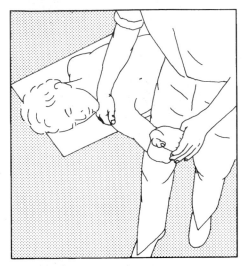

Figure 13.6 Rotation of patient's head towards shoulder during shoulder pain

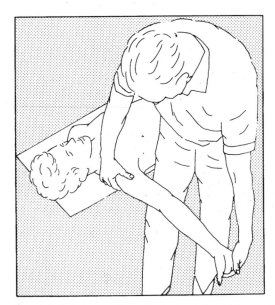

Figure 13.5 Release of lateral rotation followed by extension

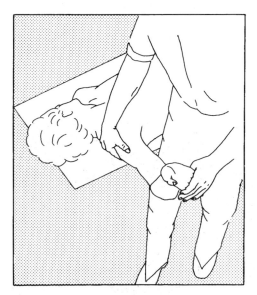

Figure 13.7 Rotation of patient's head away from shoulder during shoulder pain

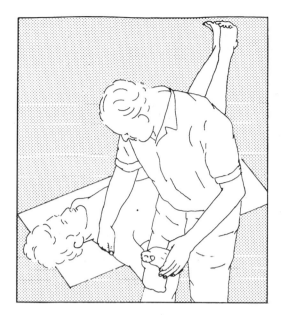

Figure 13.8 Assessment of shoulder-pain response during double straight leg raising

Although the head is to be laterally flexed to the right, the crown of the head must still remain near the midline. The examiner's hands and body fully tilt the head on the upper cervical area. As the head and neck are moved back and forth in the inner third (approximately 15 degrees) of the lateral flexion range, the thumb can feel the opening and closing of the gap between the two bony points of the transverse process of C1 and the mastoid process.

ROTATION OF THE ATLANTO-OCCIPITAL JOINT

The starting position is the same as that described for lateral flexion. With the patient's head turned fully to the right, the tip of the left thumb is positioned between the left mastoid process and the left transverse process of C1 as the head is rotated back and forth through 20 degrees in the inner third of the range. At maximum rotation, the transverse process is felt drawing nearer to the mastoid process and, as the head is brought back to the midline, it moves away (Figure 13.10).

FLEXION AND EXTENSION OF THE ATLANTO-OCCIPITAL JOINT

The patient lies supine with his or her head extending beyond the end of the couch. To feel this small movement, the examiner cradles the patient's head in his lap, holding the occiput in both hands with the thumb tips in contact with the tip of each lateral mass of C1 and the mastoid process (Figure 13.11).

The base of the skull is rocked back and forth in a nodding movement through a range of

LATERAL FLEXION OF THE ATLANTO-OCCIPITAL JOINT

The patient lies supine with the head projecting beyond the end of the couch. The examiner, standing at the head of the couch, cradles the occiput in his or her left hand and the forehead in the right. The tip of the examiner's left thumb lies between the left transverse process of C1 and the adjacent mastoid process. Pressure is applied to the crown of the head by the examiner's abdomen (Figure 13.9).

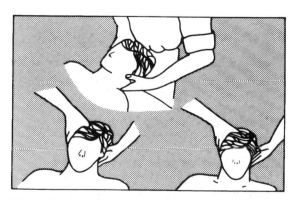

Figure 13.9 Lateral flexion at the atlanto-occipital joint

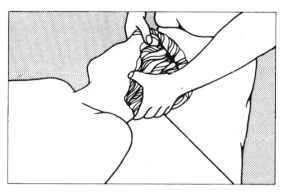

Figure 13.10 Rotation at the altanto-occipital joint

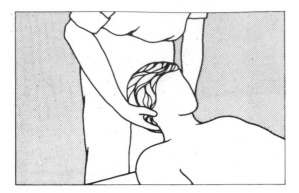

Figure 13.11 Flexion–extension at the atlanto-occipital joint

approximately 20 degrees. The crown of the head remains comparatively still. The small movement between the two bony points on each side can be assessed with the tips of the thumbs.

Atlanto-axial joint

ROTATION

The patient is seated with the examiner standing behind the left shoulder. The left hand is placed over the crown of the head, with the little finger and thumb spreading over the right and left parietal areas and hand spread backwards to its maximum over the occiput. With the right hand, the examiner grasps the spinous process of C2 in a pincer grip between the tip of the index finger and thumb (Figure 13.12).

The head is rotated back and forth from the midline to the left until the spinous process is felt to move. The lamina of C2 on the left is felt to move backwards against the thumb, and the the spinous process moves against the pad of the index finger and the range of movement assessed.

Lower cervical spine

Four movements of the cervical spine are assessed: flexion; lateral flexion; rotation; and extension.

C2–C7 flexion

The patient lies supine with the head beyond the end of the couch, and the examiner crouches at the head of the couch. The occiput is held in the heel of the right hand with fingers and thumb over the crown of the head. The left hand is placed against the left side of the neck with the thumb tip between two spinous processes, and the tips of the index and middle fingers over the anterior surface of the transverse processes.

To test movement between C3 and C4, the thumb is placed between the spinous processes, with the index and middle fingers over the anterior surface of the left transverse process of C4 and C5 (Figure 13.13).

The head is passively flexed by the right hand while the tip of the left thumb feels the opening and closing between the spinous processes as the head is moved backwards and forwards through a range of 15–20 degrees. The vertebrae below C4 are stabilized with pressure applied against the anterior surface of the left transverse processes.

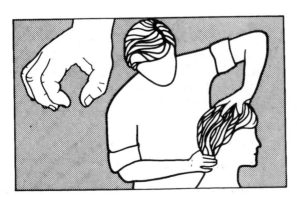

Figure 13.12 Rotation at the atlanto-axial joint

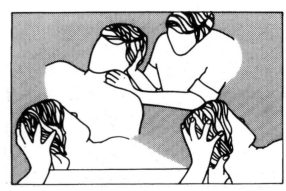

Figure 13.13 Flexion at C2–C7

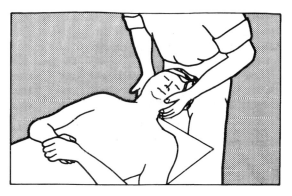

Figure 13.14 Lateral flexion at C2–C7

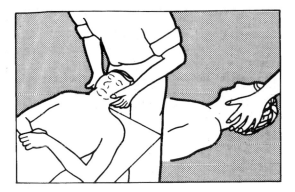

Figure 13.16 Extension at C2–C7

C2–C7 lateral flexion

The patient lies supine, head resting in the examiner's lap midway between the limits of flexion and extension. In this position both lateral flexion and rotation are most free. The tip of the index finger is placed deeply into the interlaminar space with the occiput and neck supported in both hands (Figure 13.14).

Care is necessary to ensure that the joint being tested, and not the head alone, is moved. The joint is laterally flexed towards the immobile palpating finger, assessing the extent of closing in the interlaminar space. Movement in the opposite direction is then performed.

C2–C7 rotation

The starting position is as described above for lateral flexion, except that the index finger is carried laterally, making a broader contact with the zygapophyseal joint (Figure 13.15).

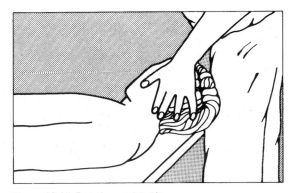

Figure 13.15 Rotation at C2–C7

The head is pivoted away from the side as the hand produces an oscillatory movement, down to, but not beyond, the joint to assess the opening between the two adjacent articular processes.

C2–C7 extension

The patient lies supine with the head resting in the examiner's lap. The examiner stands near the head, supporting underneath the head and neck to the level being tested. The tips of both index fingers are placed into the each interlaminar space on side (Figure 13.16).

The head and neck are extended down to the level being examined, while palpating with the fingertips for a closing down of the interlaminar space.

Accessory movements

These movements are tested by applying pressure against bony processes over the spinous processes and the articular pillars. They assess pain, range of movements, the end-feel of the movement, the behaviour of pain and stiffness throughout the range and muscle spasm.

Accessory movements of C1

Posteroanterior movement

The patient lies prone with the forehead resting on the hands.

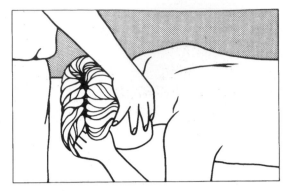

Figure 13.17 Test for accessory movements at C1. Posteroanterior pressure centrally over C1

Posteroanterior pressures are applied by the thumbs placed centrally against the posterior tubercle of the atlas first, and then laterally behind the atlanto-occipital joint (Figure 13.17).

Transverse movement

The head is rotated first to the left with the right arm by the side and the left arm level with the head, thus slightly raising the left shoulder to ease any strain. The easily palpable lateral mass of C1 will have rotated with the head.

Oscillatory pressures are applied by the thumbs directed transversely from the tip of the lateral mass of C1 on the left towards the tip of the lateral mass on the opposite side (Figure 13.18).

Accessory movements of C2

Posteroanterior pressures against the spinous process of C2 are used first, followed by

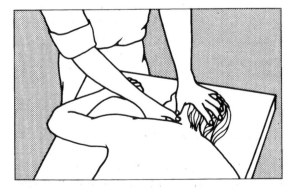

Figure 13.18 Transverse pressure against C1

posteroanterior pressure against the articular pillar of C2.

The patient lies with the head resting on the hands.

Posteroanterior pressures are applied with thumbs placed on the posterior surface of the inferior articular process of the axis.

For rotation to the left, the head is turned 30 degrees to the left with the forehead on the hands. Posteroanterior pressure on the left articular process of C2 tests rotary movement between C1 and C2 (Figure 13.19).

Accessory movements in the lower cervical spine.

Three accessory movement tests are used routinely in the lower cervical spine: posteroanterior pressures over the spinous process; posteroanterior pressures over the articular pillar; and transverse pressures against the lateral surfaces of the spinous process (Figure 13.20).

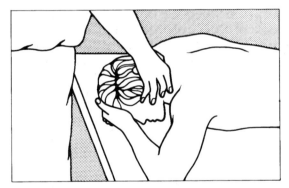

Figure 13.19 Test for for accessory movements of C2 in rotation

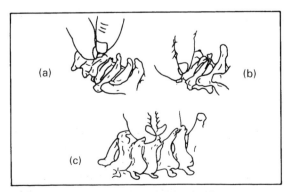

Figure 13.20 (a) Posteroanterior pressure on the spinous process; (b) posteroanterior pressure on the articular pillar; (c) transverse pressure on the lateral surface of the spinous process

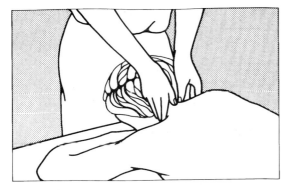

Figure 13.21 Central posteroanterior pressure over the spinous process

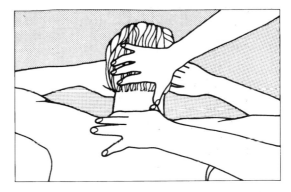

Figure 13.22 Transverse pressure against the lower cervical articular pillar

The direction given to these pressures may also be varied so that the posteroanterior pressure may also be directed towards the head or towards the feet. The direction taken by the posteroanterior pressure over the articular pillar may be further varied by directing the pressure laterally away from the spinous process, or medially towards the spinous process. Transverse pressure against the lateral surface of the spinous process may be varied by inclining the direction of pressure either toward the feet or head, or across the back of the lamina so that pressure is finally applied as a posteroanterior pressure against the articular pillar on the same side.

The patient lies prone with forehead resting on the hands and chin tucked in, avoiding a fully flexed or extended position. For posteroanterior pressures the examiner stands at the patient's head using oscillatory pressure with thumbs back to back over the spinous process (Figure 13.21). For transverse pressures against the articular process the pad of the thumb is used (Figure 13.22).

Palpation

Palpation is performed with the patient lying prone and the forehead supported by the hands to detect any alterations in bony alignments, the presence of a cervical rib, soft tissue thickening or muscle spasm. Many of the bony prominences on the back of the skull and cervical vertebrae are easily palpable. In the occiput, the inion is easily felt as a bony lump in the midline, with the nuchal lines radiating out on either side of it to end in the prominent mastoid processes. The transverse process of the atlas is readily felt between the mastoid and the angle of the jaw and can be felt to move on rotating the head.

Soft tissues are palpated next, beginning in the suboccipital areas and then down into the trough-like area between the spinous process and the lateral margin of the articular pillar. Areas of localized muscle spasm and tenderness are usually easily palpable around the scapula in the rhomboids, trapezius and levator scapulae muscles.

The spinous process of C1 is not normally easy to palpate, and C2 is the first spinous process readily felt. The spinous process from C3 to C5 cannot usually be palpated due to the cervical lordosis, although it may be possible with deep palpation, but C6 is palpable and can be felt to disappear on neck extension. The spinous process of C7 can be felt easily.

The zygapophyseal joints below C2–C3 are also palpable and can be felt to move by placing the fingers over the side of the cervical spine approximately 2–3 cm away from the midline and rotating the neck. Osteophytic lipping and tenderness about their margin may be felt occasionally.

Neurological tests

A complete assessment of the central nervous system is necessary with all cervical disorders. Motor power, sensation and reflexes are tested in

Table 13.1 Muscular weaknesses in the arm produced from lower motor neurone lesions

Movement	Main muscle involved	Nerve root	Method of testing
Abduction of arm	Deltoid	C5	The patient holds the arm abducted 45 degrees from the side while the examiner applies resistance to the lateral aspect of the arm just above the elbow
Elbow flexion	Biceps	C6	The patient holds the supinated forearm flexed at the elbow to 90 degrees. Resistance is applied against the anterior surface of the forearm just above the wrist
Elbow extension	Triceps	C7	The patient holds the elbow flexed to 90 degrees, resistance being applied against the dorsum of the forearm just above the wrist
Extension of thumb	Extensor pollicis longus	C8	The patient flexes the elbow to 90 degrees with forearm in mid-position and holds the extended thumb away from the palm and pointing towards the face. Resistance is directed against the thumbnail towards the little finger
Interphalangeal flexion	Flexor digitorum	C8	The patient flexes the elbow to 90 degrees with forearm in mid-position. The examiner stabilizes the forearm while the patient squeezes his fingers. Power of the long finger flexors is tested by resisting terminal interphalangeal flexion
Intrinsics		T1	The patient flexes the elbow to 90 degrees, extending the finger at the interphalangeal joints and flexing them at the metacarpophalangeal joints. The examiner places his or her finger between adjacent fingers of the patient in turn while the patient squeezes the extended fingers together

both upper and lower limbs. Evidence of a lower motor neurone lesion in the arm that produces muscular weakness is usually due to involvement of only one nerve root, and those of clinical significance are listed in Table 13.1. The girth of the arms is measured with a tape measure to record the presence of any muscle wasting.

Sensory disturbances to light touch and pinprick are sought in the dermatome distribution of the cervical nerves. Reflexes to be tested include the biceps jerk C5 and C6, the triceps jerk C7, and the supinator jerk C6 (Table 13.1).

Signs of an upper motor neurone lesion, including the plantar responses, are tested for in the lower limbs.

General examination

A general medical examination, including the cardiovascular system and respiratory system, is mandatory. This includes palpation and auscultation of the extracranial arteries.

14 Cervical disc degeneration

Disc degeneration commonly involves the cervical spine (Connell and Wiesel, 1992), although it differs in several important aspects from the lumbar spine. The cervical spine has a greater range of movement than the other spinal regions, and, at the same time, it has to support the weight of the head while being attached inferiorly to the relatively immobile upper thoracic segments and ribs. The greatest range of movement takes place at C5–C6, which is usually the site of the most severe degree of degeneration (Heller, 1992), followed by C6–C7 and then C4–C5 (Heller, 1992). The normal lordotic curve in the cervical spine also helps to localize these changes at the C5–C6 level.

The nucleus pulposus of the cervical disc is present at birth, but it becomes fissured with age (Bland and Boushey, 1990; Penning, 1991), and after the age of 45 years may become desiccated and absent (Bland and Boushey, 1990). The neurocentral joints occupy the posterolateral edges of the vertebra, so that the cervical discs do not extend as far posterolaterally as they do in the lumbar spine. The bony uncus may also provide some form of an anatomical barrier, and the posterior longitudinal ligament, thicker in the cervical spine than in the lumbar spine, provides stronger support. Due to these anatomical differences, cervical disc prolapse occurs much less commonly than does lumbar disc prolapse, and does not often occur after the age of 45 years.

The relationship of the nerve roots also varies. The cervical roots from C4 to C8 originate from the spinal cord at the level of the vertebral body and not at the level of the disc, so that they do not run obliquely downwards across the disc as in the lumbar spine, but are directed more laterally. Accordingly, they are protected as they run behind the vertebral body and the neurocentral joint, and they come to lie in the lower part of the foramen 4–8 mm below the disc level (Pech et al, 1985). The lower cervical nerve roots are the largest in the brachial plexus, while their intervertebral foramina tend to be smaller than in the other areas. In addition, degenerative changes in the zygapophyseal joints can result in narrowing of their intervertebral foramina, so that the C6 and C7 nerve roots will become the most commonly compromised.

Three clinical syndromes associated with disc degeneration that need to be considered are: disc prolapse; cervical spondylosis; and cervical myelopathy

Cervical disc prolapse

A cervical disc prolapse should not be looked upon as a miniature version of a lumbar disc prolapse (Kokobun et al, 1996), as they differ in several anatomical aspects. In addition, there are differences in the pathology, and cartilage endplate may be prominent in the prolapsed cervical disc material (Kokubun et al, 1996). First attacks are not at all common under the age of 30 years or over the age of 50 (Kokobun et al, 1996).

Clinically, patients present with severe pain, usually felt in the neck, scapular region and down the arm, although it may be experienced at first only in the arm. There may be a previous history of attacks of neck and interscapular pain and stiffness. Any movement of the neck may produce pain, but especially extension, a movement towards the affected side or elevation of the shoulder. Pain is made worse by neck movements, postural changes or straining, and may also be related to maintaining certain positions, for example, reading a book. Sudden straining, such as coughing or sneezing, is usually most painful. Pain is often present at night and sleep is disturbed.

Sensory changes, pins and needles or numbness in the dermatome distribution of the affected nerve root are usually present, and their distribution will vary according to the nerve root involved. Precise anatomical localization, however, may often be difficult because of several factors, such as marked anatomical variation in the brachial plexus, including the presence of a prefixed or post-fixed brachial plexus.

With C5 nerve root pressure, which exits at C4–C5, pain is felt mainly over the shoulder region, although it may also radiate down the arm.

With C6 nerve root pressure, pain usually radiates into the scapular area, the shoulder and the lateral aspect of the arm down to the thumb and index finger. Sensory disturbances may be felt in the thumb or index finger.

With C7 nerve root pressure, pain is felt over the upper border of the scapula, the shoulder and down the back of the arm and forearm to the middle fingers with sensory changes in the index and middle fingers.

With C8 nerve root pressure, pain is felt in the shoulder and medial aspect of the arm and forearm. Sensory changes are felt in the medial two fingers.

Diagnosis

Diagnosis can usually be made on the basis of a disturbance of spinal mechanics together with neurological signs. Signs of disturbed spinal mechanics include the following:

1. Disturbances of posture can often supply an important clue to diagnosis. The normal cervical lordosis is often lost and the patient stands with the head to one side, reluctant to move the neck. One of two positions may be adopted by the patient, presumably to relieve pain by shortening the distance that the nerve has to travel (Beatty et al, 1987). One is with abduction of the shoulder, so the patient may stand with the arm abducted and the palm of the hand resting on the head (Beatty et al, 1987); and the other is with the arm held by the side with the elbow flexed and supported under the elbow with the other hand.

2. Disturbances of movements. The normal range of neck movement is lost, usually with a painful limitation of extension and/or a limited lateral flexion and rotation towards the painful side. Pain may be eased on flexion, but it usually becomes worse with increasing extension (Farmer and Wisneski, 1994), since the size of the foramen decreases with extension (Yoo et al, 1992). The normal rhythm of cervical movements is commonly disturbed, so that during rotation the neck may be observed to move into flexion.

3. Other tests. Tests involving sustained pressure or overpressure in extension or to one side for approximately 20 seconds can reproduce pain, but are not usually needed to confirm the diagnosis. Pain can also be reproduced by Spurling's test, which involves rotating and laterally flexing the head to the side of pain and then compressing the vertex of the head with a downward pressure.

Neurological examination

A full neurological assessment of upper and lower limbs is undertaken. In the upper limb, this involves tests for neurological deficits, including sensory, motor and reflex changes, on a segmental basis (Table 14.1). In the lower limb, an upper motor neurone involvement is evidenced by motor weakness or reflex changes,

Table 14.1 Effects of cervical-disc prolapse

Spinal root	Muscles involved	Motor weakness	Reflex loss
C5	Deltoid, supraspinatus, infraspinatus and biceps	Glenohumeral abduction, glenohumeral lateral rotation and elbow flexion	Biceps jerk
C6	Biceps and supinator	Glenohumeral adduction, glenohumeral medial rotation and wrist supination	Biceps jerk and supinator jerk
C7	Triceps, pronators and flexor carpi radialis	Elbow extension, wrist pronation and wrist flexion	Triceps jerk
C8	Hand intrinsics, pronators, flexor digitorum and adductor pollicis	Wrist pronation, finger flexion and thumb adduction	—

including alterations in plantar responses. An EMG and nerve conduction test may be needed to confirm the presence and extent of the neurological findings.

The diagnosis of a disc prolapse can usually be made on clinical grounds, but it does need to be confirmed radiologically. Plain X-ray has little to offer, as the disc height may not be reduced on plain X-rays (Kokobun et al, 1996), so that CT, MRI (Bell and Ross, 1992; Parfenchuck and Janssen, 1994) or CT-myelography (Modic et al, 1986; Bell and Ross, 1992) may be indicated. However, a disc prolapse may be found in asymptomatic patients on MRI (Teresi et al, 1987), and a normal MRI study does not exclude the existence of clinically significant disc disease in patients with chronic neck pain (Schellhas et al, 1996).

Variations in clinical presentation

- The degree of arm pain may vary. Although usually severe, it may at times be present as a dull ache without any associated neurological symptoms.
- There may be bilateral arm pain, due mainly to a large central disc prolapse or, more rarely, to a bilateral disc prolapse.
- Distal arm pain with sensory disturbances such as numbness but without neck or proximal pain results in a clinical presentation similar to that of a peripheral entrapment neuropathy. An EMG with nerve conduction tests may be necessary to elucidate it further.

- There may be neck pain alone, due to a central disc prolapse.
- A large central disc prolapse may produce cord compression.

Management

Initial management

Most cases of cervical disc prolapse can be managed on an outpatient basis without resorting to surgery (Saal et al, 1996). The first requirement is pain relief, and this requires rest from pain producing activities, use of appropriate analgesics, pain-relieving modalities, use of a collar and cervical traction. Exercises are contraindicated at this stage.

Collars

The use of collars remains controversial (Teale and Mulley, 1990). Their main indication is pain relief (Naylor and Mulley, 1991), which can be achieved in most patients (Naylor and Mulley, 1991). The aim is not to immobilize the neck completely, for cineradiographs have demonstrated that this is most unlikely (Colachis et al, 1973; Hartman et al, 1975; Johnson et al, 1977, 1981; Fisher et al, 1977; Huston, 1988), although they may help by inhibiting spontaneous movements.

The best form of collar to use is the simplest one that best provides pain relief. They may be soft or hard, made of felt, rubber or Plastozote, or may have a brace with a chin cup as an incorporated support. A soft collar is usually found to be most comfortable (Naylor and Mulley, 1991). It is made by a physiotherapist, with the patient's neck maintained in a slight degree of flexion and incorporated in a stockinette to tie at the front. It needs to be modified or discontinued if pain or discomfort is increased. Patient compliance may be a problem. Some patients may at first be averse to wearing it, although they can be persuaded to do so if it can provide some degree of pain relief without the need for medication.

How long it needs to be worn is unanswered (Pennie and Agmar, 1990). It might be worn over a prolonged period, day or night, without causing any problem or side effects. However, a timetable should be introduced, so that the patient is weaned off it over approximately three weeks. It may then be worn only occasionally, at night or if any exertion or activity is liable to exacerbate pain.

Subsequent treatment

The severe degree of pain usually settles over approximately three weeks, and mobilization techniques can then be added to the treatment routine (see Chapter 17). Only if pain is not settling is admission to hospital with bed traction warranted.

An assessment should be made of the patient's work and recreational habits so that aggravating movements can be avoided. If excessive neck extension or flexion at work is a problem, the work level or seat is adjusted accordingly. Car driving involves rotation and often excessive vibration of the unsupported neck, and so is often a problem. Daily activities that involve extension of the neck, as in hanging clothes on the line, or in sporting activities, should be avoided until the neck has recovered normal and painless mobility.

Neck mechanics need to be assessed for the posture involved with sleep, rest, work or leisure. Neck posture during sleep is largely dependent on the type and height of pillow used. A test to determine its correct consistency may easily be performed by pushing the fist into the pillow, so making a hollow in it. After removing the fist, in pillows filled with feather or down, the hollow

should then remain for a time. The hollow is not maintained with a rubber pillow, which resumes its original shape as soon as the fist is removed. A pillow should support both the neck and head, so its height should be adjusted to the patient's posture, and in a patient with a neck deformity it is preferable to support the head with two pillows rather than one. The shape of the pillow also should be varied to increase its support. One example is a pillow made with down and separated into two compartments: the smaller part supports under the head when the patient lies down and the larger, denser portion is used for support under the cervical spine.

Ergonomics in the workplace should be reviewed to determine such problems as the eye level with the work level or a computer, and how positions involving prolonged flexion, extension, rotation or holding heavy weights can be avoided. Prolonged sitting or standing should be avoided, and rest periods enforced, as mini-breaks are important to reduce static loads (Tan and Nordin, 1992). Chairs should be chosen with a good back support and arm rests. Symptoms at rest may be exacerbated only after sitting, holding a book, or after watching television in a slumped or unsupported posture.

Exercise

Exercise to strengthen neck muscles and to increase the range of motion would appear to be logical treatment, although trials to prove their worth are lacking. Exercises are most unlikely to provide any benefit while neck pain is severe or a major problem. Nevertheless, many patients continue to perform exercises to increase range, even though they increase pain, in the mistaken belief or pious hope that they are preventing some future disability. It is more useful to commence with isometric exercises, which are of benefit in strengthening neck muscles (Ylinen and Ruuska, 1994), and can also be used while a collar is worn.

As pain settles, the aim of management is to maintain activity (Ekberg et al, 1994) with general activities such as walking, swimming, cycling, and warm pool exercises to increase aerobic fitness (Semble et al, 1990). A variety of exercises can be introduced, including flexibility, stretching and aerobic exercises (Tan and Nordin, 1992), which are used especially to maintain or increase the range of movement. The exercise regimen should involve mobility exercises into flexion, extension, lateral flexion and rotation and should be progressed in range, provided no pain is provoked. It is often useful to perform these exercises while standing under a hot shower.

Surgery should be considered if:

- Severe pain is not controlled by conservative measures
- Neurological deficit is not responding to conservative treatment
- Central disc protrusion is present with cord compression.

Cervical spondylosis

Much confusion exists about the use of the term 'cervical spondylosis', since it is used to describe two separate entities. It is used to denote a well-described degenerative pathology change, and it is also used as a diagnostic label for a less well-defined clinical syndrome. As the onset and evolution of the changes of cervical disc degeneration are gradual, the adjacent tissues can gradually adjust and any resultant symptoms are often absent or minimal. Nevertheless, cervical spondylosis is generally considered to be more common and often more severe than in the

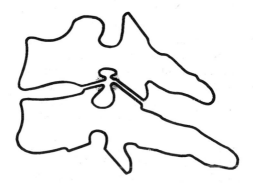

Figure 14.1 Osteophytic outgrowths from the neurocentral joint encroach upon the intervertebral foramen

lumbar spine. Accordingly, it is often used as a diagnostic label in patients with neck pain or for those in whom no alternate diagnosis is evident.

The pathological condition of spondylosis is associated with disc degeneration with loss of disc height, bony sclerosis around the vertebral endplates, hard, posterior protruding osteocartilaginous bars and osteophytic outgrowths in the zygoapophyseal joints that reduce the size of the intervertebral foramen and may compromise the nerve roots (Figure 14.1). Several additional features are present in the neck that are not present in the lumbar spine.

- Cord changes. Direct cord involvement from the hard, protruding, posterior osteocartilaginous bars may cause cord compression. In addition, occlusion of the anterior spinal artery may result in changes in the cord.
- Nerve roots may be compressed or irritated, and the radicular symptoms are increased on neck extension (Farmer and Wisneski, 1994). Thickening of the dural extension that forms the dural root sleeve may develop. This root sleeve fibrosis may also be responsible for a constriction or sharp angulation of the nerve root, rendering it more vulnerable. Inflammatory oedema (Holt and Yates, 1966) with an increase in neural connective tissue, and axonal and myelin degenerative changes, are formed as a result. An EMG is often indicated to determine the extent of these lesions.
- The diameter of the spinal canal may vary (Kamiyama et al, 1994). The smaller the diameter of the cervical spinal canal, the greater is the possibility of spinal cord compression and myelopathy.
- The neurocentral joints may be an important (Bland and Boushey, 1990), even though relatively uncommon source of symptoms (Bogduk et al, 1988a; Barnsley et al, 1993b). Degenerative changes in these joints, with rounding off of the articular surface and osteophytic outgrowths, are commonly present and further reduce the size of the intervertebral foramen.
- The vertebral artery with the postganglionic sympathetic nerve fibres may be involved in its course through the transverse processes of the cervical vertebrae (Figure 14.2).

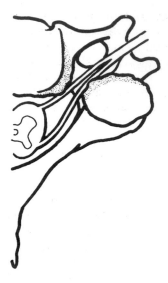

Figure 14.2 Osteophytic outgrowths from the apophyseal joint and vertebra may compress the intervertebral nerve or may even be large enough to encroach on the transverse foramen, with its vertebral artery

- Surrounding organs may be compressed by large anterior osteophytes, which may be evident during a barium swallow, and can cause hoarseness or dysphagia.

The diagnosis of spondylosis is commonly made on X-ray, even though the significance of the changes is, to say the least, doubtful. The changes are also present in asymptomatic patients (Gore et al, 1986; Teresi et al, 1987), are inevitable after the age of 40 years (Rahim and Stambough, 1992), are invariable by the age of 65 and correlate only poorly with symptoms (Heller et al, 1983). No differences could be detected between the X-ray changes seen in the necks of symptomatic patients when they were compared with control X-rays taken during a barium study (Heller et al, 1983). X-rays are, however, a help in detecting the presence of other bone disorders, as for example, a congenital block vertebra, which is often associated with degenerative changes in the surrounding discs (Figure 14.3). Since the X-ray changes have proved so unreliable, greater emphasis has been placed on CT as the major radiological investigative tool, for its value in delineating disc and bone damage. However, CT has not proved to be of any greater

benefit in most patients with neck pain, unless there is also evidence of neural compression. MRI is also used as it can depict bone and soft tissues (Kramer et al, 1991), and has a role in detecting abnormalities in the cord, although it may fail to view the course of exiting nerve roots (Russell, 1990), and it may be abnormal even in asymptomatic subjects (Boden et al, 1990b).

Management

Patients usually present with pain related to neck movements, especially extension, or extension combined with lateral flexion to the side, and pain is often related to activities such as painting ceilings, or sporting activities such as golf. A treatment programme should first provide rest from those activities known to exacerbate pain, with suitable adjustments to the patient's work, rest or sleeping habits. As with the lumbar spine, a multi-disciplinary approach to management is needed (Ekberg et al, 1994).

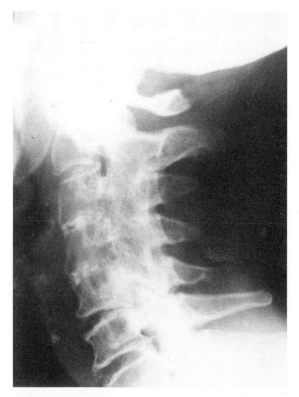

Figure 14.3 Degenerative changes associated with congenital block vertebrae

Mobilization techniques

Mobilization techniques, including traction, are usually of benefit to all patients who have no evidence of neural involvement. The more gentle mobilization techniques are usually sufficient to produce relief of symptoms (Brodin, 1985), and manipulations are only rarely indicated. Their use is considered further in Chapter 18. Exercise therapy is also needed as a follow-up.

Medications

Simple analgesics should be used for pain relief, and muscle relaxants are of no value. An inflammatory component may be present in cases of cervical disc prolapse or with synovitis involving the zygapophyseal joints. Anti-inflammatory drugs may then be used for their anti-inflammatory and analgesic effects.

Joint blocks

Degenerative changes in the cervical zygapophyseal joints may be a source of pain, and can be ameliorated by injections of local anaesthetic into the joint to anaesthetize it (Barnsley et al, 1993a; Lord et al, 1993). If this test relieves the pain, an injection of local anaesthetic and corticosteroid may then be made into the joint (Dory, 1983; Dussault and Nicolet, 1985). However, in the only controlled trial, on post-traumatic patients, no benefit was obtained (Barnsley et al, 1994b). Alternatively, a block of the medial branch of the dorsal ramus below the C2–C3 joint using percutaneous radiofrequency neurotomy can relieve pain in approximately 70 per cent of cases (Barnsley and Bogduk, 1993; Lord et al, 1995a). Problems with its use include radiation exposure, accurate placement of the electrode (Lord et al, 1995a), local trauma and cost (Swezey, 1996a).

Injections of local anaesthetic and corticosteroid into locally tender painful areas around the scapula or at muscle attachments around the nuchal line may help, although relief is usually only temporary.

Surgery

Most patients often suffer minimal symptoms or else attacks of neck and/or arm pain that respond well to conservative therapy. In addition, long periods of remission may be present and exacerbation is possibly due to a synovitis in the zygapophyseal joints after unaccustomed activities. Accordingly, since most patients with cervical spondylosis respond to conservative measures, surgery is not often indicated, and its role and results are difficult to evaluate. Operation is usually indicated, however, in patients with:

- Spinal cord compression. The cord is compromised by posterior osteocartilaginous bars often associated with a hypertrophied ligamentum flavum and narrowed spinal canal.
- Severe or progressive nerve root pressure. The lower nerve roots are compressed by osteophytic outgrowths with reduced size of the intervertebral foramen.
- Vertebral artery compression.

Preoperative assessment may require CT, CT myelography or MRI. The C5–C6 and C6–C7 discs are responsible in most cases, although some patients may have multiple levels. The choice of operative technique lies between an anterior or a posterior approach to the cervical spine. An anterior approach is the more common, as it permits disc excision and removal of osteophytes (Yamamoto et al, 1991). An interbody fusion is also usually necessary to stabilize the abnormal motion segment and prevent future deformity (Chestnut et al, 1992; Wood and Hanley, 1992; Watters and Levinthal, 1994).

The posterior approach, either through a laminectomy or a facetectomy, allows the nerve root to be examined and decompressed (Chestnut et al, 1992).

Cervical myelopathy

Cervical myelopathy is a relatively common condition (Ito et al, 1996a) in which the spinal cord becomes indented and compressed. Although it may follow an acute disc prolapse, it more commonly occurs as a cervical spondylotic myelopathy (Montgomery and Brower, 1992). This is associated with cervical disc degeneration which is complicated by a hard osteocartilaginous mass of osteophytes projecting from the posterior aspect of the vertebral body (Kurz and Herkowitz, 1992), with bulging of the ligamentum flavum into the spinal canal (Chen et al, 1994b). The normal canal is usually capacious, as the average anteroposterior dimension of the canal is about 17 mm (Edwards and LaRocca, 1985), whereas the anteroposterior dimension of the cord is 10 mm (Heller, 1992) The diameter of both the cervical and lumbar spinal canal is almost always narrowed in patients with myelopathy (Edwards and LaRocca, 1985; Penning et al, 1986; Torg et al, 1986; Parke, 1988; Bohlman, 1995). Several different clinical syndromes may result, and cord damage (Bohlman and Emery, 1988) can be further exacerbated by compression of the anterior spinal artery (Ferguson and Caplan, 1985, Bohlman, 1995).

Clinical features

The onset of symptoms is usually insidious (Heller 1992), and progression may be gradual or stepwise (Ito et al, 1996c). Symptoms arise from varying combinations of upper and lower motor neurone lesions and sensory disturbances. Anterior horn cells are involved at first, followed by the lateral and posterior funiculi (Ito et al, 1996c). Long tract signs occur below the level of the compression, so that weakness of the legs with a spastic gait is the most common presenting symptom. In the upper limbs a lower motor lesion may occur, but an upper motor neurone lesion in the arms is not common (Shinomiya et al, 1994). Sensory disturbances, pins and needles and numbness in the arms (Montgomery and Brower, 1992) and a sensation of weakness or clumsiness (Good et al, 1984) are common. Lhermitte's sign, in which flexion of the neck

exacerbates the sensory symptoms, may be present. Ultimately, if the spinal cord compression is not relieved, neural tissue will atrophy or be destroyed (Bohlman, 1995).

A full neurological examination and assessment is essential. The clinical findings and reflex changes will depend upon the level of compression, and increased tendon reflexes in the lower limbs with extensor plantar responses are usually present. If the lesion is at the C5 level, an inverted supinator reflex may be present in the upper limb. The jaw jerk is a most useful way of differentiating spinal from intracranial lesions, and is positive only in the latter. Muscle fasciculations may be evident.

The natural history of this condition without treatment is one of progressive deterioration (Sadasivan et al, 1993), and its diagnosis is often delayed because the original symptoms may be vague or overlooked (Law et al, 1993). MRI is the investigation of choice to demonstrate the degree of disc and cord damage (Boden et al, 1990b; Fukushima et al, 1991; Sadasivan et al, 1993; Okada et al, 1994; Wada et al, 1995), and also to measure the canal diameter (Bucciero et al, 1993). A rigid collar should be worn while investigations are being carried out, because neck movement, either flexion or extension, can exacerbate the degree of compression (Bohlman, 1995).

Surgery is indicated in most cases. Its main purpose is to prevent further damage to the cord (Batzdorf and Flannigan, 1991; Chestnut et al, 1992; Kurz and Herkowitz, 1992; Law et al, 1993; Sadasivan et al, 1993; Watters and Levinthal, 1994; Bohlman, 1995; Matsuyama et al, 1995) and aid recovery (Bernhardt et al, 1993), using either an anterior or posterior decompression (Cusick, 1991) and fusion.

15 Mechanical derangement of the cervical spine

Mechanical derangements of the cervical spine are a common source of symptoms, including headache, vertigo, torticollis and neck pain.

Headache

Headache is one of the most common of all human complaints (Rasmussen et al, 1991; Hasvold and Johnsen, 1993; Nilsson, 1995; Schoensee et al, 1995), with many different causes, and resulting in a large loss of productivity and high medical costs (Hurwitz et al, 1996). It commonly arises from musculoskeletal structures in the neck (Sjaastad et al, 1983, 1986; Farina et al, 1986; Fredriksen et al, 1987; Pfaffenrath et al, 1987; Edmeads, 1988; Bogduk and Marsland, 1988; Meloche et al, 1993; Nilsson, 1995; Schoensee et al, 1995), as has been recognized in the medical literature for more than 100 years (Lance, 1982; Edmeads, 1988). It was previously called 'cervical headache', but is more correctly termed 'cervicogenic headache' (Sjaastad et al, 1990) in that head pain arises in the neck, although it is not necessarily felt in the neck.

The prevalence of cervicogenic headache is uncertain, but it has been estimated to be between 14 and 30 per cent of all chronic headache patients (Sjaastad et al, 1986; Pfaffenrath and Kaube, 1990; Nilsson, 1995). In a large series of patients with neck pain, headache was reported to be present in one-third of patients (Gore et al, 1987). Although headache may, in theory, arise from any structure in the neck, it usually arises from the upper three cervical vertebral joints (Pfaffenrath et al, 1987), where the most common cause is a hypomobility lesion.

One of the main problems has been one of definition, although one definition and a set of diagnostic criteria published by the International Headache Society (1988) at least provided a starting point. Their definition (1988), 'headache arising from musculoskeletal dysfunction of the cervical spine', was inadequate as it failed to take into account its most important clinical features. A revised, lengthier definition (Sjaastad et al, 1990) also failed to take into account its major diagnostic feature: that it is associated with a movement abnormality in the upper cervical intervertebral segments. In this definition, Sjaastad et al (1990) also considered nerve root pressure to be the cause of the head pain, overlooking the fact that that is a rare cause, and that referred pain is the more important feature in these cases.

A better definition that takes in these problems is 'headache due to a disorder of the neck associated with a movement abnormality in the intervertebral segments. It may arise from the joints and surrounding soft tissues. The movement abnormality is manifested during either active or passive examination of the movement' (Bogduk

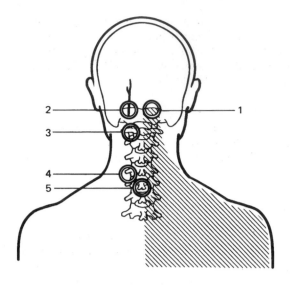

Figure 15.1 Cervical sites for the production of headache: (1) musculotendinous attachments; (2) compression of the greater occipital nerve; (3) atlanto-axial region, headache being due either to arthritis or to a hypomobility lesion; (4) involvement of the vertebral artery in the transverse foramen; (5) cervical spondylosis

et al, 1985). Other neck causes of headache are less common, and include cervical spondylosis, arthritis, nerve entrapment and musculotendinous lesions (Figure 15.1). Headache following neck trauma is a different problem, and is considered in Chapter 16.

Hypomobility lesions

Features

The clinical features of a headache associated with a hypomobility lesion in the upper cervical spine are usually so characteristic that the diagnosis should be suspected from the history alone. Pain is usually felt in the occipital region, and may radiate widely to one side of the head, behind the eyes or occasionally into the face. Pain is nearly always unilateral, does not change side during an attack ('without sideshift') (Sjaastad et al, 1990), and in any individual patient its site and radiation tends to remain constant. However, in a severe attack, it may at times also be felt across the midline, but it is still always worse on its usual side. The site of the head pain is no indication as to its site of origin in the neck. Pain, usually

described as dull and aching or as a sensation of soreness, is typically worse in the morning or immediately after first raising the head from the pillow. When severe, it may be also felt during the night, and the patient may not be able to bear the presence of the head against the pillow. The headache usually eases as the day goes on, but may be aggravated by neck and head movements or by jolting, such as riding in a bus, sneezing, coughing or straining. Some patients notice that their headache can be relieved or exacerbated by posturing the neck, and that headache tends to come on with sustained postures such as holding the neck in flexion or extension. Reversing a car or painting a ceiling is usually difficult. In some patients, pain may have been present for years, while in others pain tends to come on in attacks, although the attacks may vary in their duration and frequency. Patients frequently complain of these symptoms, but it is just as common to have them ignored.

Pain in the face may also be due to lesions of the upper cervical spine. Pain, often deep-seated, dull and aching, is usually unilateral, tends to be constant in site, may be made worse by neck movements and may be associated with unusual facial sensations such as a coldness. Pain may be sited in the supra- or infraorbital region, behind the eyes, or around the ear, but not in the jaw. Pain in the infraorbital region is often mistaken for sinusitis, so forming the basis for cases of 'sinusitis' that are said to have been cured by manipulation of the neck.

In addition to head and neck pain, vertigo or vague symptoms, such as feelings of being generally unwell, nausea, depression, or a feeling of uncertainty (Bogduk et al, 1985) may rarely be present. They may be due to sympathetic nervous system involvement (Heller, 1992), and are at times be difficult to differentiate from a psychosomatic disorder.

Diagnosis

The cardinal feature of cervicogenic headache is that there is a movement abnormality in the upper neck, hypomobility, which is responsible for the pain, and clinical examination should confirm that certain neck movements reproduce the head pain. Accordingly, the important criteria for the diagnosis of cervicogenic headache due to a hypomobility lesion are:

- Pain is felt mainly in the occipital region with radiation into the head or face
- The presence of a typical history, as above
- Neck movements reproduce the patient's pain, but particularly with testing of the passive and accessory movements of the upper cervical joints
- X-rays are of no special value in confirming the diagnosis
- Other diagnoses may need to be excluded.

Examination

A general examination is performed, followed by examination of the neck.

INSPECTION

Posture is assessed with the patient first standing and then sitting to examine spinal curves and look for any muscle weakness, asymmetry or tightness. The neck muscles are tested by an isometric contraction.

MOVEMENTS

Active and passive movements of flexion, extension, lateral flexion and rotation are tested to assess their range (Pfaffenrath et al, 1988), any restriction in or disturbance of movement, reproduction of pain and the presence of muscle spasm.

In patients with cervical spondylosis, some degree of restriction of neck movements is to be expected, but in hypomobility lesions the overall physiological range may appear to be normal. However, testing the passive intervertebral movements in the upper cervical joints will reveal that their range is restricted, and that they reproduce the pain. The sensitivity and specificity of these manual examination tests in the cervical spine were assessed by Jull et al (1988), who reported 100 per cent accuracy in detecting abnormal movement in the upper cervical spine, validated by diagnostic nerve blocks, and concluded that these tests could reliably discriminate a symptomatic joint and that they could reproduce the pain. These signs may be present at one or more levels from C1 to C3, but usually at C2–C3, and

may be associated with local tenderness and thickening on palpation. Restriction of movement may be found at two levels but on opposite sides; such as, the right side of C1–C2, and the left side at C2–C3.

PALPATION

The patient lies prone, supporting the forehead on the hands while the bony outlines and soft tissues are palpated for any tenderness or muscle spasm.

Neural mechanisms

The neural pathways forming the basis of cervicogenic headaches have been well described by Bogduk (1989). The spinal nucleus of the trigeminal nerve is its nociceptive centre, and it descends from the pons to become continuous with the dorsal horns of the upper cervical spinal cord. There they are indistinguishable from each other, as they form a continuous column of grey matter extending from the brainstem into the upper spinal cord. Afferent neurones of the three divisions of the fifth cranial nerve form its spinal tract, which also descends caudally into the upper cervical cord. Here they anastomose with and converge upon afferent fibres from the upper three cervical segments, which supply the joints and ligaments of the upper three vertebrae. The multisegmental, overlapping distribution is such that the first division of the trigeminal nerve descends as far as the C3 segment of the spinal cord. Hence, nociceptive impulses from the upper cervical segments may be referred to the head. The trigeminocervical nucleus also receives afferents from the seventh, ninth and tenth cranial nerves (Bogduk, 1989).

The upper cervical joints with their ligaments and muscles are supplied by C1 to C3 cervical nerves. C1 has a sensory but not a cutaneous branch. Its posterior primary ramus supplies mainly the suboccipital muscles, but it also supplies a filament to the greater occipital nerve. The posterior primary ramus of C2 divides into a lateral and a medial branch. The latter, known as the greater occipital nerve, receives a communication from the first and third cervical nerves and supplies the scalp. The anterior primary ramus of C2 may receive a branch from C3, then ascends as the lesser occipital nerve and also supplies the scalp. Accordingly, the scalp is supplied mainly by branches of the posterior primary rami of the upper cervical nerves, which may radiate as far as the frontal region (Bradley, 1977). Branches from the C1–C3 sinuvertebral nerves arise from the ventral rami and distribute sensory and sympathetic fibres to the dura mater, periosteum and blood vessels in the floor of the posterior cranial fossa (Bogduk, 1982).

The basis for cervicogenic headaches is that it is a referred pain from the neck, and direct nerve compression is not involved as its cause (Bogduk et al, 1985). As in other sites, the distance that pain is referred may reflect the severity of the underlying lesion. Referred pain into the head from stimulation of neck structures, including injections of hypertonic saline, has been described in various experiments (Campbell and Parsons, 1944; Feinstein et al, 1954; Kerr and Olafson, 1961; Kerr, 1972). Electrical stimulation of the C3 dorsal ramus (Bogduk and Marsland, 1986) evoked pain in the occiput, mastoid area and forehead regions.

Differential diagnosis

The typical form of cervicogenic headache, as described above, is usually so characteristic that it can, and should, be suspected on clinical grounds alone. The other causes of cervical headache are discussed below. However, it may also be necessary to exclude other, more serious, causes such as a tumour of the posterior fossa or skull, or congenital anomalies at the craniovertebral junction, which may be associated with an Arnold-Chiari malformation or Paget's disease, any of which may present with neck pain and headache. They may be associated with other symptoms and signs, and require appropriate investigations.

Management

A hypomobility lesion of the upper cervical spine is the most common cause of cervicogenic headache, and it usually responds well to mobilization techniques (Turk and Ratkolb, 1987; Bellavance et al, 1989; Jensen et al, 1990; Schoensee et al, 1995). Substantial relief of pain may be expected after a few treatments, even if the headache has been present for some time. Traction may be added for those patients who do not respond fully, and only occasionally is a manipulation indicated (Vernon, 1991). Pain relief may also be obtained with the use of a collar, especially if worn at night to ease the typical early morning pain, and it will need to be worn for a short period of time only. Active exercises do not have a role to play in the initial management, but isometric exercises can be prescribed. After the headache starts to settle, the patient is encouraged to become as active as possible and range of movement exercises are instituted.

Cervical spondylosis

Headache is a common symptom in patients with cervical spondylosis (Brain, 1963; Chirls, 1975; Peterson et al, 1975; Pawl, 1977; Michler et al, 1991; Bovim et al, 1992; Heller, 1992), and it often has the typical characteristics that have been described above for cervicogenic headaches. Since it seems most unlikely that the neural mechanisms in the upper spine would also be acting in the lower spine, an alternative explanation is necessary. One possibility is that there is an associated hypomobility lesion, or perhaps joint degeneration in the upper cervical spine (Holt and Yates, 1966). Another possibility is that pain originates in the muscles (Peterson et al, 1975; Pawl, 1977), and is associated with postural changes, or perhaps muscle spasm.

Management

Headaches associated with cervical spondylosis usually respond well to traction and manipulative therapy. A collar may also be used, especially if head or neck pain is severe or a problem at night. Locally tender areas around the musculotendinous attachments to the skull may also be infiltrated with local anaesthetic and corticosteroid if a patient is slow to respond. While it is not at all common to have a cervical fusion performed because of the headaches alone, it is not uncommon for patients who have undergone this surgery to report that their headache has now resolved.

Arthritis

Both inflammatory and degenerative types of arthritis may involve joints in the upper cervical spine and craniovertebral junction and can produce head pain (*see* Chapter 12). Arthritis of the atlanto-occipital or atlanto-axial joints may occur in patients with either rheumatoid arthritis, spondyloarthritis or osteoarthritis. Pain arising from post-traumatic degenerative changes at the C2–C3 zygapophyseal joint has been described (Bogduk and Marsland 1986, Lord et al, 1995b) (*see* Chapter 16).

The diagnosis of arthritis is confirmed by suitable tests, including X-rays. Management should consist of general medical management of the arthritis and use of a collar. Manual methods, traction and active exercises are contraindicated.

Entrapment neuropathy

An entrapment neuropathy of the greater occipital nerve, the medial branch of the posterior primary ramus of C2, may occur, but it is rare, and its proposed site of entrapment is still conjectural. It was not recognized as a cause of headache by the International Headache Society (1988), although diagnostic criteria have been proposed for it subsequently (Sjaastad et al, 1990). It was first described in 1821 (quoted in Horowitz and Yonas, 1993), and later by Hunter and Mayfield (1949) who believed it to be due to bony compression of the nerve following neck movements. Surgeons operated on this site enthusiastically, but usually with disastrous results (Weinberger, 1978). The anatomy was described in detail by Bogduk (1980, 1982), who demonstrated that the nerve could not be entrapped as it had been previously described.

Although entrapment of the nerve is rare, it is a commonly made diagnosis, and is also often used to describe any form of cervical headache. The nerve runs through the semispinalis capitis muscles (Anthony, 1989; Rifat and Lombardo, 1995) and a tendinous sling arising from the trapezius (Bogduk, 1980). It crosses the nuchal line with the occipital artery, and is distributed to the scalp as far as the frontal and temporal regions (Bradley, 1977). It remains a possibility for the nerve to be entrapped (Evans, 1992) in

the soft tissues, especially following a forceful extension injury.

Pain has been described as severe, intermittent, burning, throbbing or piercing, radiating from the neck to the head, and often present at night. Associated hyperalgesia or paraesthesia of the scalp may be reproduced by direct pressure or tapping (Tinel's sign) over the nerve just distal to the nuchal line. It may also be possible to demonstrate sensory disturbances over the skin of the scalp.

Treatment is best with non-steroidals (Rifat and Lombardo, 1995) and injection with local anaesthetic and corticosteroid (Bovim and Sand, 1992). Surgery has been advocated (Dubuisson, 1995), although results are not usually impressive.

Musculotendinous lesions

Lesions of the musculotendinous attachment of the cervical muscles to the nuchal line of the skull, although not common, may also result in pain in the head. One of three causes may be present:

1. Alteration in the patient's posture, which itself may be associated with an underlying hypomobility lesion or cervical spondylosis.
2. An underlying tension state causing muscular tension in the neck muscles. Patients may complain of neck or head pain alone, but more commonly complain of head and neck pain together.
3. An area of enthesopathy may occasionally occur as the sole clinical finding and without any evidence of other associated conditions.

Tendinitis in this area is tested by an isometric contraction of the neck muscles, which should also reproduce pain, and a localized area of tenderness on palpation. Infiltrating the locally tender area with local anaesthetic and corticosteroid should relieve the symptoms, at least temporarily, and may be repeated from time to time as indicated.

Manual therapy techniques are indicated when there is an associated hypomobility lesion of the cervical spine, and may be used together with the injection therapy.

Migraine

Migraine is due to a disturbance of cranial blood flow. Its clinical features are well described and it clearly represents a different clinical picture to that of cervicogenic headaches, and it is not directly related to lesions of the cervical spine. Accordingly, the failure of a controlled clinical trial of manipulation to diminish the frequency and duration of migraine attacks (Parker et al, 1978) was entirely predictable. However, considerable confusion exists about the relationship between migraine and the cervical spine, and for several reasons.

First, the diagnosis of migraine may have been incorrect. This is a commonly made mistake with patients who have a severe degree of headache from any cause, especially if it has a throbbing quality, to be diagnosed as having migraine. Accordingly, a diagnosis of migraine may be applied incorrectly to a severe cervicogenic headache, and appears to be the most common reason to explain migraine being 'cured' after manipulation of the neck.

Second, migraine may occur coincidentally with a cervical lesion. One possibility is that the neck lesion could be a non-specific triggering mechanism, capable of inducing an attack of migraine. If so, treatment to the neck with mobilization techniques could help to abort an attack.

Third, migraine may very rarely be produced by compression of the vertebral artery in the neck, described by Dutton and Riley (1969) as cervical migraine. In their case report, a 54-year-old-man complained of severe attacks of recurrent headaches of a migrainous nature. Arteriography during an attack demonstrated compression of the left vertebral artery due to degenerative changes at the C6–C7 level. The patient was cured with surgery. In addition, patients with vertebrobasilar insufficiency due to atheroma may complain of attacks of headaches associated with visual disturbances and vertigo.

Vertigo

The causes of vertigo are many and include disturbances of the inner ear, neurological lesions and vascular disorders. Attempts have been made to differentiate between the terms 'vertigo' and 'dizziness', but the terms are now usually used interchangeably. The differential diagnosis is long, and only those directly related to the cervical spine are considered here. Five disorders arising in the cervical spine, either vascular or musculoskeletal, may be associated with vertigo.

Vascular causes

The blood supply to the brain is supplied by the carotid and vertebrobasilar arteries, with approximately 20 per cent of its supply supplied through the latter. Vertebrobasilar insufficiency occurs when a reduction in its blood flow results in ischaemia in the tissues it supplies (Bogduk, 1981; Thiel, 1991), and vertigo is usually its first and major symptom. Atheroma involving the vertebral artery is the most common cause, although congenital anomalies are not uncommon. In addition, any alteration in the carotid system due to atheroma or other vascular abnormalities may affect the vertebrobasilar supply. Investigations of the blood flow, including angiography and Doppler sonography, may be necessary.

The vertebral artery may be conveniently divided into four segments and different problems may arise at the different sites along its course.

The first segment runs from the subclavian artery to the transverse foramen of the sixth cervical vertebra. Musculoskeletal structures such as the surrounding muscles or bands may cause an extrinsic compression of the artery.

The second segment runs a straight course to the second cervical vertebra, protected within the transverse foramina of the cervical transverse processes. It lies in close proximity to the zygapophyseal joints posterolaterally and to the neurocentral joints on its medial side, and may be compromised by any osteophytes that develop from degenerative changes in these joints.

In the third segment, the course of the artery now changes from its vertical direction through the transverse foramina to emerge through the transverse foramen of the atlas. It passes horizontally through the oblique ligament on the atlas in a groove on the upper surface of the posterior arch of the atlas. Here it is relatively fixed between the transverse foramina of C1 and the atlanto-occipital membrane (Bogduk, 1981; Kunnasmaa and Thiel, 1994). In this region, it is in danger of being damaged by movement of the atlas on the axis, as occurs in rotation and/or extension of the head (de Kleyn and Nieuwenhuyse, 1927; Husni and Storer, 1967; Simeone and Goldberg, 1968; Nagler, 1973; Sherman et al, 1981; Danek, 1989; Stevens, 1991; Thiel, 1991; Kunnnasmaa and Thiel, 1994; Refshauge, 1994). These movements may cause arterial damage by stretching or compressing the vertebral artery on the opposite side. This causes a reduction in its flow, so that it can then become obstructed (Brain and Wilkinson, 1967; Thiel, 1991; Kunnasmaa and Thiel, 1994). This may happen following a neck manipulation, or with a subluxation of the joint in rheumatoid arthritis.

In the fourth segment, the artery unites with its opposite number about the level of the foramen magnum as it enters the cranium to become the basilar artery. It also may be compromised here during head extension. When there is marked inequality in the vertebral arteries, the basilar artery supply becomes dependent upon the dominant artery (Kreuger and Okazaki, 1980).

Cervical spondylosis

Cervical spondlyosis may also cause an alteration in the vertebral artery flow in the presence of:

- Osteophytes arising from the neurocentral or zygapophyseal joints that may encroach on the artery in its transverse foramen (Hutchinson and Yates, 1956; Sheehan et al, 1960). The alteration in flow becomes more marked with head movement, but it may occur even with the head in the neutral position.
- Kinking and distortion of the vertebral artery.

Patients with cervical spondylosis may have vertebrobasilar symptoms such as vertigo, but without any direct evidence of vertebral artery compression. The cause is unknown, but it may be due to an associated hypomobility lesion or related to alterations in postural reflexes.

Trauma

Vertigo and other symptoms may occur after either direct trauma to the neck or more commonly after indirect trauma due to motor-vehicle accidents, when dizziness is a common complaint (*see* Chapter 16).

Rheumatoid arthritis

Patients with rheumatoid arthritis involving the upper cervical spine may also complain of vertigo. It may follow atlanto-axial subluxation with distortion of the vertebral artery, surgery (Rogers et al, 1994) or, more rarely, it may be produced by occlusion of the vertebral artery (Webb et al, 1968).

Cervical vertigo

Vertigo due to a cervical lesion was first described by Barré (1926), whose original theory, that a lesion of the cervical sympathetic nerves was responsible, has long been discarded. The term 'cervical vertigo' was first used by Ryan and Cope (1955) to describe a relatively uncommon cause of vertigo and nystagmus in patients with neck pain. Vertigo was relieved with the use of a collar. Wing and Hargrave-Wilson (1974) reviewed 80 patients, mostly women between the ages of 40 and 60 years, who had no history of neck trauma, who developed cervical vertigo and in whom the only abnormal finding was a hypomobility lesion of the upper three cervical joints. They reported that their cases responded well to neck manipulation.

Clinical features

Patients describe vertigo with rotary movements of objects and a sense of falling to one side. Nausea or vomiting, coming on in attacks and lasting a variable length of time, is almost always present. Other symptoms include unsteadiness, diplopia, blurring of vision and facial paraesthesia, and nystagmus is usually present. Attacks may be brought on by sudden changes in head position, and often occur on looking up, reversing a car, after changing a position that has been maintained for some time, or getting out of bed in the morning. There may be a short latent period between the neck and head movement and the onset of vertigo.

The essential clinical feature is the demonstration of a hypomobility lesion, with restriction in the range of passive intervertebral movements in one or more of the upper three cervical vertebrae. The restriction may involve either rotation, flexion, extension or lateral flexion, and is usually associated with spasm and tenderness in the upper cervical muscles.

Mechanism

In patients with cervical hypomobility lesions, the restriction in movement may cause a disturbance of normal proprioception, which is made worse on neck movements or after a sustained movement towards the affected side. Also, alterations in the proprioceptive impulses that arise with stretching musculoskeletal structures in the upper cervical spine could produce vertigo (Cope and Ryan, 1959). The upper cervical joints are richly supplied with mechanoreceptors responsible for joint, ligament and muscle proprioception, and impulses from them provide tonic neck-righting reflexes, of major importance in normal balance control (deJong et al, 1977; Abrahams, 1981; Richmond, 1988). They are carried along nerve fibres that connect to centres in the brain stem. Stimulation of the muscles supplied by C1 and C2, but not by C3–C5, causes nystagmus in humans (Vidal et al, 1982).

Vertebral artery testing

Testing of the vertebrobasilar system is part of the general examination of the cervical spine (*see* Chapter 13), but it becomes even more necessary if there are any symptoms that could be attributed to it (Australian Physiotherapy Association, 1988). It is also important to perform these tests before any neck treatment is undertaken, but most especially before any manual therapy. The tests may provide an indication that these procedures should not be carried out, although they cannot guarantee that no untoward effects could eventuate following any treatment. The following tests are carried out as a routine, while enquiring with each one whether or not any vertigo or other

related symptoms are produced. If any test does so, the head is immediately returned to the resting position. If pain or stiffness restricts full rotation or extension of the cervical spine, assessment of the artery cannot then be complete.

With the patient standing, first test one side and then the other. The head is turned from side to side through a full range. The test is repeated while holding the head steady, and the trunk is twisted fully from side to side while the head and feet remain stationary. With the patient first seated, test one side and then the other, followed by sustained rotation. The head is rotated to one side and maintained there for at least 10 seconds. Extension is added and the position is maintained for at least 10 seconds, followed by sustained extension. Gentle overpressure is applied for 10 seconds.

If these tests are negative, further tests are carried out with the patient supine and with the head and neck extended over the end of the couch. Nystagmus is looked for at the conclusion of each test. The sustained rotation position is maintained for at least 10 seconds. Sustained rotation with extension is added. Extension is sustained for 10 seconds.

Neck pain

Neck pain due to a mechanical derangement of a cervical intervertebral joint is usually localized to one side only. The essential clinical finding is a painful restriction of the active and passive range of movement in certain directions only. The common pattern is a restriction of extension and lateral flexion and rotation towards the painful side. Less commonly, movements away from the painful side are restricted, and only rarely is flexion restricted. Ancillary tests using overpressure, sustained pressure or the quadrant position may reproduce the pain. Passive intervertebral joint movements are restricted in range, and should reproduce pain. Tenderness and a sensation of thickening may be found over interspinous ligaments in the midline or over the zygapophyseal joints, and tender painful areas with palpable spasm are found around the scapula on the affected side.

There are no abnormal neurological signs. X-rays are consistent with aging changes alone. Mobilization and/or manipulative techniques are the treatment of choice in patients with a cervical hypomobility lesion involving the neck and referred pain.

Torticollis

Torticollis is a descriptive title for a lateral deformity of the cervical spine. The most common form is an acute torticollis, also called an acute wry neck, which may need to be differentiated from several other causes of torticollis that have similar clinical presentations.

Acute torticollis

This common, painful deformity usually occurs in young females aged from about 15 to 25 years, who present with unilateral neck pain and deformity. The onset is usually sudden, and the patient often awakes with neck pain in the morning or during the night. Alternatively, the neck becomes painfully 'stuck' during a sudden spontaneous movement during the day. The neck is flexed to one side and the patient is unable to return the head to its normal position, and any attempts to do so will exacerbate the pain. The unilateral pain is felt on the convex side of the curve, and rarely may radiate either up the neck or down into the interscapular region. There are no neurological symptoms or signs.

Examination reveals that the head and neck are held to one side in lateral flexion with a slight degree of rotation and flexion. The neck is usually flexed away from the painful side. Both active and passive movements are painfully limited, the usual pattern being restriction of lateral flexion and rotation towards the painful side and loss of extension. The most painful and restricted movement is to attempt to return the lateral flexion back towards the painful side. The passive intervertebral movements and accessory movements are always found to be limited by pain and marked spasm.

The severity of the attacks may vary, and minor degrees of this condition can also occur. Its underlying pathology is not known, although the natural history and the age of onset would seem to rule out disc degeneration as its cause. This condition represents a mechanical derangement of intervertebral joint movement in which the zygapophyseal joint is the most likely site of restriction. It may, however, need to be differentiated from disc prolapse or destructive or traumatic disorders of the cervical spine.

Management

Acute torticollis is best treated with mobilization techniques. These techniques are performed by a lateral gliding away from the painful side, to produce restoration of the normal movement. Most patients usually require a few treatments and manipulation is rarely needed.

Congenital (infantile) torticollis

This deformity, more common in boys, is usually apparent soon after birth, when a hard lump, the so-called sternomastoid tumour, may be visible in that muscle. A lateral flexion deformity of the neck develops due to contracture of the sterno-mastoid muscle with limitation of neck movement. It may be caused by ischaemia following birth trauma, such as a difficult labour due to the intrauterine position (Chen and Au, 1994). As the infant grows, the muscle fails to elongate and facial asymmetry may develop. The hard, cord-like fibrous tissue that replaces the muscle may cause the degree of rotation to become increased (Singer et al, 1994). CT and MRI may be used to demonstrate the increased fibrous tissue (Singer et al, 1994).

Treatment consists of daily muscle stretching and overcorrection, undertaken at first by a physiotherapist, who can then teach the procedure to the parents. This is usually successful, but if it is not, surgery may be indicated (Chen and Au, 1994).

Traumatic torticollis

Children may develop torticollis after a rotational subluxation of the atlanto-axial joint, which may be idiopathic or follow minor trauma or an upper respiratory infection. The posture of the head is typical, but X-ray changes are difficult to interpret (Grogaard et al, 1993), and CT or MRI are more of a help (Bredenkamp and Maceri, 1990; Scapinelli, 1994). Fractures or fracture dislocations of the cervical spine may present with a similar clinical picture and need to be excluded by X-ray. Treatment consists of manipulation under general anaesthetic followed by immobilization.

Spasmodic torticollis

This rare but most distressing condition (van Herwaarden et al, 1994) is a focal form of dystonia in which the patient suffers recurrent attacks of rotation or lateral flexion of the head. It may come on at any age (Greene et al, 1995), more commonly in women, and a family history may be present. It was previously considered to be a form of hysterical torticollis, although the attacks are sufficiently different not to cause confusion.

Management consists of injections of Botulinum toxin type A , which provide the most benefit (Blackie and Lees, 1990; Hughes, 1994). It is injected intramuscularly every three to four months, producing a chemical denervation by blocking the release of acetycholine at the neuromuscular junction (Hughes, 1994). Many other treatments have previously been advocated. Splinting with collars, muscle relaxants, manipulations and surgery, including division of peripheral nerves (Braun and Richter, 1994) or the accessory nerve, have all been tried without any success.

Hysterical torticollis

Hysterical torticollis, with its repetitive tic-like movements, is rare, but is usually easy to diagnose. The patient usually forcibly hunches his shoulders while laterally flexing the head to one side and the neck muscles can be felt to be actively and rigidly contracted.

16 Whiplash injuries

Motor vehicle accidents involving either a rear-end or a head-on collision can cause considerable trauma to the neck. Although fractures or dislocations may occur, injuries involve mainly the soft tissues, ligaments, joint capsules, discs and muscles. The term 'whiplash' was first used by Crowe in 1928, although he subsequently stated that he regretted its widespread acceptance. One problem is that it has no pathological connotation, but with its strong emotional overtones it has now become firmly entrenched in medical, lay and legal minds. Further, it is not an accurate description of the mechanism of injury, because the action of the neck differs from that of a whip. Since the neck damage occurs as the result of the abruptly forced stopping, alternative terminology such as 'deceleration injury', or 'whiplash syndrome' (MacNab, 1971b) or 'whiplash associ-

ated disorders' (Spitzer et al, 1995) might also be preferable.

Whiplash does not constitute a single disorder, but is a constellation of disorders with varying degrees of severity. The Quebec Classification, based on the scientifically admissible studies available, grouped them according to the degree of their symptoms and signs in a scale of 0–4 (Spitzer et al, 1995) (Table 16.1).

Its exact prevalence has not been determined (Barnsley et al, 1994a), but acute neck injuries from motor-vehicle accidents involve about one million people each year (Evans, 1992). The extent of damage that is produced will vary according to whether the collision is rear-end, head-on or side-on, and also to the degree of hyperextension or hyperflexion involved. Hyperextension occurs much more commonly with

Table 16.1 The Quebec classification of whiplash-associated disorders (Spitzer et al, 1995)

Grade	Clinical presentation
0	No complaint about the neck and no physical signs
1	Complaint of neck pain, stiffness and tenderness, and no physical signs
2	Neck complaint and musculoskeletal signs
3	Neck complaint and neurological signs
4	Neck complaint and fracture or dislocation

rear-end collisions and it usually produces the greater degree of injury, since flexion injuries can be limited by the chin hitting the chest.

Rear-end collision

The typical history is that a stationary car is hit from behind by another car, which may be travelling at any rate. The usual sequence of events is that:

1. At impact, the vehicle is suddenly accelerated forwards
2. The front seat is then accelerated forward, taking the lower part of the trunk and shoulders with it, although much more rapidly than the head, which initially does not move from its rest position (Figure 16.1)
3. As the shoulders travel forward, the neck becomes suddenly forcibly hyperextended, until
4. Reflex muscular contraction of the stretched anterior cervical muscles produces flexion of the head and neck
5. This is followed by significant deceleration of the head.

The forces involved are considerable since this sequence all takes place over some 500 milliseconds (Barnsley et al, 1994a). If the car is stationary and is hit by another car from behind, a 40-kg force can be suddenly exerted on the head and neck, and the head can reach an acceleration of 12–15G (Severy et al, 1955;

Bogduk, 1988; Hirsch et al, 1988; Barnsley et al, 1994a).

Degree of injury

The degree of injury is influenced by many factors, including the degree and direction of forces applied, whether the collision is rear-end or head-on, if the head is held in rotation (Sturzenegger et al, 1995), as might happen if the driver were talking to the other front-seat occupant, and the impact causes further rotation and side bending, the angle of the seat, and whether or not a seat belt is worn (Porter, 1989; Bourbeau et al, 1993) or a head rest fitted (Morris, 1989). A seat belt can add a rotational force to the injury, aggravating the damage, especially if a headrest is not fitted (MacNab, 1971b; Kesuib et al, 1985; Deans et al, 1987; Sumchai et al, 1988; Porter, 1989; Newman, 1990; Svensson et al, 1996). A properly fitted headrest can reduce the severity of the injury (Svensson et al, 1996), although in most cars they are not fitted properly. The headrest needs to be in line with the seat, positioned as close as possible to the head, strong enough to resist impact, but yielding enough to avoid rebound. If the seat is broken, less damage may be produced (MacNab, 1971b). The degree of damage to the neck can be positively correlated with crash severity (Ryan et al, 1993), although it may be mitigated by awareness of the impending collision (Ryan et al, 1993). It is an advantage if the crash is anticipated and the muscles braced, as ligament damage is greater with the muscles relaxed (Dvorak, 1988a).

Injuries

A rear-end collision can result in injuries to several neck structures.

Soft tissues

Hyperextension of the neck results in injuries to the soft tissues (Hohl, 1974; Barnsley et al, 1994a), while compression forces applied to the

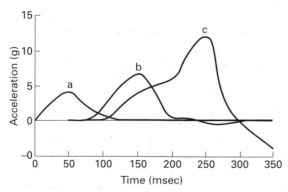

Figure 16.1

posterior soft tissue may include ligament tears, especially of the anterior longitudinal ligament (Davis et al, 1991), tears of the neck muscles (Jonsson et al, 1991) or haematoma involving especially the sternomastoid muscle. Diagnosis may be difficult, although ultrasound may be a good diagnostic tool for muscle injuries.

Zygapophyseal joints

Injuries to the zygapophyseal joints are common (Barnsley et al, 1995). At postmortem, contusions, haemarthrosis, fractures of the tips of the facets, and compression fracture of the articular column are seen (Jonsson et al, 1991; Taylor and Finch, 1993). Fractures may be occult (Abel, 1975; Binet et al, 1977; Woodring and Goldstein, 1982; Jonsson et al, 1991), and may result in subsequent degenerative joint changes (Watkinson et al, 1991). Chronic pain in these joints has been investigated by the use of selective blocks to the joints, and from 25 to 62 per cent of subjects were found to be suffering zygapophyseal joint pain (Aprill et al, 1990; Aprill and Bogduk, 1992; Barnsley and Bogduk, 1993; Barnsley et al, 1993a,b). A prevalence of 60 per cent was found by Lord et al (1996), who looked specifically at post-traumatic chronic zygapophyseal joint pain.

Intervertebral discs

Injuries to the discs are also common, and more than one disc may be involved. Three main types of injury have been described (Taylor and Kakulas, 1991; Taylor and Finch, 1993; Taylor and Twomey, 1993).

1. The most common is a rim lesion, which is a transverse tear near the anterior vertebral rim, caused by distraction and shear during the sudden extension (Davis et al, 1991)
2. The posterior portion of the disc is compressed, contused and may be ruptured (Jonsson et al, 1994)
3. Another characteristic lesion, avulsion of the disc from the vertebral endplate, may occur, especially in adolescents (MacNab, 1971b; Davis et al, 1991; Jonsson et al, 1991).

A complication of disc injury is that the incidence of disc degeneration and spondylosis are increased as a consequence (MacNab, 1971b; Hohl, 1989; Davis et al, 1991; Watkinson, et al, 1991).

Other injuries

Temporomandibular joint injury may occur as the mouth is flung open and then forcibly shut (Weinberg and Lapointe, 1987; Epstein, 1992; Brooke and Lapointe, 1993; Kronn, 1993; Benoliel et al, 1994; Magnusson, 1994), although it is not certain how often it occurs (Heise et al, 1992).

Injury to the vertebral artery and its sympathetic nerve supply may be the cause of a range of eye, ear and vestibular symptoms.

Clinical findings

Neck pain is felt as a muscular pain soon after the accident, although it is not necessary to experience severe pain immediately, and it usually becomes worse on the following day (Jonsson et al, 1994). Neck pain and stiffness then progressively worsen, often radiating up into the head or down across the shoulders into the arms, although not commonly felt in more distal sites. The patient may be most unwilling to move the neck, and marked muscle spasm can be detected. The anterior neck muscles are often involved, causing pain and stiffness, which can interfere with activities such as raising the head from the pillow in the morning. Symptoms may be influenced by age, sex, and the presence of any degenerative changes in the spine before the accident.

Headache is one of the most common symptoms (Balla and Karnaghan, 1987; Radanov et al, 1992, 1993), and may be the main reason for protracted disability (Radanov et al, 1993). Vertigo may develop (Dvorak et al, 1989; Bring and Westman, 1991; Chester, 1991; Pennie and Agambar, 1991; Magnusson, 1994), and three theories have been proposed to explain it: sympathetic nerve involvement, vertebral artery damage, or abnormality in the neck reflexes. Investigations, including electronystagmography, may be necessary (Pang, 1971; Rubin, 1973; Chester, 1991; Oosterveld et al, 1991).

Cognitive complaints, such as loss of attention or impaired memory, are not uncommon (Schwartz et al, 1987; Yarnell and Rossie, 1988; Olsnes, 1989; Kischka, et al, 1991; Radanov et al, 1992; Radanov and Dvorak, 1996), although follow-up studies detailing their persistence are rare (Ettlin et al, 1992; Radanov and Dvorak, 1996). Imaging techniques such as PET or SPECT may increase their recognition (Radanov and Dvorak, 1996). Symptoms may also be related any associated head injury.

Nerve root compression has been described (Jonsson et al, 1994), although it is not common (Keith, 1986; Tamura, 1989; Newman, 1990), even in the presence of cervical spondylosis (Newman, 1990). Decrease in the sagittal width of the spinal canal correlates with the likelihood of developing neurological symptoms (Eismont et al, 1984; Pettersson et al, 1995). Paraesthesia along the ulnar border of the hand could be related to thoracic outlet involvement (Bring and Westman, 1991; Pennie and Agambar, 1991), with a reflex spasm of the scalene muscles (Magnusson, 1994).

Other symptoms (Hildingsson et al, 1989; Claussen and Claussen, 1995), including tinnitus, visual disturbances, hoarseness, dysphagia, Horner's syndrome, or a strange feeling of uncertainty or depression, may be present. They have been presumed to be due to an autonomic nervous system disturbance (Tamura, 1989).

Diagnosis

Diagnosis rests upon a detailed history regarding the mechanism of injury, including a description of the force of impact, the speed of the cars, the damage they sustained, damage to the seat, seat moorings or steering wheel, whether or not a seat belt was being worn or an air bag in place, details of related injuries, such as lacerations or bruising, concussion, whether knocked unconscious, and for how long.

X-rays taken soon after the accident are usually unhelpful (Pearce, 1989), as they are most likely to be normal for the patient's age (Miles et al, 1988), and routine X-rays do not demonstrate

soft tissue changes. Nonetheless, they are needed to exclude any associated bone damage (Abel, 1975; Maimaris et al, 1988; Davis et al, 1993). Special views may be necessary to demonstrate zygapophyseal joint fractures, and flexion–extension views may be indicated to reveal any segmental cervical spine instability (Dvorak et al, 1988b). Bone damage is best demonstrated by CT or bone scan. MRI is not a great help in demonstrating the soft tissue changes (Schippel and Robinson, 1986; Davis et al, 1991), although it may be indicated with persistent symptoms (Jonsson et al, 1994), if disc injury is suspected or if neural structures are involved (Goldberg et al, 1988; Davis et al, 1991).

Management

Initial care

Management remains difficult and controversial, as improvement may be slow (Pearce, 1989) and uncertain (Gargan and Bannister, 1994), and there is no simple way to estimate prognosis (Norris and Watt, 1983).

Reassurance to patients is most important (Newman, 1990). Most studies now agree that in most patients, whiplash is a relatively benign condition, and the majority of patients will recover (Deans et al, 1987; Maimaris et al, 1988; Hohl, 1989). Most of this recovery takes place over the first three months (Deans et al, 1987; Barry, 1992; Pearce, 1994), but the longer it takes, the poorer the prognosis becomes (Gargan and Bannister, 1990).The patient can be informed that the injury usually involves soft tissues whose natural process is one of repair, although it may take some time to complete. Pain relief is also important, and may be helped by rest from any activities known to provoke pain, and suitable analgesics given in appropriate doses. Sedation, muscle relaxants and heat (Foley-Nolan et al, 1992) are of little or no value, although antidepressant tablets taken at night may help with pain and sleep. Manual methods including traction, mobilization, manipulation and exercises are contraindicated at this stage.

A collar may be worn. Although it is not capable of providing complete immobilization of the neck, it can prevent sudden movements (Huston, 1988) and does provide a degree of pain relief. It should be fitted by and adjusted by a physiotherapist, usually as a soft or moulded collar with the neck maintained in a non-painful posture, typically either in slight flexion or neutral (Pennie and Agambar, 1990). Unfortunately, it is often fitted in neck extension, which can cause increased pain (Pennie and Agambar, 1990). A collar should be discarded if it produces discomfort or fails to relieve pain. There is no consensus as to how long it should be worn (Pennie and Agambar, 1990). Patients should be weaned off it as soon as possible because prolonged use could delay the time taken for recovery (Mealy et al, 1986; McKinney, 1989; McKinney et al, 1989), and the patient may become psychologically dependent upon it (Balla, 1980).

Subsequent course

The aim at this stage is to mobilize the patient so as to allow a return to full activity as soon as is practicable (Mealy et al, 1986; McKinnney et al, 1989; Pennie and Agambar, 1990; Evans, 1992; Jonsson et al, 1994). Patients should be advised that pain should ultimately settle, provided forced or extreme neck movements are avoided, although complete control of pain is often unlikely for some time. They are also advised on how to live within the means of the altered spinal mechanics; and that pain associated with daily activities does not necessarily represent any worsening of the underlying condition. The collar should now be used only intermittently, such as when the patient is engaged in activities known to produce pain or at the end of the day.

Maitland mobilization techniques with posteroanterior pressure may be used at this stage of management, provided they do not exacerbate pain. These techniques have been shown to be a help in one prospective trial, although it contained only a few patients (Mealy et al, 1986). Forcible manipulation is never indicated. Isometric neck exercises are taught and performed each day, within the limits of pain. Pain relieving modalities such as TENS or acupuncture are always worth a trial for pain relief. Injection of local anaesthetic and cortico-

steroid into the zygapophyseal joint does not provide any long-lasting benefit, since the joint problem is a traumatic and not an inflammatory one. It has been used in one randomized, controlled trial (Barnsley et al, 1994b), but it was not shown to be a help, and it was not recommended by Spitzer et al (1995). Locally tender areas in muscles or at the musculotendinous attachment to the occiput may be infiltrated with local anaesthetic and corticosteroid injections. Chronic problems may be best helped by referral to a pain clinic with its multidisciplinary approach to improving coping skills.

Late chronic syndrome

Six months after an accident, as the chances of further recovery become limited, a proportion of patients, variously estimated to be between 10 and 25 per cent (Wallis, et al, 1996), might then develop a late whiplash syndrome (Balla, 1980). It is characterized by prolonged suffering and disabling symptoms (Norris and Watt, 1983; Maimaris et al, 1988; Bring and Westman, 1991; Johnssonn et al, 1994), with inevitable involvement in costly insurance litigation (Norris and Watt, 1983; Yarnell and Rossie, 1988; Claussen and Claussen, 1995).

Allthough it is true that whiplash patients do have genuine pathology (Barnsley et al, 1994a), it is also true that some develop psychological problems associated with chronic pain (Merskey, 1993). Almost all activities of daily living involve some degree of neck movement, and if these are painful or if symptoms are widespread, patients may easily become fearful, anxious, depressed and worried about the implications for the future (Kischka et al, 1991; Lee et al, 1993b; Radanov et al, 1991, 1992, 1993). Malingering is most rare, but problems of compensation, secondary gain and exaggerated pain responses can be present (Lee et al, 1993b), and are exacerbated by the differences between the insurers and the plethora of conflicting medicolegal opinions (Claussen and Claussen, 1995).

The paper by Gotten (1956) that threw the legal cat among the compensation pigeons stated that recovery mainly occurred after a payout settlement had been made. This view became commonplace, especially among medical people, although it has often since been refuted (Norris and Watt, 1983; Mendelson, 1982, 1984, 1992; Merskey, 1984; Bogduk, 1988; Maimaris et al, 1988; Pennie and Agambar, 1991; Shapiro and Roth, 1993; Swartzman et al, 1996; Wallis et al, 1996). Swartzman et al (1996) suggest that if litigation is pending, disability is not affected, but that litigants do report more pain. In a prospective trial of 78 patients (Radanov et al, 1991), no psychological factors were found that could predict the persistence of symptoms at six months. A paper from Lithuania (Schrader et al, 1996), where there is no injury insurance or personal compensation, compared 202 whiplash victims with 202 controls, and found that none of them had persistent or disabling symptoms. Their conclusion was that the late symptoms described in other countries are due to the expectation of disability compensation. Pain and psychological symptoms were assessed in 137 whiplash patients, 52 male and 85 female, aged 21–69 years, using SCL-90-R and a McGill Pain Questionairre (Wallis et al, 1996). This yielded a homogeneous pattern of pain response that did not describe any diagnostic personality or neurotic disorder, and concluded that psychological symptoms were secondary to the chronic pain (Wallis et al, 1996).

Surgery

Surgery could be indicated in cases that are classified as Quebec grade 4 (Spitzer et al, 1995) with fractures or dislocations. Otherwise, in their absence, surgery in the early stages is not indicated. It may subsequently be indicated if instability or neurological deficits develop (Tamura, 1989; Algers et al, 1993; Jonsson et al, 1994).

Prevention

The provision of headrests to the back of car seats has been of some benefit (Svensson et al, 1996), but need to be better made and used as an extension of the seat to provide stability. To prevent any backward movement of the head if the car is hit from behind, they need to project further forward than do most presently available headrests do. The use of the newer type of seat belts has not resulted in any decreased incidence of this injury, and indeed could result in increased damage resulting from hyperflexion injuries of the neck.

17 Manual therapy for the cervical spine

Manual therapy techniques used on the cervical spine include mobilization, manipulation and traction.

Manipulation of the cervical spine involves a small but definite risk of damage to the vertebral artery and spinal cord, whereas mobilization techniques are usually very effective and much safer. Accordingly, manipulation is rarely indicated and should never be performed under a general anaesthetic. The incidence of complications following cervical manipulation is difficult to estimate (Assendelft et al, 1996; Hurwitz et al, 1996), as controlled trials are few (Brodin, 1985; Sloop et al, 1982), and no systematic or prospective studies have been undertaken. Moreover, they are probably underreported in the literature (Frisoni and Anzola, 1991; Powell et al, 1993; Assendelft et al, 1996).

The estimates that have been given range from one per 20 000 patients up to one per million cervical manipulations (Powell et al, 1993; Assendelft et al, 1996). In one large series detailing the randomized controlled trials that used conservative management for neck disorders, including manual therapy, only 1.3 per cent (16 out of 1254 subjects) had any side effects or increase in symptoms, and no serious complications or deaths were reported (Gross et al, 1996). Another survey of more than two million treatments (Dvorak and Orelli, 1985) found 1255 complications of cervical manipulation with no deaths, no patients required surgery, and vertigo was the most frequent complaint. Based on Canadian insurance estimates, the risk of developing serious injury is estimated to be 5–10 per 10 million manipulations, with the risk for major neurological impairment between 3 and 6 per million manipulations (Hurwitz et al, 1996). The risk of death was given as less than 3 per 10 million manipulations (Hurwitz et al, 1996).

The major complication of manipulation is damage to the vertebrobasilar artery which may result in brainstem dysfunction or death (Lee et al, 1995b). The course of the vertebral artery is described in Chapter 15. It is most vulnerable to damage in its third segment during neck movements. This occurs, usually on rotation, as a shearing force is produced at the atlanto-axial joint, as the range of neck rotation, of the order of 35–45 degrees, is greatest here (see Chapter 11). As the atlas on one side pivots on the atlanto-axial joint, the opposite side moves anteriorly. This allows the contralateral artery to be kinked, commencing at about 35 degrees of rotation, and it can become markedly affected at about 45 degrees. Damage may follow a sudden abrupt turning of the neck, with or without its being manipulated (Sherman et al, 1981).

The vascular accidents most commonly reported relate to the vertebrobasilar system, tend to occur more commonly in younger patients (Miller and Burton, 1974; Kreuger and Okazaki, 1980), and are most common after chiropractic manipulations (Frumkin and Baloh,

1990; Lee et al, 1995b). An acute intimal tear in the endothelial surface of the artery is produced, so that blood can track into the arterial wall, leading to its dissection and to thrombus formation. Other predisposing vascular disorders, including atheroma, hypertension, or congenital lesions such as a single vertebral artery, may occur, although they are not commonly found in these cases (Teasell and Marchuk, 1994). When there is marked inequality in the vertebral arteries, the basilar artery supply becomes dependent upon the dominant artery (Kreuger and Okazaki, 1980). Although carotid artery damage is much less common than vertebral artery damage (Beatty, 1977; Hart and Easton, 1983), it may also occur following neck rotation and results in a reduced carotid blood flow.

The first report of ischaemic brainstem damage following cervical manipulation was of two patients who died within a day following chiropractic manipulation (Pratt-Thomas and Berger, 1947). Since then, there have been many reports, mainly single case reports, in the literature. In a detailed literature review (Assendelft et al, 1996), 165 vertebrobasilar accidents, 13 other cerebral complications and 39 deaths were recorded. In an earlier review of 139 cases of cerebrovascular accidents following cervical manipulation (Kunnasmaa and Thiel, 1994), approximately half of the patients were considered to have had an underlying neck abnormality that predisposed them to arterial damage. However, whether these abnormalities provided any causal relationship was not clear, and could well be a rationalization.

Symptoms are usually brought on immediately after the manipulation, although in some 20 per cent their onset may be delayed or symptoms may be only mild. Problems that have been described include vertigo, transient loss of consciousness, dysarthria, paralysis, quadraparesis, nausea and vomiting, visual disturbances or loss of vision, stroke and death (Kreuger and Okazaki, 1980). Wallenberg's syndrome (lateral medullary infarction) was described in four patients (Frumkin and Baloh, 1990). Injuries to other structures (Patijn, 1991) include bone, disc or cord damage, meningeal haematoma, compression neuropathy, and diaphragmatic palsy (Sivakumaran and Wilsher, 1995).

Controlled trials

Seven controlled clinical trials dealing with acute and chronic mechanical neck pain, and excluding whiplash injuries, that have used manipulation and mobilization have been reported (Nordemar and Thorner, 1981; Sloop et al, 1982; Howe et al, 1983; Brodin, 1985; Cassidy et al, 1992a,b; Koes et al, 1992, 1993). Ancillary treatments were also used in some trials. However, they have in general demonstrated some increase in mobility and decrease of pain, especially in the short-term. No side effects were reported. Nevertheless, the number of trials and the number of their patients are small, so no definite result can be reached (Hurwitz et al, 1996). There is also obviously a need for more and larger trials to be carried out.

Manual therapy techniques

These may be either: mobilization; manipulation; or traction, and techniques may differ between the upper and the lower cervical spine.

Mobilization

Mobilization of the upper cervical spine

In the upper cervical spine the three main techniques used are: longitudinal movement; posteroanterior central pressure; and posteroanterior unilateral pressure. The main indications for these techniques are unilateral upper cervical pain or head pain arising from C1–C2.

LONGITUDINAL MOVEMENT
The patient lies supine, head supported over the end of the couch, neck midway between full extension and flexion and the head in a straight line. The therapist stands at the end of the couch, supporting the head in the right hand with fingers spread out over the patient's occiput to behind the left ear and the thumb placed behind the right ear. The therapist grasps the patient's chin with the left hand, with the forearm alongside the patient's face (Figure 17.1).

An oscillatory movement is produced in the intervertebral joints by a gentle longitudinal pull

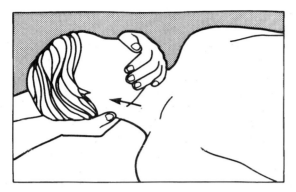

Figure 17.1 Cervical mobilization: longitudinal movement

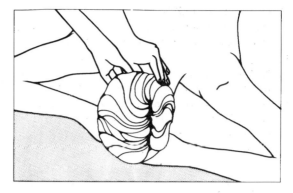

Figure 17.3 Cervical mobilization: posteroanterior unilateral vertebral pressure

elongating the neck. The forearms produce a slight backward movement of the body followed by a controlled relaxation back to the starting position.

POSTEROANTERIOR CENTRAL VERTEBRAL PRESSURE

The patient lies prone with the chin tucked in. The therapist stands at the patient's head with thumb-tips back to back over the vertebra to be mobilized, fingers around the patient's neck (Figure 17.2). The spinous process of C2 is usually easy to palpate but the spinous processes of C1 and C3 are usually difficult to palpate. The oscillatory pressure should be very gentle.

POSTEROANTERIOR UNILATERAL VERTEBRAL PRESSURE

Posteroanterior unilateral pressure applied to C2 with the patient's head kept straight mobilizes the C2–C3 joint (Figure 17.3). If the head is rotated to the left and a similar pressure applied to the left side of C2, the C1–C2 joint is mobilized in rotation. In this position, C1 is fully rotated to the left on C2, so that posteroanterior pressure on the left articular pillar of C2 further increases the rotation.

The patient lies prone with the head turned to the left supported in the palms. The therapist stands at the head with the tips of his or her opposed thumbs against the left articular pillar of C2. The long axis of each thumb is directed posteroanteriorly and tilted slightly towards the head.

Movement produced by the therapist's trunk and arm is transmitted to the thumbs. Posteroanterior pressure against C2 increases the rotation between C1 and C2.

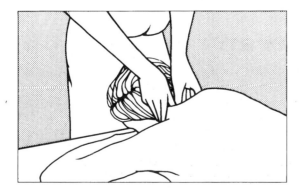

Figure 17.2 Cervical mobilization: posteroanterior central vertebral pressure

Mobilization of the lower cervical spine

Seven techniques are used

LONGITUDINAL MOVEMENT

This is used for most painful cervical conditions and acute torticollis. As it helps the therapist to gain the patient's confidence, it serves as a guide, since patients who improve are likely to respond to other techniques.

The patient lies supine with the head in a neutral position over the end of the couch, supported by the therapist's hands. The therapist grasps the occipital area in his or her right hand

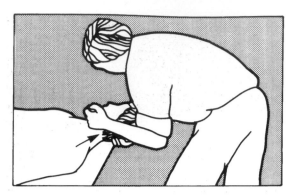

Figure 17.4 Mobilization of the lower cervical spine: longitudinal movement

and supports the chin with the left hand, with the left forearm along the left side of the patient's face (Figure 17.4).

Oscillatory movements elongating the patient's neck are produced at the intervertebral joints by a gentle longitudinal movement of the forearm and body.

POSTERANTERIOR CENTRAL VERTEBRAL PRESSURE
Indications are midline or unilateral pain, especially with muscle spasm.

The patient lies prone, forehead resting on the hands, chin slightly tucked in. The therapist stands at the patient's head, thumbs over the spinous process to be mobilized and fingers straddling the neck (Figure 17.5).

Pressure is applied through the thumbs by movement of the therapist's arms and trunk.

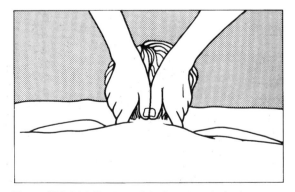

Figure 17.5 Mobilization of the lower cervical spine: posteroanterior central vertebral pressure

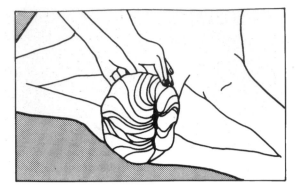

Figure 17.6 Mobilization of the lower cervical spine: posteroanterior unilateral vertebral pressure

POSTEROANTERIOR UNILATERAL VERTEBRAL PRESSURE
This is used for unilateral neck pain.

The patient lies prone with the forehead resting on the hands and the therapist stands to the side of the head with his thumbs back to back on the articular pillar of the side to be mobilized (Figure 17.6).

Oscillatory pressure is directed posteroanteriorly against the articular pillar.

LATERAL FLEXION
This is used for painfully restriction cervical rotation with unilateral pain.

The patient lies supine with head and neck over the end of the couch. To produce lateral flexion to the right, the therapist stands alongside the patient's right shoulder, his or her right arm lying across the shoulder. The patient's head is then laterally flexed. The movement can be localized to one intervertebral level by pressure of the palmar surface of the left index finger against the articular pillar (Figure 17.7).

Oscillatory movements are produced by rocking the hips from side to side with a forward movement of the right side of his pelvis. The head is held firmly to the therapist's body. For the upper cervical regions, the patient's head is held in the neutral flexion–extension position; for the lower cervical regions, the head is held slightly flexed.

TRANSVERSE VERTEBRAL PRESSURE
This is used for cervical pain, especially if unilateral and very localized.

The patient lies prone with the head on the

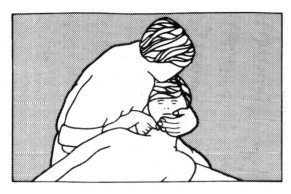

Figure 17.7 Mobilization of the lower cervical spine: lateral flexion

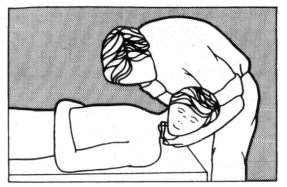

Figure 17.9 Mobilization of the lower cervical spine: rotation

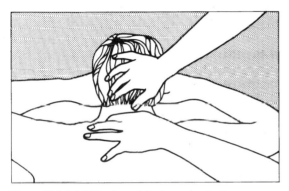

Figure 17.8 Mobilization of the lower cervical spine: transverse vertebral pressure against spinous processes

hands and chin tucked in. The therapist stands on the patient's right side with the pad of his or her thumbs against the right side of the spinous process (Figure 17.8). Gentle pressure is needed since only a small oscillation can be produced.

ROTATION
This is used to treat unilateral neck pain.

The patient lies with head and neck over the end of the couch. To rotate the patient's head to the left, the therapist crouches at the end of the couch, his or her right hand supporting the head, left hand under the chin and left arm lying alongside the head (Figure 17.9).

Rotation of the head is produced by an arm movement using a synchronous action of both hands. For the upper cervical spine, the patient's

neck is held on the same plane as the body; the lower the cervical level to be mobilized the greater the degree of neck flexion necessary.

ANTEROPOSTERIOR UNILATERAL VERTEBRAL PRESSURE
This is performed for pain in the front or side of the neck reproduced by anterpostrior pressures.

The patient lies supine without a pillow to support the head. The therapist stands by the head with both thumbs over the transverse process of the vertebra to be mobilized, fingers spread around the adjacent neck area (Figure 17.10).

The oscillatory anteroposterior pressures are performed by the therapist's arms and trunk. The anterior neck muscles make direct contact with the transverse process rather difficult, so the thumbs must be carefully positioned.

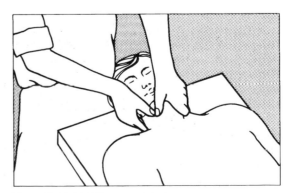

Figure 17.10 Mobilization of the lower cervical spine: anteroposterior unilateral vertebral pressure

Manipulation

Non-specific techniques

ROTATION

The starting position is the same as illustrated in Figure 17.9.

This technique is never performed as a large movement by putting the neck through a full range from the central position. Rather, the head and neck are rotated to the limit of their range and then a quick rotary movement is given through a further 3 degrees.

Specific techniques

ATLANTO-OCCIPITAL JOINT ROTATION

The patient lies supine with the therapist standing towards the left shoulder, with the patient's chin in his or her right hand and the atlas grasped with the left hand. The patient's head is rotated to the right until about 20 degrees short of full rotation (Figure 17.11).

Sudden rotation of the patient's head to the right through a few degrees by the right hand is effected while the left hand rotates the patient's atlas to the left.

Atlanto-axial joint rotation

The patient lies supine, head over the end of the couch. The chin and head are held in the left arm and the head rotated through 40 degrees. C2 is firmly cradled by supporting the left articular pillar with the metacarpophalangeal joint of the index finger and the right transverse process of

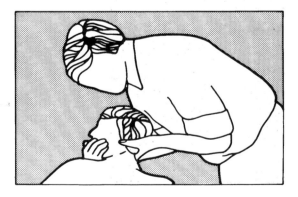

Figure 17.11 Manipulation of the atlanto-occipital joint: rotation

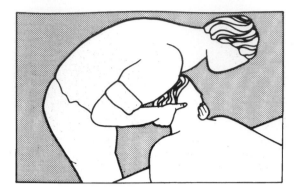

Figure 17.12 Manipulation of the atlanto-axial joint: rotation

C2 supported with the left thumb. The therapist stands behind the head with the left elbow pointed towards the floor (Figure 17.12).

The manipulation is carried out by a small rotary movement of the head to the left by the left hand, together with a small amplitude unilateral posteroanterior thrust against the left side of C2 as it is rotated by the right hand.

Lower cervical spine

LATERAL FLEXION

The patient lies supine with the head over the end of the couch, chin supported by the left arm and the proximal phalanx of the right index finger placed against the articular pillar. The neck is displaced to the left and the head is laterally flexed to the right. The head is next rotated to the left by the left hand until the joint is felt to be at full stretch. The forearm is kept in line with the plane of the zygapophyseal joint (Figure 17.13).

A sudden thrust is given with the right index finger, stretching the zygapophyseal joint, while an equal pressure is applied with the left arm on the head and neck.

ROTATION

The patient lies supine with the neck and head beyond the end of the couch. The therapist, at the head of the couch, places his or her right hand under the head with the palmar surface of the index finger against the articular pillar of the vertebra to be manipulated. The chin is grasped

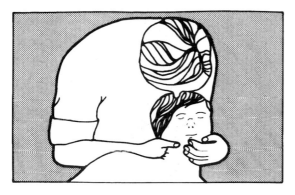

Figure 17.13 Manipulation of the lower cervical spine: lateral flexion

- The presence of structural abnormalities in the cervical spine, whether due to disease, trauma or congenital anomalies
- The site of pain. With the lower cervical spine the neck is positioned more towards flexion; for the upper spine, it is positioned in the neutral position
- The rate of subsequent improvement.

Whether the patient sits or lies down is governed by his or her comfort and the ease of administration. In general, traction in neutral for the upper cervical spine is best given with the patient sitting, and traction in flexion for the lower cervical spine with the patient lying down. Traction may be given either in the neutral position or in flexion.

by the left hand and the head is comfortably supported. The head is turned to the left by the left hand until the articular pillar is felt to move under the right index finger. The vertebrae above the index finger are held together so that they all move as a unit with the patient's head (Figure 17.14).

The patient's head is sharply rotated to the left through a tiny range with the therapist's right index finger emphasizing the movement at the one joint being manipulated.

Cervical traction

The joint to be treated is positioned approximately midway between its position of flexion and extension. This is further influenced by:

Traction in neutral

The patient sits comfortably slumped in a chair, with the back and arms supported and the head halter adjusted so that traction lifts the head off the neck in a neutral position. The occipital strap is used to lift under the occiput, not under suboccipital structures (Figure 17.15).

After determining the site and severity of symptoms, the therapist places the tip of the index or

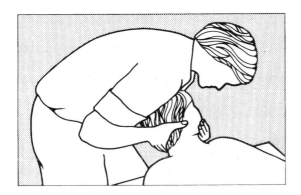

Figure 17.14 Manipulation of the lower cervical spine: rotation

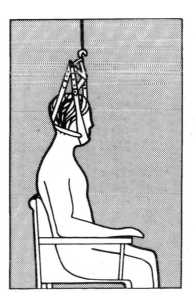

Figure 17.15 Cervical traction in neutral: starting position

middle finger against the side of the interspinous space of the affected joint. Traction is then applied and relaxed in an oscillatory movement, very gently at first but gradually increasing, until movement in the interspinous space can be felt with the minimum of pressure. Symptoms are reassessed after 10 seconds. Subsequent alterations are influenced if:

- Severe symptoms are completely relieved. The pressure is reduced by half for less than five minutes to minimize any exacerbation
- Symptoms have been partly relieved. Traction should be maintained at this level for five minutes with severe pain and 10 minutes for more moderate degrees of pain
- Symptoms have not altered; the amount of traction can be increased by a small amount for 10 minutes
- Symptoms are made slightly worse, then the weight is halved.

If symptoms persist, the head–neck relationship is changed by altering the harness or sitting position before reapplying gentler traction. If symptoms still persist one of two courses remain: either traction is discontinued or gentle traction is maintained for up to five minutes. If this produces some improvement, traction can be continued, but if symptoms become worse, traction is discontinued.

The position chosen for treatment is governed not by the relief of symptoms but by the movement produced at the relevant intervertebral joint. The amount and duration of traction are guided by any alteration of symptoms. Whether traction is indicated and whether the position, weight and duration chosen are correct is indicated by any change in symptoms or signs. When traction has been applied in the chosen position, it should not be altered in an attempt to influence symptoms.

Method of progression

Treatment is guided by a continuous reassessment of symptoms and signs. Changes in techniques, as with mobilization, are guided by the patient's movements after treatment and also by the improvement between treatments. With severe pain, treatment should be progressed very slowly by small increases in duration of the traction rather than increases in weight. With little or no reaction, the weight also can be increased gradually. However, if initial symptoms are moderate, progression can be both by poundage and by duration. The total treatment time is rarely more than 15 minutes, since longer periods do not produce better results. Traction should be discarded after four treatments if symptoms and signs remain unchanged.

The amount of traction given is governed by assessing symptoms and signs before, during and after traction. The application of pressure is first governed by the movement at the intervertebral segment being treated: 4 kg traction applied to a 102-kg patient will produce less movement than in a 42-kg patient.

Traction in flexion

The patient lies comfortably on the back, one or two pillows supporting the neck in slight flexion so that the joint being treated is midway between flexion and extension. Hips and knees are flexed to rest the lower back. The halter is applied and the occipital strap positioned. Because the head is rested on this strap on the pillows, it will remain in position while the side straps and chin strap are being adjusted. To ensure that the harness is correctly adjusted, the therapist applies some traction via the spreader bar while ensuring that the head–neck relationship remains constant (Figure 17.16).

The operator alternately applies and relaxes pressure through the pulley system while

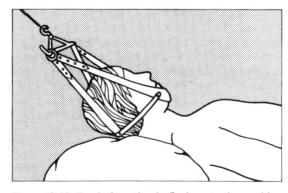

Figure 17.16 Cervical traction in flexion: starting position

watching and palpating for movement at the relevant intervertebral level. Pressure is sustained at the lowest value needed to produce joint movement. After approximately 10 seconds symptoms are reassessed. Subsequent treatment is as described for traction in neutral.

Complications

- Discomfort or pain in the temporomandibular joints may be relieved by altering the position of the straps or placing a pad between the molars. However, traction of this magnitude should not be required
- Thoracic or lumbar pain may be induced by cervical traction
- Traction in neutral may induce nausea usually only after prolonged or strong traction or with excessively apprehensive patients
- Traction should be released slowly and the patient allowed to rest for a time, as some may feel giddy on its release
- Traction in flexion can produce a burning feeling or pain in the suboccipital area; if so, the harness is adjusted to extend the head

slightly on the upper neck while maintaining the neck in flexion.

Indications

- Traction is of value in almost all cases of cervical joint pain. However, the rate of improvement is slower than with mobilization
- Patients with arm pain and restriction of lateral flexion and rotation of the neck towards the painful side are best treated by traction in flexion
- Traction is the treatment of choice with recent neurological changes
- When intervertebral joint movement is restricted, traction may be ineffective unless preceded by a manipulation
- Intermittent variable cervical traction can be applied in neutral or in flexion for similar indications, using the same weights and duration of treatment. But with severe symptoms, the amount of movement should be decreased with longer hold and rest periods. As symptoms abate, the rest period can be reduced and the hold period maintained for approximately three to five seconds.

18 The thoracic spine

Musculoskeletal lesions in the thoracic spine are a common source of pain, which may be felt in any part of the chest wall, and symptoms may mimic those of various visceral, especially cardiac, disorders. No detailed studies of its prevalence and incidence have been carried out, but in one large emergency room series, one-quarter of admissions with chest pain had a musculoskeletal cause (Karlson et al, 1991). Two other series (Levine and Mascette, 1989; Wise et al, 1992) found definite evidence of musculoskeletal involvement in 11 and 16 per cent of patients, respectively.

Thoracic and chest wall pain

Thoracic pain may arise from either visceral diseases, which are not discussed further here, or musculoskeletal disorders, which are a common and important source of thoracic pain (Wise et al, 1992; Wise, 1994), and may at times closely mimic the pain of visceral diseases, such as cardiac (Epstein et al, 1979; Peyton, 1983; Assey, 1993; Disla et al, 1994; Martin et al, 1996), pulmonary (Donat, 1987) or abdominal diseases (Maigne, 1980; Richter, 1991; Benahamou et al, 1993; Whitcomb et al, 1995), leading to incorrect diagnosis and treatment. Further confusion may arise if breathing, coughing or alteration in posture aggravates the pain. It is obviously important not to miss the diagnosis of any of these visceral disorders, but it is also important to recognize a musculoskeletal disorder, if present, as a cause of chest or chest wall pain, for it is so often amenable to appropriate treatment.

Two of the most common causes of musculoskeletal chest pain are a referred pain from the thoracic or lower cervical intervertebral joints and a thoracic hypomobility lesion. To confirm the first diagnosis it is necessary to reproduce pain by testing the appropriate spinal joints. Mobilization of the appropriate spinal segment should then improve the pain. However, in the older age groups degenerative changes may involve both musculoskeletal structures and the coronary arteries, and so more difficulty may be experienced in determining the exact cause of pain. Moreover, it is not uncommon that a patient who has had a previous coronary occlusion will subsequently develop chest wall pain. After finding no evidence of any current cardiac disease, the chest wall pain will invariably be ignored or labelled as being psychogenic. However, in these patients, it may often be possible to find a thoracic segmental hypomobility lesion, and treatment with appropriate mobilizations should relieve the pain. The reason that this common type of hypomobility lesion develops is not understood, although abnormal viscerosomatic reflexes have been postulated.

Examination of the thoracic spine

First carry out an inspection: observe the patient's build, posture, bony contours, deformities, and gait. Then test active movements: flexion; extension; lateral flexion; and rotation. Observe range, rhythm and any reproduction of pain.

Auxiliary tests include: overpressure; repeating movements quickly; sustained pressure; cervical spine movements; and neural tension tests.

Test passive movements: passive range at each joint; and accessory movements.

Test costochondral and costovertebral joints, plus intercostal movement, followed by palpation, neurological testing and radiological examination.

Inspection

Spinal deformity due to a kyphosis or a scoliosis, or a combination of the two, is readily apparent on inspection. Kyphosis may be generalized or localized. The most common cause of a generalized, smooth, rounded kyphosis in adolescents is Scheuermann's disease, and in the elderly patients, intervertebral disc degeneration. One or more fractured and collapsed thoracic vertebrae, due to trauma, osteoporosis or a secondary deposit, usually produce a localized kyphosis. Scoliosis is gauged by inspecting the spinal processes, with minor deviations being relatively common. It may be associated with asymmetry of musculoskeletal structures, including the shoulder levels with relative prominence of one scapula and ribcage. With a structural scoliosis these deformities become more prominent on forward flexion.

Active movements

Movements of the thoracic spine form part of a continuous, coordinated pattern with the lumbar spine movements, and so they are assessed together. The patient is tested first while

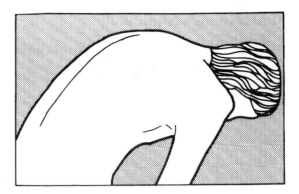

Figure 18.1 Limitation in the range of forward flexion at two levels of the thoracic spine: between about T5 and T8 forward flexion is very limited, whereas between T10 and L1 the movement appears less limited

standing, and asked if any symptoms are experienced in this position. He or she is asked to flex and then extend the spine, followed by lateral flexion and then rotation to both sides. The normal active range of flexion is to approximately 90 degrees, while the normal active range of extension, lateral flexion and rotation is to approximately 30 degrees. Flexion may be measured by the distance the fingertips reach form the floor, and side bending by the distance of the fingers from the knees, at the same time observing the relative movement of the spinous processes and record any loss of range (Figure 18.1). Rotation is tested by bending forward to 45 degrees with the hands behind the head, feet together and rotating fully to right and left. It is further tested while the patient is seated, and the trunk is moved first into flexion and then into extension. Overpressure can also be easily applied in this position to test for any reproduction of pain.

Note is taken of the range of each of these movements, whether or not symptoms are reproduced, disturbances in the normal synchronous rhythm and the presence or not of any muscle spasm.

In thoracic spine hypomobility lesions, the usual pattern is that a painful restriction on lateral flexion and/or rotation to the painful side is associated with a restriction of either flexion or extension.

Auxillary tests

Auxiliary tests include:

- Overpressure, in which small oscillatory movements are applied in each direction at the end of the painless range
- Performing the test movements repeatedly and at an increasing speed
- Application of sustained pressure at the limit of the range of relevant movements for approximately 10 seconds
- The neck movements are tested to determine if thoracic pain is referred from the lower cervical intervertebral joints. However, pain arising in thoracic spinal joints may also be exacerbated on neck flexion.

Passive movement tests

These tests assess:

- The passive range of intervertebral joint movement at each individual joint level by feeling the movement between the adjacent spinal processes
- The accessory movements.

Passive range at individual joints

The passive movements of flexion, extension, lateral flexion and rotation are tested separately in the upper (T1–T4), and lower, (T5–T11), spines.

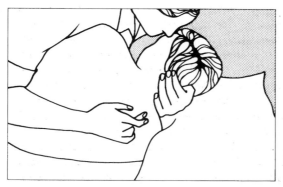

Figure 18.2 Intervertebral movement between T1 and T4 (flexion–extension)

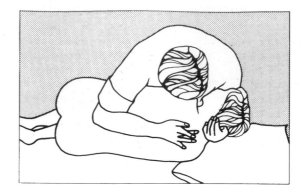

Figure 18.3 Intervertebral movement between T1 and T4 (lateral flexion)

T1–T4 flexion–extension

The patient lies on the right side and the examiner stands in front. The patient's head is grasped by the examiner's left hand and moved into flexion and extension while thoracic intervertebral movement is felt by the middle finger of the right hand placed between the spinous processes (Figure 18.2).

T1–T4 lateral flexion

The patient lies on the right side near the edge of the couch, with the head resting on pillows. The examiner stands facing the patient, the head cradled in his or her left arm. The examiner leans across the patient to palpate the interspinous space and lateral flexion is obtained by lifting the patient's head and neck upward (Figure 18.3).

T1–T4 rotation

The starting position is as above. Rotation is difficult to produce accurately without producing some degree of flexion or lateral flexion, but it may be felt by placing the index finger on the side of the patient's interspinous space. The examiner cradles the patient's head and rotates the lower cervical spine towards him or her by elevating the scapula to its highest point, with counter-pressure applied over the thorax (Figure 18.4).

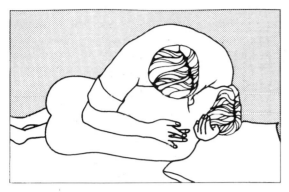

Figure 18.4 Intervertebral movement between T1 and T4 (rotation)

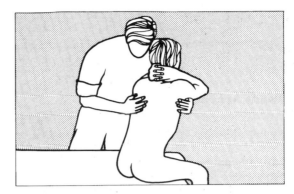

Figure 18.5 Intervertebral movement between T5 and T11 (lateral flexion)

T5–T11 Flexion–extension

This is tested with the patient sitting, hands clasped behind the head. The examiner, standing by the left side of the patient, places his or her left arm under the patient's left upper arm to grasp the right upper arm. The examiner places his or her right hand across the spine just below the level to be tested and, with the pad of the tip of the middle finger in the far side of the interspinous space, palpates between adjacent spinous processes.

To test flexion, the trunk is lowered from the neutral position until movement can be felt under the examiner's right middle finger. The patient is then returned to the neutral position by lifting under the arms, so producing an oscillatory movement through an arc of approximately 20 degrees.

Extension is similarly produced by the examiner assisting trunk extension with the heel and ulnar border of the right hand, and maintaining the pad of his or her middle finger between adjacent spinous processes. Movement at only one joint is examined, so large trunk movements are unnecessary.

T5–T11 lateral flexion

The patient sits with the hands clasped behind the neck. The examiner stands side-on behind the patient's left side and reaches with the left arm to hold behind the patient's right shoulder. He or she grips the patient's trunk firmly between his or her left arm and left side. As the movement extends below T8, this grasp is moved to the lower scapular area. The examiner places the heel of the right hand on the left side of the back and places the tip of the pad of his or her flexed middle finger in the far side of the interspinous space of the joint to be tested (Figure 18.5).

The examiner laterally flexes the patient's trunk towards him or her with the heel of the right hand, and laterally flexes the upper trunk by lifting his or her left arm and pressing downwards with his or her left axilla. Interspinous movement is palpated through the pad of the middle finger.

T11 rotation

This is tested with the patient lying on the right side with hips and knees flexed while the examiner, standing in front of the patient, leans over the patient's trunk and cradles the pelvis between his or her right side and right upper arm. The examiner's forearm is then in line with the patient's spine and his or her hand is placed at the level to be moved. The pad of the right middle finger palpates the undersurface of the interspinous space. The examiner's left hand grasps as far medially as possible over the suprascapular area with the forearm over the sternum (Figure 18.6). The patient's trunk is rotated back and forth repeatedly by the examiner's left forearm and hand through an arc of approximately 25 degrees, and the palpating finger follows the patient's trunk movement. When movement occurs at the joint being examined, the upper spinous process will be felt to press into the pad of the upwardly directed middle finger.

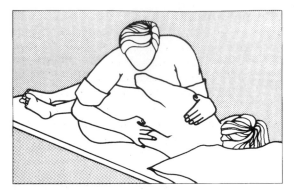

Figure 18.6 Intervertebral movement between T5 and T11 (rotation)

Accessory movements

These passive movements are produced by the pressure of the thumbs against the two accessible bony vertebral processes, the spinous process and the transverse process. Spinous processes are tested using posteroanterior and transverse pressures, which may be varied by angling the direction of the pressure towards the head or feet. This is then followed by posteroanterior pressures against the transverse processes. These tests have been described in detail above for the cervical and lumbar spines.

Costovertebral joints

The costovertebral joints and intercostal movements are tested using an oscillatory posteroanterior pressure applied by the thumbs over the angle of the rib, which can be varied by directing the pressure in a cephalic or caudal direction to reproduce pain.

Palpation

The spinous processes of C7 and T1 are easily palpated. The upper four thoracic spinous processes tend to lie somewhat horizontally, but the next four run obliquely downwards, their tip at the level of the lower border of the subjacent vertebra.

The transverse processes of the thoracic vertebrae are usually readily palpable with the patient lying prone. The region of the costotransverse joint, formed by a facet on the rib articulating with the transverse process, is palpable two finger breadths laterally to a spinous process. The angle of the rib is found at the lateral border of the spinal extensor muscles. The scapula is easily palpable; its spine lies subcutaneously at the level of T3 and its lower angle lies opposite the spine of T7. Anterior structures such as the sterno-clavicular joint, manubrium sterni, ribs and costochondral junctions are also subcutaneous, and so are readily identifiable.

The thoracic spine is palpated for any alteration in bony misalignment, muscle spasm and any localized tenderness, which is best felt over the supraspinous ligaments or to the side of the interspinous space. Tapping sharply with the finger or a percussion hammer on the spinous processes, with the patient standing and fully flexed, may elicit local tenderness over an affected level.

Neurological testing

A full neurological asessment of upper and lower limbs is undertaken, and the sensation in the skin over the dorsal spine is also assessed.

Routine radiological examination

Radiological examination includes a chest X-ray and AP and lateral X-rays of the thoracic spine.

Classification

Classification of musculoskeletal thoracic problems is made according to the structure involved. Thoraic intervertebral disc lesions include: intervertebral disc prolapse; thoracic spondylosis; senile kyphosis; and localized intervertebral disc degeneration. Thoracic hypomobility lesions include the T4 syndrome. Thoracic rheumatological diseases are discussed, followed by discussion of the thoracic joints: costochondral joints (including Tietze's syndrome and slipping rib); costovertebral joints; zygapophyseal joints; manubriosternal joints; sternoclavicular joints; xiphoid process; and scapulothoracic joints. The lower cervical spine, ribs and muscular lesions are also discussed.

Thoracic intervertebral disc lesions

Thoracic intervertebral disc prolapse

This is an uncommon condition, which may occur in either sex (Carson et al, 1971; Benson and Byrnes, 1975; Benjamin, 1983; O'Leary et al, 1984; Arce and Dohrmann, 1985; Ridenour et al, 1993; Schellhas et al, 1994; Wood et al, 1995). Any level of the thoracic spine may be involved (Winter and Siebert, 1993), but it more commonly involves only one disc and that in the lower thoracic spine. Pain may involve one spinal level with a radicular pain, but it may at times be diffuse. Cord compression, with a resultant upper motor neurone lesion in the lower limbs, sensory loss and bladder or bowel symptoms, is the most obvious complication. An accurate neurological assessment, including demonstration of a sensory spinal level, is mandatory. MRI is the best investigative tool, as CT is not so useful in this region. However, similar changes on MRI may also be present in normal people (Awwad et al, 1991; Wood et al, 1995).

Management is generally considered to be surgical (Albrand and Corkill, 1979; Bohlman and Zdeblick, 1988; Otani et al, 1988; Simpson et al, 1993), usually by an endoscopic anterior fusion (McAfee et al, 1995). However, in a retrospective study, only one-quarter of 55 patients was found to require surgery (Brown et al, 1992). Major postoperative complications are common (Wood et al, 1995). At times, at operation, the nuclear material present may be found to be calcified. Disc calcification also occurs in children, is rare, involves the nucleus and presents with severe back pain.

Thoracic spondylosis

Degenerative changes in the thoracic intervertebral discs are similar to those in other spinal areas, with loss of disc space and reactive changes in surrounding structures. Patients with a scoliosis or kyphosis develop similar changes, which occur on the concave side of the curvature.

Patient's present with thoracic pain (Skubic, 1993; Schellhas et al, 1994), usually related to exercise, but it may also be present on lying down. Stiffness is also present, often worse in the morning but wearing off during the day. Nerve root involvement may also be a complication with pain radiating around the chest wall about the line of the rib, and may be associated with sensory changes over the same distribution. Pain may also be referred from the lower thoracic vertebrae into the abdomen as far as the iliac crest (Whitcomb et al, 1995), where it is often misdiagnosed as being due to various intra-abdominal disorders, and patients often undergo repeated and expensive tests to no avail.

The aim of management is to control pain and increase spinal mobility and muscle control. This is achieved by analgesics, pain-relieving modalities, mobilization techniques, and exercises to increase postural control. It is common for patients with thoracic spondylosis to be told, after X-rays have been taken, that they have arthritis of the spine. This will render any patient very difficult to cure, since he or she will now have become convinced that he or she will be permanently crippled in a wheelchair, living a life of unremitting pain. Even worse off are those who come bearing X-rays with arrows pointing to some minor alteration or osteophyte, for it is impossible to cure arrows.

Senile kyphosis

This common postural condition occurs in older patients, and is associated with degenerative changes, sometimes severe, in the mid-thoracic intervertebral discs, with its summit about T7 (Larouche et al, 1995). As a result, the anterior part of the disc and bodies become more compressed, resulting in increased degeneration and osteophytic changes. It needs to be differentiated from similar appearances that occur with osteoporosis and X-rays are helpful as they (Osman et al, 1994) mirror the degenerative changes, with loss of disc space and bony fusion, especially anteriorly.

Senile kyphosis is characterized clinically by rounded shoulders with a forward carriage of the head and development of a dowager's hump. It is often asymptomatic, although some patients may present with severe aching pain, present for many years, worse after activity, disturbing sleep at night, with a tendency to be episodically worse, and difficult to control. Patients may be helped with the use of a brace and back-strengthening exercises (Itoi and Sinaki, 1994).

Localized degenerative disc lesion

This usually involves the lower thoracic spine, as thoracic spine movement is maximal at the thoracolumbar junction. It occurs especially in sports people (Sward et al, 1990a) such as professional golfers or cricketers, or in workers, whose occupation involves repeated thoracic rotation (Figure 18.7). Nerve root involvement with pain radiating around the chest wall follows the line of the ribs, and may be associated with paraesthesia over the same distribution. Pain is made worse by movement, and is often worse on lying down.

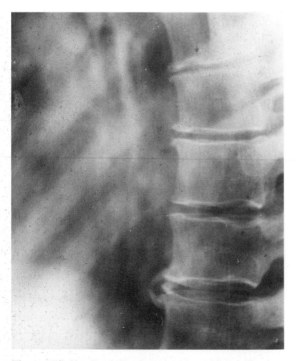

Figure 18.7 Localized disc degeneration with calcification and osteophyte formation

Treatment is often difficult. Rest from the particular activity is necessary, and mobilization and traction, together with some form of back support, are needed.

Thoracic hypomobility syndromes

A hypomobility lesion is relatively common finding in the thoracic spine. Pain arising from these lesions is usually of sudden onset, may be severe at times, and is often aggravated by movement or by breathing, so that it can often be difficult to differentiate from heart or lung disease. It is characterized by pain in several different sites.

- Pain is commonly localized posteriorly to one or other side of the midline. It may be felt over one or several segmental levels, but it radiates out along the chest wall for only a few centimetres.
- Chest wall pain is more common, and it may be felt anywhere around the chest wall. It may be present with or without posterior pain, and is felt to radiate around the chest wall or passing through to the front of the chest. The most common site for this referred pain to be experienced is anteriorly over the region of the costochondral junction. Since a localized lesion of the costochondral joints may also cause similar anterior pain, it may be difficult at times to differentiate the exact cause of the symptoms. In addition, a common cause of persistent chest wall pain after a cardiac infarct or a coronary artery bypass operation is the presence of a thoracic hypomobility lesion. Other causes of costochondral pain need to be differentiated.
- Low back pain may rarely result from referred pain due to a thoracic hypomobility lesion.

Examination

Routine testing of active and passive spinal movements should reveal a limited range, usually painful, of either flexion or extension, combined with a restriction of rotation and/or lateral flexion towards the painful side. The restriction may become evident while these movements are being carried out. The altered movement may also be associated with either a localized area of scoliosis or an arc of pain felt in the mid-range of spinal flexion. The diagnosis is confirmed clinically by testing passive joint movements, in which intervertebral movement in the affected segment is restricted and reproduces the patient's pain. Tenderness over the interspinous ligament and localized muscle spasm to one side of the affected segment help to confirm these findings.

Management

This condition usually responds very well to treatment, especially with mobilization techniques.

- With back, or back plus chest wall pain, mobilization of the affected segment usually produces marked relief after only a few sessions.
- With anterior pain in the costochondral region, treatment is to mobilize the affected thoracic intervertebral joint and assess its effect on the anterior pain. In a proportion of cases, it will also be necessary to inject the locally tender area with local anaesthetic and corticosteroid, for one to three times over several weeks.
- Stretching and strengthening exercises are necessary when pain is relieved to help prevent recurrences.

The T4 syndrome

This refers to a group of diffuse symptoms, of unknown aetiology, associated with the finding of a hypomobility lesion at the T4 level. Pain or a vague sensation of discomfort with paraesthesia or numbness, which does not follow any dermatome pattern, is felt in the arm or posterior neck. A hypomobility lesion at the T4 or T3 level is the only positive sign to be elicited. There is doubt if this condition really exists (Dreyfus, 1994d), and so, if mobilization of the involved area does not relieve the symptoms after a few treatments, the diagnosis should be discarded.

Rheumatological diseases

The thoracic spine is a common site for rheumatological disorders to occur, including:

- Inflammatory diseases such as spondyloarthritis or, rarely, rheumatoid arthritis
- Malignancies, especially secondary deposits (Figure 18.8)
- Metabolic bone diseases such as osteoporosis
- Degenerative changes may be due to ankylosing hyperostosis (DISH) or to Scheuermann's disease
- Infective discitis, due to many organisms, including tuberculosis
- Viral diseases such as herpes zoster or Bornholm's disease.

Spondyloarthitis

The chest wall is a common site of involvement of the seronegative group of spondyloarthritis (Jurik, 1992) and the rare SAPHO (synovitis, acne, pustulosis, hyperostosis and osteitis) syndrome (Katz et al, 1989).

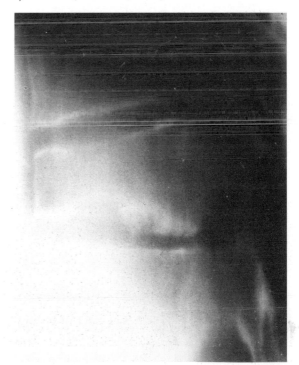

Figure 18.8 Secondard deposit in a thoracic vertebra

Rheumatoid arthritis

Rheumatoid arthritis may involve the thoracic and lumbar spines, although it is not common (Sims-Williams et al, 1977; Cohen et al, 1978). The essential lesion is a rheumatoid discitis, spreading from adjacent costovertebral or zygapophyseal joints (Bywaters, 1981). In the lumbar spine, rheumatoid discitis may occur in a normal or degenerated disc, resulting in discovertebral destruction and vertebral instability.

Thoracic joints

Costochondral joints

Pain in this anterior chest wall region due to a so-called costochondritis is quite common, and has been given other names, for example, the costosternal syndrome (Wolf and Stern, 1976; Flynn, 1981). Two common mistakes are made here, particularly with anxious patients. One is to misdiagnose this pain as being due to cardiovascular disease; alternatively, to label all pain in this region as being due to Tietze's syndrome.

The upper seven ribs articulate anteriorly with the sternum through their costal cartilages. The costochondral junction forms a fibrocartilaginous joint in which the rib and cartilage slot in together. With the exception of the first rib, these costal cartilages also articulate with the sternum through a synovial sternocostal joint. The eighth, ninth and tenth ribs articulate through their costal cartilage with the rib above it, whereas the last two ribs are unattached.

Pain may involve either the upper or lower costochondral region. Pain in the upper costochondral region of musculoskeletal origin may arise from one of four sources. It may be referred; due to a polyarthritis; post-traumatic; or due to a Tietze's syndrome. The most common cause of upper costochondral pain is referred pain from thoracic or cervical spinal lesions, as described above. Inflammatory polyarthritis, such as spondyloarthritis or rheumatoid arthritis, may at times produce pain in the sternocostal joint. Pain may follow trauma or surgery (Schmidt et al, 1994), may occur after a burst of coughing or be due to local trauma or other rare causes (Schmidt

et al, 1994). It may be associated with some degree of prominence of one or two costochondral joints and is commonly wrongly diagnosed as being due to Tietze's syndrome. Treatment consists of reassurance as to its benign nature, injections with local anaesthetic and corticosteroid (Wolf and Stern, 1976) and mobilizations.

Tietze's syndrome

This is quite a rare condition, which presents as an acute, painful swelling usually involving the upper costal cartilages (Aeschlimann and Kahn, 1990). It occurs mainly in young adults of either sex, who complain of upper chest pain, sometimes diffuse, which is made worse by activity or sudden strain such as coughing or sharp inspiration. Either one of the second costochondral cartilages may be involved, while the next most common is the third costochondral cartilage, but other costal cartilages or the sternoclavicular joint have very rarely been described. The attack lasts for a varying length of time, usually days, although it may last for months or years or recur at intervals. X-rays are normal, thus differentiating it from other diseases that may involve this area.

Its pathogenesis is unknown. It is a benign condition with no systemic manifestations and no known relationship with any other inflammatory disease. A biopsy of the costal cartilage is basically normal, although minor inflammatory changes have been described in the surrounding perichondrium. It has been suggested that this condition is only a form of post-traumatic prominence of the costochondral cartilage, although it is considered unlikely. Echography may demonstrate the localized swelling (Martino et al, 1991).

DIFFERENTIAL DIAGNOSIS

Other disorders or swellings that may be found in this area include: congenital deformities; infections, including sexually transmitted diseases; post-traumatic causes, including callus formation; primary tumours, including multiple myeloma; and secondary deposits, especially from thyroid, breast, bronchus, kidney or prostate. X-rays (Jurik et al, 1987) and bone scans may be necessary to differentiate between them.

Slipping rib

In this condition, pain is felt in the lower costo-chondral region of the eighth, ninth or tenth ribs, where the cartilaginous rib tip is loosely joined anteriorly to the one above it. A slipping or clicking rib is caused by either direct or indirect trauma, which causes a subluxation of the interchondral joint associated with a painful clicking (Spence and Rosato, 1983; Broadhurst, 1989a; Arroyo et al, 1995). It may occur at any age (Wright, 1980; Porter, 1985), and is felt as a sharp or dull aching pain, localized in the epigastrium or hypochondrium, usually made worse with movement, slumping, while lying down, or with direct pressure. Without treatment, pain can persist for a long time, even years.

Diagnosis is made by hooking the fingers under the ribcage and pulling it anteriorly (Figure 18.9), thus reproducing the pain (Heinz and Zavala, 1977). To confirm the diagnosis, pain can also be abolished by infiltrating the area with local anaesthetic. X-rays are normal (Copeland et al, 1984). This condition is very slow to resolve, but it may respond to an injection with local anaesthetic and corticosteroid, plus the use of non-steroidal anti-inflammatory agents. Surgery with resection of the anterior rib margin has been reported (Copeland et al, 1984), but is not often necessary.

Costovertebral joints

The costovertebral joints may be a source of thoracic pain (Arroyo et al, 1992), as they may be involved in inflammatory or degenerative joint disease. Pain in this joint is common in ankylosing spondylitis (Pascual et al, 1992), and examination reveals local tenderness and a reduced chest expansion, a useful measure which can be used to assess disease progress. Degenerative changes may also occur (Nathan et al, 1964; Bywaters, 1981), and commence during the fourth decade of life. Although they are usually asymptomatic, and often only a chance finding on X-ray, symptoms such as localized pain, stiffness and tenderness may occur following some form of local trauma. Degenerative changes were described in about half of 345 skeletons, and also in 17 per cent of 100 random chest X-rays, by Nathan et al (1964). Their distribution was related to anatomical factors, so that joints with a single facet, namely, T1, T11 and T12, (Figure 18.10) have a much higher incidence of degenerative changes than the remainder of the joints, which have two hemi-facets. The inferior joint facets, rather than the superior ones, are the usual site of involvement.

Treatment for pain and stiffness with mobilization techniques and/or injection with local anaesthetic and corticosteroid into the joint is usually quite successful in relieving symptoms.

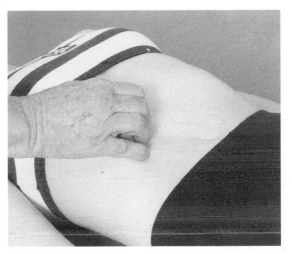

Figure 18.9 The hook test

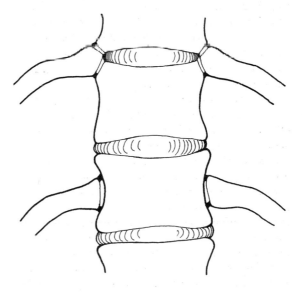

Figure 18.10 Costovertebral joints

Zygapophyseal joints

The thoracic zygapophyseal joints are set obliquely. The facets are slightly convex so that the superior facet faces posterior, superior and lateral, whereas the inferior facet faces anterior, inferior and medial. Rotation is greater here than in the lumbar spine, and flexion–extension is maximal in the lower thoracic spine. It appears that the joints are innervated similarly to those of the lumbar vertebrae (Bogduk and Valencia, 1994).

These joints can be a source of pain (Wilson, 1987; Stolker et al, 1993; Dreyfus et al, 1994; Chua and Bogduk, 1995), although it is difficult to diagnose or confirm clinically. They may develop changes of osteoarthritis (Malmivaara, et al, 1987; Sanzhang and Rothschild, 1993), or spondyloarthritis (Sanzhang and Rothschild, 1993). Pain was produced experimentally (Dreyfus et al, 1994d) by injecting 40 zygapophyseal joints, distending the joint capsule with contrast medium. They charted a consistent pain response producing local and some referred pain in 29 joints. Stolker et al (1993) anaesthetized the nerve supply to these joints and performed percutaneous radiofrequency denervation of the joints. Local anaesthetic with corticosteroid was injected into these joints in 17 patients (Wilson, 1987); 13 of them obtained immediate pain relief, nine of whom obtained long-term relief.

Manubriosternal joints

These joints are usually classified as being cartilaginous, although a synovial cavity is present in approximately 30 per cent of people. Inflammatory lesions occur in both spondyloarthritis and rheumatoid arthritis. It is more commonly involved in ankylosing spondylitis with joint erosion and enthesitis, which may lead ultimately to bony fusion. It is a common site for infections in intravenous drug users.

Sternoclavicular joints

Pain from these joints may be referred into the upper costochondral region. These synovial joints can be the site of degenerative changes that result in an upward subluxation of the clavicle (van Holsbeeck et al, 1992). An inflammatory synovitis may occur in rheumatoid arthritis (Dura et al, 1993), but is more common in patients with spondyloarthritis. Trauma may lead to dislocation (Jougon et al, 1996). Hyperostosis is a rare X-ray finding.

Xiphoid process

Pain here is commonly post-traumatic, but it may be a neurotic symptom. A painful tenderness to this structure occurring as a separate condition has been described (Fyler, 1980), but it is most rare (Howell, 1992).

Scapulothoracic joints

The gliding plane between the scapula and thorax, lined by thin muscles, is necessary for the considerable range of scapular movement. Two lesions are described here: snapping scapula and scapulocostal tendinitis.

Snapping scapula

Patients, usually young, present with pain along the medial scapular border, associated with a loud cracking or snapping sound as the arm is abducted. Patients can soon learn to perform the snapping as a trick movement, and may then habitually click the scapula back and forth. Pain is felt as a dull ache, usually constantly present, along the medial border of the scapula, although patients often do not associate the pain with the disturbance of scapular movement.

A generalized hypermobility syndrome is often present. Shoulder examination reveals the abnormality of scapular movement, which may be felt and seen as the scapula moves. With the shoulder full abducted, tenderness may be palpated along the medial scapular border. X-rays should include a lateral view of the scapula, to detect any underlying bony abnormality that may be present, such as an osteoma or a bony spur.

Patients must be taught to avoid this trick movement. The tender area in the muscle may be injected with local anaesthetic and corticosteroid, which affords at least temporary relief. If a local bony abnormality is demonstrated, and if symptoms persist, bone resection can be curative.

Scapulocostal tendinitis

Localized pain and tenderness, sometimes quite severe, may be found along the upper part of the medial scapular border. Pain usually gets worse as the day goes on or after use of the shoulders. It is commonly found in typists or in sports people, and may be associated with postural faults such as sagging shoulders. However, the constancy of the site, its localized nature and the ability to reproduce the pain on resisted scapular movement make it more likely to be due to an enthesitis than to a postural disturbance alone.

Treatment consists of avoiding movements known to produce pain, deep-friction massage, injection with local anaesthetic and corticosteroid into the painful area, and re-education exercises.

Lower cervical spine

Pain referred from the cervical spine is most commonly felt between or above the scapulae. It may, however, be felt anywhere over the upper anterior chest wall; occasionally it is episodic or related to exertion, when it is difficult to distinguish from angina. Pain is reproduced on movement of the cervical spine.

Ribs

A fractured rib following direct trauma is usually easy to diagnose on clinical grounds alone. A bone scan is necessary if there is any doubt about the diagnosis. An X-ray is necessary to confirm the diagnosis and to exclude other problems such as a pneumothorax.

Stress fracture of the rib is a not uncommon sporting injury, probably caused by overuse with excessive muscle traction on the ribs. Diagnosis is best made by bone scan.

Muscular lesions

Injuries to the chest wall muscles are not particularly common, but in sports people may involve the serratus anterior, intercostal muscles or the musculotendinous origins of the abdominal muscles. Pain due to overuse of the intercostal muscles, in sport or as a result of coughing, is often associated with a stress fracture of the rib, and should be investigated with a bone scan. One not uncommon condition is a periodic attack of a sudden, sharp, momentary, cramp-like muscular pain in the anterior chest wall, which often follows a sudden movement or after slouching in a chair. Its mechanism is unknown but it may be that it is caused by a mechanical derangement in a costal joint.

Postural pain

Muscular pain without any underlying lesion of the cervical or thoracic joints is usually related to abnormal posture. The patient, usually a woman, often middle-aged, complains of stiffness and tenderness of muscle groups related to the shoulder girdle and thorax. The pain usually becomes worse as the day goes on and the patient is often conscious that pain may be related to postural activities, such as sitting for prolonged periods, with keyboard activities or other types of continuous work. Pain may be also made worse by fatigue, emotional stress or, at times, by changes in the weather. In some women there is a marked postural sagging of the shoulders or the presence of heavy, pendulous breasts.

Ancillary tests such as X-rays and blood tests are normal, but other conditions, such as fibromyalgia, psychogenic rheumatism, hypomobility or hypermobility lesions, need to be excluded. Treatment is with simple measures, such as reassurance, heat, analgesics, exercises and stretching, and injections with local anaesthetic and corticosteroid into the locally tender areas.

Manual therapy techniques for the thoracic spine

The three techniques described are: mobilization; manipulation; and and traction.

Mobilization techniques

Three mobilization techniques (Tables 18.1 and 18.2) commonly used are:

1. Posteroanterior central vertebral pressure
2. Transverse vertebral pressure
3. Posteroanterior unilateral vertebral pressure.

Table 18.1 Manipulation of the thoracic spine, sequence of selection of techniques

Unilateral symptoms	Bilateral symptoms
Posteroanterior central vertebral pressure	Posteroanterior central vertebral pressure
Transverse vertebral pressure	Transverse vertebral pressure to each side
Posteroanterior unilateral vertebral pressure	Traction
Traction	

Table 18.2 Indications for thoracic spine mobilization techniques

Technique	Main indications
Posteroanterior central vertebral pressure	Bilateral pain, poorly defined or widespread unilateral pain
Transverse vertebral pressure	Unilateral pain
Posteroanterior unilateral vertebral pressure	Unilateral pain
Traction	Widely distributed pain, especially if associated with disc degeneration; or hypomobility lesions

Posteroanterior central vertebral pressure

The patient lies prone. Techniques vary according to the site in the thoracic spine.

- Upper thoracic spine: the therapist stands at the patient's head with the pads of the thumbs over the spinous process. Pressure is directed initially at right angles to the area being mobilized (Figure 18.11a).
- Mid-thoracic spine: the therapist stands by the patient's side with his thumbs placed along the spine, pointing towards each other. The fingers spread out on either side of the vertebral column (Figure 18.11b).

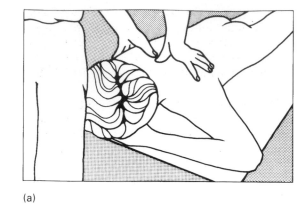
(a)

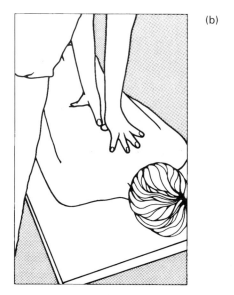
(b)

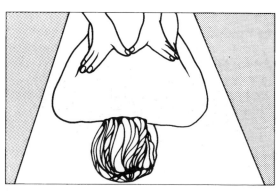
(c)

Figure 18.11 Posteroanterior central vertebral pressure: (a) upper thoracic; (b) mid-thoracic; and (c) lower thoracic

● Lower thoracic spine: the direction of pressure must initially be at right angles to the body surface at the level being treated, so that the therapist's shoulders are either over the thoracic spine or the sacrum (Figure 18.11c).

Oscillatory pressure on the spinous process is produced by the body and then transmitted through the arms to the thumbs. Pressure is achieved by body weight, not by the thumbs.

This is the best technique for all cases of thoracic pain, especially with midline or bilateral pain.

Transverse vertebral pressure

This is used for unilateral thoracic pain.

The patient lies prone. The therapist stands on the right side at the level of the vertebra to be mobilized, thumbs against the side of the spinous process and fingers spread over the chest wall. One thumb is reinforced by placing the other thumb over it (Figure 18.12). Pressure is applied through trunk movement. The upper thoracic region is readily accessible but has only limited movement, whereas the lower thoracic region is easily moved without much pressure. The mid-thoracic spinous processes are relatively inaccessible.

Posteroanterior unilateral vertebral pressure

This technique is also used for unilateral thoracic pain.

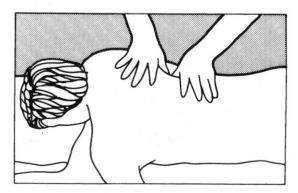

Figure 18.12 Transverse vertebral pressure: thoracic region

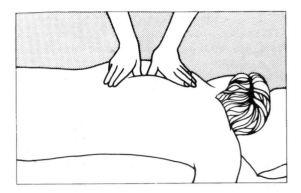

Figure 18.13 Posteroanterior unilateral vertebral pressure: thoracic region

The patient lies prone, head to one side and arms over the sides of the couch. For the lower thoracic spine, the therapist stands by the patient's side with the pads of the thumbs pointing towards each other over the transverse process. Pressure is applied in a direct line through the shoulders and arms and at right angles to the body (Figure 18.13).

Oscillation is produced with trunk movements and firm pressure from the thumbs, but only a little movement can be obtained.

Manipulation

Non-specific technique

POSTEROANTERIOR PRESSURE
With the patient lying prone, the therapist, using the pisiform bone of his or her right hand against the patient's spinous process, stretches the intervertebral joint to its limit and then produces a sudden movement of very small range.

Specific techniques

ROTATION
The patient sits on the edge of the couch, hugs his or her arms to the chest and turns the trunk to the left. The therapist reaches around with his or her left arm to the patient's right side, cradling the left shoulder in his axilla. With the right hand, the therapist puts pressure over the line of the ribs (Figure 18.14).

A synchronous movement of the therapist's trunk together with pressure through the right hand is produced. With the trunk, the therapist

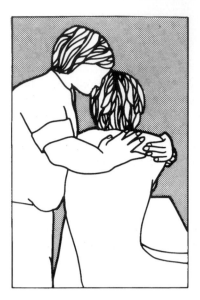

Figure 18.14 Rotation or intervertebral joints T3–T10 (mid-thoracic area)

produces an oscillatory movement at the limit of the range of rotation. Manipulation consists of an overpressure at the limit of the range.

POSTEROANTERIOR CENTRAL PRESSURE

The patient lies supine with hands linked behind the head. The therapist stands by the patient's right side with his or her right hand made into a fist by flexing the ulnar three fingers into the palm, leaving the thumb and index finger extended. The lower spinous process is grasped between the terminal phalanx of the middle finger and the palmar surface of the head of the first metacarpal. The patient is then lowered until the right hand is wedged between the patient and the couch, with the therapist's forearm projecting laterally. The patient's elbows are grasped and the upper trunk gently moved back and forth in flexion and extension to obtain the mid position of this movement (Figure 18.15).

Manipulation consists of a downward thrust directed through the patient's elbows and upper arms.

Thoracic traction

Traction can be administered to the thoracic spine as readily as in the cervical and lumbar areas, and the guiding principles are similar. However, thoracic traction is less often successful, partly due to the thoracic cage limiting the degree of movement. The vertebral column is so positioned that the treated joint is relaxed midway between all ranges. The amount of pressure used is guided first by movement in the joint, and further changes in tension are made in response to changes in symptoms. Further treatment is guided by any changes in the symptoms and signs.

Upper thoracic spine

The patient lies on his or her back with one or two pillows under the head to flex the neck with the level to be treated positioned midway between flexion and extension. A cervical halter is applied and counter-traction may be needed. A belt fitted around the pelvis is attached to the foot end of the couch to stabilize the distal end of the vertebral column. The halter is then attached to its fixed point so that the angle of its pull on the neck is approximately 45 degrees from the horizontal. The angle used varies with the degree of kyphosis present in the upper thoracic spine but should allow the thoracic joint to be stretched longitudinally in a position midway between its limit of flexion and extension. The hips and knees may be flexed to relieve the strain on the lower back.

Traction may be adjusted from either or both ends. Whatever type is used friction between the trunk and the couch must be reduced to a minimum by gently allowing the traction to relax

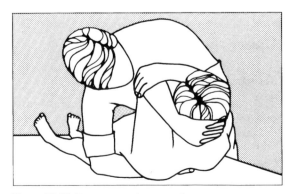

Figure 18.15 Posteroanterior central pressure on intervertebral joints T3–T10

back into a new position. Friction is virtually eliminated by use of a couch with its surface in two halves free to roll longitudinally. Releasing the traction is relatively easy but should be done slowly.

Lower thoracic spine

Traction is usually more effective with the patient supine, although it may also be used with the patient prone. For the lower thoracic spinal conditions, a thoracic belt similar to that used for lumbar traction replaces the cervical halter. The thoracic belt is applied above the spinal level being treated to hold the chest and is then attached to its fixed point. The direction of the pull is longitudinal in the line of the patient's trunk, but pillows may be used to adjust the position of the spine with the joint being stretched relaxed midway between flexion and extension.

Traction is applied from either end or from both ends but care is necessary to reduce friction to a minimum. This may be achieved with a roll top couch. The traction is released gradually and the patient rests for a time before standing up.

Intermittent variable traction can also be used in the thoracic spine and the times for 'rest' and 'hold' periods are similar to those used for the cervical spine.

LOCAL VARIATIONS
Positioning the patient is controlled by the degree of thoracic kyphosis, which varies considerably, especially in the upper thoracic spine. Theoretically, the direction of pull should be at right angles to the upper and lower surfaces of the intervertebral disc of the level that is being stretched.

PRECAUTIONS
Traction should not cause any low back pain. It may cause occipital headache, which can be prevented as previously described for cervical traction in flexion.

INDICATIONS
Mobilization techniques are usually used before traction, but if these fail, traction can be used and may still prove successful. It is of most value to patients with a wide distribution of thoracic pain due either to hypomobility or to disc degeneration, even if neurological changes or nerve root pain are present.

References

Abbott, G. T. and Carty, H. (1993). Pyogenic sacroiliitis, the missed diagnosis. *British Journal of Radiology*, **66**, 120–122.

Abel, M. S. (1975). Occult traumatic lesions of the cervical vertebrae. *Critical Review Clinical Radiology*, **6**, 469–553.

Abrahams, V. C. (1981). Sensory and motor specialization in some muscles of the neck. *Trends in Neurosciences*. **1**, 24–27.

Abumi, K., Panjabi, M. M., Kramer, K. M. et al. (1990). Biomechanical evaluation of lumbar spinal stability after graded facetectomies. *Spine*, **15**, 1141–1147.

Acaroglu, E. R., Iatridis, J. C., Setton, L. A. et al. (1995). Degeneration and aging affect the tensile behavior of human lumbar anulus fibrosus. *Spine*, **20**, 2690–2701.

Adams, M. A., Dolan, P. and Hutton, W. C. (1986). The stages of disc degeneration as revealed by discograms. *Journal of Bone and Joint Surgery*, **68B**, 36–41.

Adams, M. A., Dolan, P. and Hutton, W. C. (1987). Diurnal variations in the stresses on the lumbar spine. *Spine*, **12**, 130–137.

Adams, M. A. and Hutton, W. C. (1982). Prolapsed intervertebral disc: a hyperflexion injury. *Spine*, **7**, 184–191.

Adams, M. A. and Hutton W. C. (1983). The effect of posture on the fluid content of lumbar intervertebral discs. *Spine*, **8**, 665–671.

Adams, M. A., McMillan, D. W., Green, T. P. and Dolan, P. (1996). Sustained loading generates stress concentrations in lumbar intervertebral discs. *Spine*, **21**, 434–438.

Adams, M. A., McNally, D. S., Chinn, H. and Dolan, P. (1994). Posture and the compressive strength of the lumbar spine. *Clinical Biomechanics*, **9**, 5–14.

Aeschlimann, A. and Khan, M. F. (1990). Tietze's Syndrome: a critical review *Clinical and Experimental Rheumatology*, **8**, 407–412.

Ahles, T. A., Yunus, M. B. and Masi, A. T. (1987). Is chronic pain a variant of depressive disease? The case of fibromyalgia syndrome. *Pain*, **29**, 105–111.

Ahlstrom, H., Feltelius, N., Nyman, R and Hallgren, R. (1990). Magnetic resonance imaging of sacroiliac joint inflammation. *Arthritis Rheumatism*, **33**, 1763–1769.

Ahmed, A. M., Duncan, N. A., and Burke, D. L. (1990). The effect of facet geometry on the axial torque-rotation response of lumbar motion segments. *Spine*, **15**, 391–401.

Alaranta, H., Rytokoski, U., Rissanen, A. et al. (1994). Intensive physical and psychosocial training program for patients with chronic low back pain. A controlled clinical trial. *Spine*, **19**, 1339–1349.

Albrand, O. W. and Corkill, G. J. (1979). Thoracic disc herniation: treatment and prognosis. *Spine*, **4**, 41–46.

Alderink, G. J. (1991). The sacroiliac joint: review of anatomy, mechanics, and function. *Journal of Orthopedic and Sports Physical Therapy,* **13**, 71–84.

Algers, G., Peteresson, K., Hildingsson, C. and Toolanen, G. (1993). Surgery for chronic symptoms after whiplash injury. *Acta Orthopaedicia Scadinavica,* **64**, 654–656.

Aliabadi, P. and Nikpoor, N. (1991). Imaging evaluation of sacroiliitis. *Rheumatic Diseases Clinics of North America,* **17**, 809–812.

Aloia, J. F., Cohn, S. H., Ostuni, J. A. et al. (1978). Prevention of involutional bone loss by exercise. *Annals of Internal Medicine,* **89**, 356–358.

Althoff, B. and Goldie, I. F. (1980). Cervical collars in rheumatoid atlanto-axial subluxaton: a radiographic comparison. *Annals of the Rheumatic Diseases,* **39**, 485–489.

Altmaier, E. M., Lehmann, T.R., Russell, D.W. et al. (1992). The effectiveness of psychological interventions for the rehabilitation of low back pain: a randomized controlled trial evaluation. *Pain,* **49**, 329–335.

Amundsen, T., Weber, H., lilleas, F. et al. (1995). Lumbar spinal stenosis. Clinical and radiological features. *Spine,* **20**, 1178–1186.

An, H. S., Andreshak, T. G., Nguyen, C. et al. (1995). Can we distinguish between benign versus malignant compression fractures of the spine by magnetic resonance imaging? *Spine,* **20**, 1776–1782.

Andersen, K. H. and Mosdal, C. (1987). Epidural application of corticosteroids in low back pain and sciatica. *Acta Neurochirurgica,* **87**, 52–53.

Andersson, G. B. J. (1983). The biomechanics of the posterior elements of the lumbar spine. Introductory remarks. *Spine,* **8**, 326.

Annear, P., Chakera, T., Foster, D. and Hardcastle, P. (1994). Pars interarticularis stress and disc degeneration in cricket's potent strike force, the fast bowler. *Australian and New Zealand Journal of Surgery,* **62**, 768–773.

Anthony, N. (1989). Occipital neuralgia. *Cephalalgia,* **9**, 174–175.

Aprill, C. and Bogduk, N. (1992). The prevalence of cervical zygapophyseal joint pain; a first approximation. *Spine,* **17**, 744–747.

Aprill, C., Dwyer, A. and Bogduk, N. (1990). Cervical zygapophyseal joint pain patterns. 11. A clinical evaluation. *Spine,* **15**, 453–457.

Arce, C. A. and Dohrmann, G. J. (1985).

Herniated thoracic disks. *Neurologic Clinics,* **2**, 383–392.

Arnoldi, C. C., Brodsky, A. E., Cauchoix, J. et al. (1976). Lumbar spinal stenosis and nerve root entrapment syndromes. *Clinical Orthopaedics and Related Rearch,* **115**, 4–5.

Arntz, A., Dreessen, L. and DeJong, P. (1994). The influence of anxiety on pain: attentional and attributional mediators. *Pain,* **56**, 307–314.

Arroyo, F. J., Jolliet, P. and Junod, A. F. (1992). Costovertebral joint dysfunction: another misdiagnosed cause of atypical chest pain. *Postgraduate Medical Journal,* **68**, 655–659.

Arroyo, F. J., Vine, R., Reynaud, C. and Michel, J. P. (1995). Slipping rib syndrome: do not be fooled. *Geriatrics,* **50**, 46–49.

Asfour, S. S., Khalil, T. M., Waly, S. M. et al. (1990). Biofeedback in back muscle strengthening. *Spine,* **15**, 510–513.

Assendelft, W. J., Bouter, S. M. and Knipschild, P. G. (1996). Complications of spinal manipulation: a comprehensive review of the literature. *Journal of Family Practice,* **42**, 475–480.

Assendelft, W. J. J., Koes, B., Knipschild, P. G. and Bouter, L. M. (1995). The relationship between methodological quality and conclusions in reviews of spinal manipulation. *Journal of the American Medical Association,* **274**, 1942–1948.

Assey, M. E. (1993). The puzzle of normal coronary arteries in the patient with chest pain: what to do? *Clinical Cardiology,* **16**, 170–180.

Aufdermaur, M. and Spycher, M. (1986). Pathogenesis of osteochondritis juvenilis Scheuermann. *Journal of Orthopaedic Research,* **4**, 452–457.

Auld, A. W., Perlmutter, I. and Dooley, D. M. (1969). Normal leg raising tests with herniated lumbar disk. *Journal of the American Medical Association,* **207**, 2104.

Australian Physiotherapy Association. (1988). Protocol for premanipulative testing of the cervical spine. *Australian Journal of Physiotherapy,* **34**, 97–100.

Avrahami, E., Frishman, E., Fridman, Z. and Azor, M. (1994). Spina bifida occculta of S1 is not an innocent condition. *Spine,* **19**, 12–15.

Awad, E. A. (1973). Interstitial myofibrositis: a hypothesis of the mechanism. *Archives of Physical Medicine and Rehabilitation,* **54**, 449–453.

Awwad, E. E., Martin, D. S., Smith, K. R. and

Baker, B. K. (1991). Asymptomatic versus symptomatic herniated thoracic discs: their frequency and characteristics as detected by computed tomography after myelography. *Neurosurgery*, **28**, 180–186.

Bakland, O. and Hansen, J.H. (1984). The axial sacroiliac joint. *Anatomia Clinica*, **6**, 29–36.

Balla, J. I. and Karnmaghan, J. (1987). Whiplash headache. *Clinical and Experimental Neurology*, **23**, 179–182.

Balla, J. I. (1980). The late whiplash syndrome. *Australian and New Zealand Journal of Surgery*, **50**, 610–614.

Barnsley, L. and Bogduk, N. (1993). Medial branch blocks are specific for the diagnosis of cervical zygapophyseal joint pain. *Regional Anesthesia*, **18**, 343–350.

Barnsley, L., Lord, S. M. and Bogduk, N. (1993a). Comparative local anaesthetic blocks in the diagnosis of cervical zygapophyseal joint pain. *Pain*, **55**, 99–106.

Barnsley, L., Lord, S. M., Wallis, B. and Bogduk, N. (1993b). False-positive rates of cervical zygapophyseal joint blocks. *Clinical Journal of Pain*, **9**, 124–130.

Barnsley, L., Lord, S. M. and Bogduk, N. (1994a). Whiplash injury. *Pain*, **58**, 283–307.

Barnsley, L., Lord, S. M. and Bogduk, N. (1994b). Lack of effect of intra-articular corticosteroids for chronic zygapophyseal joint pain. *New England Journal of Medicine*, **330**, 1047–1050.

Barnsley, L., Lord, S. M. Wallis, B. J. and Bogduk, N. (1995). The prevalence of chronic cervical zygapophyseal joint pain after whiplash. *Spine*, **20**, 20–25.

Barré, N. (1926). Sur un syndrome sympathique cervical posterieure et sa course frequente: L'arthrite cervicale. *Revue Neurologique*, **33**, 1246–1248.

Barrett-Connor, E. (1995). The economic and human costs of osteoporotic fracture. *American Journal of Medicine*, **98** suppl 2A, 3S–8S.

Barry, M. (1992). Whiplash injuries. *British Journal of Rheumatology*, **31**, 579–581. Editorial.

Barry, M. and Jenner, J. R. (1995). Pain in the neck, shoulder, and arm. *British Medical Journal*, **310**, 183–186.

Bartelink, D. L. (1957). The role of abdominal pressure in relieving the pressure on the lumbar intervertebral discs. *Journal of Bone and Joint Surgery*, **39B**, 718–725.

Bartlett, R. M., Stockill, N. P., Elliott, B. C. and Burnett, A. F. (1996). The biomechanics of fast bowling in men's cricket: a review. *Journal of Sports Sciences*, **14**, 403–424.

Barton, P. M. (1991). Piriformis syndrome: a rational approach to management. *Pain*, **47**, 345–352.

Battafarano, D. F., West, S. G., Rak, K. M. et al. (1993). Comparison of bone scan, computed tomography, and magnetic resonance imaging in the diagnosis of active sacroiliitis. *Serminars in Arthritis and Rheumatism*, **23**, 161–176.

Battie, M., Bigos, S., Fisher, L. et al. (1989). A prospective study of raising the role of cardiovascular risk factors in fitness in industrial back pain complaints. *Spine*, **14**, 141–144.

Battie, M., Bigos, S., Fisher, L. et al. (1990). Anthropometric and clinical measures as predictors of back pain complaints in industry: a prospective study. *Journal of Spinal Disorders*, **3**, 195–204.

Battie, M., Videman, T., Gill, K. et al. (1991). Smoking and lumbar intervertebral disc degeneration: an MRI study of identical twins. *Spine*, **16**, 1015–1021.

Battie, M. C., Videman, T., Gibbons, L. E. et al. (1995). Determinants of lumbar disc degeneration. A study relating lifetime exposures and magnetic resonance imaging findings in identical twins. *Spine*, **20**, 2601–2612.

Batzdorf, U. and Flannigan, B. (1991). Surgical decompressive procedures for cervical spondylitic myelopathy: a study using magnetic resonance imaging. *Spine*, **16**, 123–127.

Baumstark, K. E., Buckelew, S. P., Sher, K. J. et al. (1993). Pain behavior predictors among fibromyalgia patients. *Pain*, **55**, 339–346.

Beal, M. C. (1989). Incidence of spinal palpatory findings: an overview. *Journal of the American Osteophathic Association*, **89**, 1027–1035.

Beaman, D. N., Graziano, G. P., Glover, R. A. et al. (1993). Substance P innervation of lumbar spine facet joints. *Spine*, **18**, 1044–1049.

Beattie, P. F., Brooks, W. M., Rothstein, J. M. et al. (1994). Effect of lordosis in the position of the nucleus pulposus in supine subjects. *Spine*, **19**, 2096–2102.

Beatty, R. A. (1977). Dissecting hematoma of the

internal carotid artery following chiropractic cervical manipulation. *Journal of Trauma*, **17**, 248–249.

Beatty, R. A. (1994). The piriformis muscle syndrome: a simple diagnostic maneuver. *Neurosurgery*, **34**, 512–514.

Beatty, R. M., Fowler, F. D. and Hanson, E. J. (1987). The abducted arm as a sign of ruptured cervical disc. *Neurosurgery*, **21**, 731–732.

Beks, J. W. F. (1989). Kisssing spines: fact of fancy? *Acta Neurochirurgical*, **100**, 134–135.

Beliveau, P. (1971). A comparison between epidural anaesthesia with and without corticosteroid in the treatment of sciatica. *Rheumatology and Physical Medicine*, **11**, 40–43.

Bell, D. F., Ehrlich, M. G. and Zaleske. D. J. (1988). Brace treatment for symptomatic spondylolisthesis. *Clinical Orthopaedics and Related Research*, **236**, 192–198.

Bell, G. R. and Ross, J. S. (1992). Diagnosis of nerve root compression. Myelography, computed tomograyhy and MRI. *Orthopedic Clinics of North America*, **23**, 410–419.

Bell, P. S. (1992). Spondylolysis in fast bowlers: principles of prevention: a survey of awareness among cricket coaches. *British Journal of Sports Medicine*, **26**, 273–275.

Bellah, R. D., Subbervile, D. A., Treves, S. T. and Micheli, L. J. (1991). Low back pain in adolescent athletes: detection of stress injury to the pars interarticularis with SPECT. *Radiology*, **180**, 509–512.

Bellamy, N., Park, W. and Rooney, P. J. (1983). What do we know about the sacroiliac joint? *Seminars in Arthritis and Rheumatism*, **12**, 282–313.

Bellavance, A., Belzile, G., Bergeron, Y. et al. (1989). Letter. Cervical spine and headaches. *Neurology*, **39**, 1269.

Bengtsson, A., Henriksson, K. G. and Larson, J. (1986a). Muscle biopsy in primary fibromyalgia: light-microscopical and histochemical findings. *Scandinavian Journal of Rheumatology*, **15**, 1–6.

Bengtsson, A., Henriksson, K. G., and Larson, J. (1986b). Reduced high-energy phosphate levels in painful muscle in patients with primary fibromyalgia. *Arthritis and Rheumatism*, **29**, 817–821.

Benhamou, C. L., Roux, C., Touliere, D. et al.

(1993). Pseudovisceral pain referred from costovertebral arthropathies. Twenty-eight cases. *Spine*, **18**, 790–795.

Benjamin, V. (1983). Diagnosis and management of thoracic disc disease. *Clinical Neurosurgery*, **30**, 577–605

Bennett, R. M. (1981). Fibrositis: misnomer for a common rheumatic disorder. *Western Journal of Medicine*, **134**, 405–413.

Bennett, R. M. (1987). Fibromyalgia. *Journal of the American Medical Association*, **257**, 2802–2803.

Benoliel, R., Eliav, E., Elishoov, H. and Sharov, Y. (1994). Diagnosis and treatment of persistent pain after trauma to the head and neck. *Journal of Oral and Maxillofacial Surgery*, **52**, 1138–1147.

Benson, M. K. D. and Byrnes, D. P. (1975). The clinical syndromes and surgical treatment of thoracic intervertebral disc prolapse. *Journal of Bone and Joint Surgery*, **57B**, 471–477.

Berg, G., Hammer, M. Moller-Neilsen, J. et al. (1988). Low back pain during pregnancy. *Obstetrics and Gynecology*, **71**, 71–75.

Bernard, T. N. (1990). Lumbar discography followed by computered tomography. Refining the diagnosis of low back pain. *Spine*, **15**, 690–707.

Bernard, T. N. and Cassidy, J. D. (1991). The sacroiliac joint syndrome. In *The Adult Spine: Principles and Practice*. (J. W. Frymoyer, ed.) pp. 2107–2130, Raven Press.

Bernard, T. N. and Kirkaldy-Willis, W. H. (1987). Recognizing specific characteristics of non-specific low back pain. *Clinical Orthopaedics and Related Research*, **217**, 266–280.

Bernhardt, M., Hynes, R. A., Blume, H. W. and White, A. A. (1993). Current concepts review: cervical spondylotic myelopathy. *Journal of Bone and Joint Surgery*, **75A**, 119–128.

Best, B. A., Guilak, F. and Setton, L. A. (1994) Compressive mechanical properties of the human anulus fibrosus and their relationship of biochemical composition. *Spine*, **19**, 212–221.

Bhojraj, S. Y. and Dandawate, A. V. (1994). Progressive cord compression secondary to thoracic disc lesions in Scheuermann's kyphosis managed by posterolateral decompression, interbody fusion and pedicular fixation. A new approach to management of a rare clinical entity. *European Spine Journal,* **3**, 66–69.

Biering-Sorensen, F., Hansen, F., Schroll, M. and Runeborg, O. (1985). The relation of spinal x-ray to low back pain and physical activity among 60-year-old men and women. *Spine,* **10**, 445–449.

Biering-Sorensen, F., Thomsen, C. and Hillden, J. (1989). Risk indicators for low back pain. *Scandinavian Journal of Work, Environment and Health,* **17**, 420–424.

Bigos, S., Spengler, D., Martin, N. et al. (1986). Back injuries in industry: a retrospective study. 11. Employee-related factors. *Spine,* **11**, 252–256.

Binet, E. F., Moro, J. J., Marangola, J. P. and Hodge, C. J. (1977). Cervical spine tomography in trauma. *Spine,* **2**, 163-172.

Bird, H. A. and Barton, L. (1993). Joint hyperlaxity and its long-term effects on joints. *Journal of the Royal Society of Health,* **113**, 327–329.

Bjarnason, K., Hassager, C., Svendsen, O. L. et al. (1996). Anteroposterior and lateral spinal DXA for the assessment of vertebral body strength: comparison with hip and forearm measurement. *Osteoporosis International,* **6**, 37–42.

Bjersand, A. J. (1980). Juvenile kyphosis in identical twins. *American Journal of Roentgenology,* **134**, 598–599.

Blackie, J. D. and Lees, A. J. (1990). Botulinum toxin treatment in spasmodic torticollis. *Journal of Neurology, Neurosurgery and Psychiatry,* **53**, 640–643.

Bland, J. H. and Boushey, D. R. (1990). Anatomy and physiology of the cervical spine. *Seminars in Arthritis and Rheumatism,* **20**, 1–20.

Block, A. R., Vanharanta, H., Ohnmeiss, D. D. and Guyer, R. D. (1996). Discographic pain report—influence of psychological factors. *Spine,* **21**, 334–338.

Blomberg, S., Svardsudd, K. and Mildenberger, F. (1992). A controlled, multi-centre trial of manual therapy in low back pain. *Scandinavian Journal of Primary Health Care,* **10**, 170–178.

Blumenthal, S. L., Roach, J. and Herring, J. A. (1987). Lumbar Scheuermann's. A clinical series and classification. *Spine,* **12**, 929-932.

Boden, S. D. (1994). Rheumatoid arthritis of the cervical spine. Surgical decision making based on predictors of paralysis and recovery. *Spine,* **19**, 2275–2280.

Boden, S. D. (1996). The use of radiographic imaging studies in the evaluation of patients who have degenerative disorders of the lumbar spine. *Journal of Bone and Joint Surgery,* **78A**, 114–124.

Boden, S. D., Davis, D. O., Dina, T. S. et al. (1990a). Abnormal magnetic resonance scans of the lumbar spine in asymptomatic subjects: a prospective investigation. *Journal of Bone and Joint Surgery,* **72A**, 403–408.

Boden, S. D., McCowin, P. R., Davis, D. O. et al. (1990b). Abnormal magnetic resonance scans of the cervical spine in asymptomatic subjects. A prospective investigation. *Journal of Bone and Joint Surgery,* **72A**, 1178–1184.

Bogduk, N. (1980). The anatomy of occipital neuralgia. *Clinical and Experimental Neurology,* **17**, 167–184.

Bogduk, N. (1981). Dizziness and the vertebral artery. In *The Cervical Spine and Headache Symposium.* pp. 61–82, Manipulative Therapists' Association of Australia.

Bogduk, N. (1982). The clinical anatomy of the cervical dorsal rami. *Spine,* **7**, 319–330.

Bogduk, N. (1983). The innervation of the lumbar spine. *Spine,* **8**, 286–293.

Bogduk, N. (1988). The anatomy and pathophysiology of whiplash. *Clinical Biochemistry,* **1**, 92–101.

Bogduk, N. (1989). Anatomy of headache. Proceedings of a symposium on headache and face pain. pp. 1–16, Manipulative Physiotherapists Association of Australia.

Bogduk, N. (1991). The lumbar disc and low back pain. *Neursurgery Clinics of North America,* **2**, 791–806.

Bogduk, N. (1994). Point of view. *Spine,* **19**, 2824–2825.

Bogduk, N. and Aprill, C. (1993). On the nature of neck pain, discography and cervical zygapophyseal joint blocks. *Pain,* **54**, 213–217.

Bogduk, N. and Engel, R. (1984). The menisci of the lumbar zygapophoseal joints. A review of their anatomy and clinical significance. *Spine,* **9**, 454–460.

Bogduk, N. and Jull, G. (1985). The theoretical pathology of acute locked back: a basis for manipulative therapy. *Manual Medicine*, **1**, 78–82.

Bogduk, N. and Long, D. M. (1980). Percutaneous lumbar medial branch neurotomy; a modification of facet denervation. *Spine*, **5**, 193–200.

Bogduk, N. and Marsland, A. (1986). On the concept of third occipital headache. *Journal of Neurology, Neurosurgery and Psychiatry*, **49**, 775–780.

Bogduk, N. and Marsland, A. (1988). The cervical zygapophyseal joint as a source of neck pain. *Spine*, **13**, 610–617.

Bogduk, N. and McIntosh, J. (1984). The applied anatomy of the thoracolumbar fascia. *Spine*, **9**, 164–170.

Bogduk, N. and Modic, M. T. (1996). Controversy. Lumbar discography. *Spine*, **21**, 402–404.

Bogduk, N. and Schwarzer, A. C. (1995). Facet joint pain (letter). *Australian Family Physician*, **24**, **924**.

Bogduk, N. and Twomey, L. T. (1991). *Clinical Anatomy of the Lumbar Spine*, 2nd edn. Churchill Livingstone.

Bogduk, N. and Valencia, F. (1994). Innervation and pain patterns of the thoracic spine. In *Physical Therapy of the Cervical and Thoracic Spine*, 2nd edn. pp. 77–87, Churchilll Livingstone.

Bogduk, N., Tynan, W. and Wilson A. S. (1981). The nerve supply to the human lumbar intervertebral discs. *Journal of Anatomy*, **132**, 39–56.

Bogduk, N., Wilson A. S. and Tynan, W. (1982). The human lumbar dorsal rami. *Journal of Anatomy*, **134**, 383–397.

Bogduk, N., Corrigan, A. B., Kelly, P. et al. (1985). Cervical headache. *Medical Journal of Australia*, **143**, 202–207.

Bogduk, N., MacIntosh, J. and Marsland, A. (1988a). Technical limitations to the efficacy of radiofrequency neurotomy for spinal pain. *Neurosurgery*, **20**, 529–535.

Bogduk, N., Windsor, M. and Inglis, A. (1988b). The innervation of the cervical intervertebral discs. *Spine*, **13**, 2–8.

Bogduk, N., Brazenor, G., Christophidis, N. et al. (1994). *Epidural use of steroids in the management of back pain.* pp. 1–76, National Health and Medical Research Council, Canberra.

Bohay, D. R. and Gray, J. M. (1993). Sacroiliac joint pyoathrosis. *Orthopaedic Review*, **22**, 817–823.

Bohlman, H. H. (1995). Multilevel cervical spondylosis. Laminoplasty versus anterior decompression. Controversy. *Spine*, **20**, 1733–1734.

Bohlman, H. H. and Emery, S. E. (1988). The pathophysiology of cervical spondylosis and myelopathy. *Spine*, **13**, 843–846.

Bohlman, H. H. and Zdeblick, T. A. (1988). Anterior excision of herniated thoracic discs. *Journal of Bone and Joint Surgery*, **70A**, 1038–1047.

Bolender, N. F., Schonstrom, N. S. R. and Spengler, D. M. (1985). Role of computed tomography and myelography in the diagnosis of central spinal stenosis. *Journal of Bone and Joint Surgery*, **67A**, 240–245.

Bollow, M., Braun, J., Hamm, B. et al. (1995). Early sacroiliitis in patients with spondyloarthritis: evaluation with dynamic gadolinium-enhanced MR imaging. *Radiology*, **194**, 529–536.

Bongers, P. M., Boshuizen, H. C., Hulshof, C.T.J. and Koemeester, A. P. (1988). Back disorders in crane operators exposed to whole body vibration. *International Archives of Occupational and Environmental Health*, **60**, 129–137.

Bongers, P., Hulshof, C., Boshuizen, H. et al. (1990). Back pain and exposure to whole body vibration in helicopter pilots. *Ergonomics*, **33**, 1007–1026.

Boos, N., Wallin, A., Schmucker, T. et al. (1994). Quantitative MR imaging of lumbar intervertebral disc and vertebral bodies: methodology, reproducibility, and preliminary results. *Magnetic Resonance Imaging*, **12**, 577–587.

Booth, R. E. and Rothman, R. H. (1976). Cervical angina. *Spine*, **1**, 28–32.

Boshuizen, H., Bongers, P. and Hulshof, C. (1992). Self-reported back pain in fork-lift, truck and freight-container tractor drivers exposed to whole body vibration. *Spine*, **17**, 59–65.

Boshuizen, H., Verbeek, J., Broersen, J. and Weel, A. (1993) Do smokers get more low back pain? *Spine*, **18**, 35–49.

Bostman, O. (1993). Body mass index and height in patients requiring surgery for lumbar intervertebral disc hernation. *Spine*, **18**, 851–854.

Botsford, D. J., Esses, S. I. and Ogilvie-Harris, D. J. (1994). In vivo diurnal variation in intervertebral disc volume and morphology. *Spine*, **19**, 935–940.

Bough, B., Thakore, J., Davies, M. and Dowling, F. (1990). Degeneration on the lumbar facet joints. Arthrography and pathology. *Journal of Bone and Joint Surgery*, **72B**, 275–276.

Bourbeau, R., Desjardins, D., Maag, U. et al. (1993). Neck injuries among belted and unbelted occupants of the front seat of cars. *Journal of Trauma*, **35**, 794–799.

Bouxsein, M. L. and Marcus, R. (1994). Overview of exercise and bone mass. *Rheumatic Diseases Clinics of North America*, **20**, 787–802.

Bovenzi, M. and Zadini, A. (1992). Self-reported low back symptoms in urban bus drivers exposed to whole-body vibration. *Spine*, **17**, 1048–1059.

Bovim, G. and Sand, T. (1992). Cervicogenic headaches, migraine without aura and tension type headache: diagnostic blockade of greater occipital and supra-orbital nerves. *Pain*, **51**, 43–48.

Bovim, G., Berg, R. and Dale, L. G. (1992). Cervicogenic headache: anesthetic blockades of cervical nerves (C2–C5) and facet joint. *Pain*, **49**, 315–320.

Bovim, G., Schrader, H. and Sand, T. (1994). Neck pain in the general population. *Spine*, **19**, 1307–1309.

Bowen V. and Cassidy, J. D. (1981). Macroscopic anatomy of the sacroiliac joint from embryonic life until the eighth decade. *Spine*, **6**, 620–628.

Bozzao, A., Galluca, M., Masciocchi, M. et al. (1992). Lumbar disk herniation: MR imaging assessment of natural history in patients treated without surgery. *Radiology*, **185**, 135–141.

Bradbury, N., Wilson, L. F., and Mulholland, R. C. (1996). Adolescent disc protrusions. A long-term follow-up of surgery compared to chymopapain. *Spine*, **21**, 372–377.

Bradley, K. (1977). Communication to the Australian Association of Manipulative Medicine, Melbourne. Unpublished.

Bradshaw, C., Watling, B., Bryce, C. and Steen, I. N. (1995). Manipulative physiotherapy for spinal problems in primary care: outcomes of care. *British Journal of Rheumatology*, **34**, 1070–1073.

Brain, W. R. (1963). Some unsolved problems of cervical spondylosis. *British Medical Journal*, **1**, 771–777.

Brant-Zawadzki, M. N., Jensen, M.C., Obuchowski, N. et al. (1995). Interobserver and intraobserver variability and interpretation of lumbar disc abnormalities. *Spine*, **20**, 1257–1264.

Braun, J., Bollow, M., Eggens, U. et al. (1994). Use of dynamic magnetic resonance imaging with fast imaging in the detection of early and advanced sacroiliitis in spondyloarthropathy patients. *Arthritis and Rheumatism*, **37**, 1039–1045.

Braun, V. and Richter, H. P. (1994). Selective peripheral denervation for the treatment of spasmodic torticollis. *Neurosurgery*, **35**, 58–62.

Bredenkamp, J. K. and Maceri, D. R. (1990). Inflammatory torticollis in children. *Archives of Otolaryngology Head and Neck Surgery*, **116**, 310–313.

Brendstrup, P., Jespersen, K. and Asboe-Hansen, G. (1957). Morphological and chemical connective tissue changes in fibrositic muscles. *Annals of the Rheumatic Diseases*, **16**, 438–440.

Brieg, A. and Troup, J.D.G. (1979). Biomechanical considerations in the straight leg raising test: cadaveric and clinical studies of medial hip rotation. *Spine*, **4**, 242–250.

Brightbill, T., Pile, N., Eichelberger, R. P. and Whitman, M. (1994). Normal magnetic resonance imaging and abnormal discography in lumbar disc disruption. *Spine*, **19**, 1075–1077.

Bring, G. and Westman, G. (1991). Chronic post-traumatic syndrome after whiplash injury. A pilot study of 22 patients. *Scandinavian Journal of Primary Health Care*, **9**, 135–141.

Brinkman, P. (1986). Injury to the annulus fibrosus and disk protrusions, an in vitro investigation on human lumbar disks. *Spine*, **11**, 149–153.

Broadhurst, N. (1989a). Slipping rib syndrome – a review. *Australian Association of Manual Medicine Bulletin*, **5**, 16–19.

Broadhurst, N. A. (1989b). Sacroiliac dysfunction as a cause of low back pain. *Australian Family Physician*, **18**, 623–628.

Broadhurst, N. A. (1990). Piriformis syndrome

and buttock pain. *Australian Family Physician,* **19**, 1754.

Brodeur, R. (1995). The audible release associated with joint manipulation. *Journal of Manipulative and Physiological Therapeutics,* **18**, 155–164.

Brodin, H. (1985). Cervical pain and mobilization. *Manual Medicine,* **2**, 18–22.

Brooke, R. I. and Lapointe, H. J. (1993). Temporomandibular joint disorders following whiplash. *Spine: State of the Art Reviews,* **7**, 443–454.

Brown, C. W., Deffer, P. A., Akmakjian, J. et al. (1992). The natural history of thoracic disc herniation. *Spine,* **17** suppl 6, S97–S102.

Brown, M. (1971). The pathophysiology of disc disease. *Orthopedic Clinics of North America,* **2**, 359–370.

Brunner, C., Kissling, R. and Jacob, H. A. C. (1991). The effects of morphology and histopathologic findings on the mobility of the sacroiliac joint. *Spine,* **16**, 1111–1117.

Bruusgaard, D., Evensen, A. R. and Bjerkedal, T. (1993). Fibromyalgia – a new cause for disability pension. *Scandinavian Journal of Social Medicine,* **21**, 116–119.

Bucciero, A., Vizioli, L. and Tedeschi, G. (1993). Cord diameters and their significance in prognostication and decision about management of cervical spondylotic myelopathy. *Journal of Bone and Joint Surgery,* **37**, 223–228.

Buckwalter, J. A. (1995). Aging and degeneration of the human intervertebral disc. *Spine,* **20**, 1307–1314.

Buckwalter, J. A., Woo, S. L.Y., Goldberg, V. M. et al. (1993). Current concepts review. Soft tissue aging and musculoskeletal function. *Journal of Bone and Joint Surgery,* **75A**, 1533–1548.

Bulos, S. (1973). Herniated intervertebral lumbar disc in the teenager, *Journal of Bone and Joint Surgery,* **55B**, 273–278.

Burdof, A. and Zondervan, H. (1990). An epidemiological study of low back pain in crane operators. *Ergonomics,* 33, 981–987.

Burton, A. and Tillotson, K. (1991). Does leisure sports activity influence lumbar mobility or the risk of low back trouble? *Journal of Spinal Disorders,* **4**, 329–336.

Burton, A., Tillotson, K. and Troup, J. (1989).

Prediction of low back trouble frequency in a working poulation. *Spine,* **14**, 939–946.

Burton, A. K., Clarke, R. D., McClune, T. D. and Tillotson, K. M. (1996). The natural history of low back pain in adolescents. *Spine,* **21**, 2323–2328.

Burton, C. V. (1976). Percutaneous radiofrequency facet denervation. *Applied Neurophysiology,* **39**, 80–86.

Busch, E. and Wilson, P. R. (1989). Atlanto-occipital and atlantoaxial injections in the treatment on headache and neck pain. *Regional Anesthesia,* **14**, 45.

Bush, K. and Hillier, S. (1991). A controlled study of caudal epidural injection of triamcinolone plus procaine for the management of intractable sciatica. *Spine,* **16**, 572–575.

Bush, K., Cowan, N., Katz, D. E. and Gishen, P. (1993). The natural history of sciatica associated with disc pathology. *Journal of Orthopaedic Medicine,* **15**, 31–37.

Buswell, J. (1982). Low back pain: a comparison of two treatment programmes. *New Zealand Journal of Physiotherapy,* **10**, 13–17.

Butler, D., Trafimow, J. H., Andersson, G. B. J. et al. (1990). Discs degenerate before facets. *Spine,* **15**, 111–113.

Bywaters, E. G. L. (1981). Thoracic intervertebral discitis in rheumatoid arthritis due to costovertebral joint involvement. *Rheumatology International,* **1**, 83–97.

Cady, J. M. and Trier ,K. K. (1987). Exercise and smoking habits in patients with and without low back and leg pain. *Journal of Manipulative and Physiological Therapeutics,* **10**, 239–245.

Cady, J. M., Bischoff, D. P., O'Connell, E. R. et al. (1979). Strength and fitness related to subsequent back injuries in firefighters. *Journal of Occupational Medicine,* **21**, 269–272.

Cahill, D. W., Love, L. C. and Rechtine, G. R. (1991). Pyogenic osteomyelitis of the spine in the elderly. *Journal of Neurosurgery,* **74**, 878–886.

Callahan, E. P. and Aguillera, H. (1993). Complications following minor trauma in a patient with diffuse idiopathic skeletal hyperostosis. *Annals of Emergency Surgery,* **22**, 1067–1070.

Cameron, D. M., Bohannon, R. W. and Owen, S. V. (1994). Influence of hip position on measurements of the straight leg raising test.

Journal of Orthopedic and Sports Physical Therapy, **19**, 168–172.

Cameron, H. U. and Noftal, F. (1988). The piriformis syndrome. *Canadian Journal of Surgery,* **31**, 210

Campbell, D. G. and Parsons, C. M. (1944). Referred head pain and its concomitants. *Journal of Nervous and Mental Disease,* **99**, 544–551.

Campbell, S. M. (1986). Is the tender point concept valid? *American Journal of Medicine,* **81**, suppl 3A, 33-37.

Campbell, S. M., Clark, S., Tindall, E. A. et al. (1983). Clinical characteristic of fibrositis: I 'blinded', controlled study of symptoms and tender points. *Arthritis and Rheumatism,* **26**, 817–824.

Caputy, A. and Luessenhop, A. (1992). Long-term evaluation of decompressive surgery for degeneration lumbar stenosis. *Journal of Neurosurgery,* **77**, 669–706.

Carette, S., Marcoux, S., Truchon, R. et al. (1991). A controlled trial of corticosteroid injections into facet joints for chronic low back pain. *New England Journal of Medicine,* **325**, 1002–1007.

Carette, S., Leclaire, R , Marcoux, S. et al. (1997). Epidural corticosteroid injections for sciatica due to herniated nucleus pulposus. *New England Journal of Medicine,* **336**, 1634–1640.

Carlson, S. A. and Jones, J. S. (1994). Pyogenic sacroiliitis. *American Journal of Emergency Medicine,* **12**, 639–642.

Carrera, G. F. (1980a). Lumbar facet joint injection in low back pain and sciatica. Preliminary results. *Radiology,* **137**, 665–667.

Carrera, G. F. (1980b). Lumbar facet joint in low back pain and sciatica. Description of technique. *Radiology,* 661–664.

Carrera, G. F. and Williams, A. L. (1984). Current concepts in evaluation of the lumbar facet joints. *Critical Reviews in Diagnostic Imaging,* **21**, 85–104.

Carson, J., Gumpert, J. and Jefferson, A. (1971). Diagnosis and treatment of thoracic intervertebral disc protrusions. *Journal of Neurology, Neurosurgery and Psychiatry,* **34**, 68–77.

Casey, A. T. H. and Crockard, A. (1995). In the rheumatoid patient: surgery to the cervical spine. *British Journal of Rheumatology,* **34**, 1078–1086.

Casez, J. P., Fischer, S., Stussi, E. et al. (1995). Bone mass at lumbar spine and tibia in young males – impact of physical fitness, exercise, and anthropometric parameters: a prospective study in a cohort of military recruits. *Bone,* **17**, 211–219.

Caspar, W., Cambell, B., Barbier, D. et al. (1991). The Caspar microsurgical discectomy and comparison with a conventional standard lumbar disc procedure. *Neurosurgery,* **28**, 78–87.

Cassidy, J. D., Yong, H. K., Kirkaldy-Willis, W. and Wilkinson, A. A. (1988). A study of the effects of bipedism and upright posture on the lumbosacral spine and paravertebral muscles of the Wistar rat. *Spine,* **13**, 301–308.

Cassidy, J. D., Loback, D., Yong-Hing, K. and Tchang, S. (1992a). Lumbar facet joint asymmetry. Intervertebral disc herniation. *Spine,* **17**, 570–574.

Cassidy, J. D., Lopes, A. A., Yong-Hing, K. (1992b). The immediate effect of manipulation versus mobilizatiion on pain and range of motion in the cervical spine. *Journal of Manipulative and Physiological Therapeutics,* **15**, 570–575.

Cavanaugh, J. M. (1995). Neural mechanisms of lumbar pain. *Spine,* **20**, 1804–1809.

Chan, F., Ho, E. K. W. and Chau, E. M. T. (1988). Spinal pseudarthrosis complicating ankylosing spondylitis: comparison of CT and conventional tomography. *American Journal of Roentgenology,* **150**, 611–614.

Chapuy, M. C., Arlot, M. E., Duboeuf, F. et al. (1992). Vitamin D3 and calcium to prevent hip fractures in elderly women. *New England Journal of Medicine,* **327**, 1637–1642.

Charnley, J. (1951). Orthopedic signs in the diagnosis of disc protrusion with special reference to the straight leg raising test. *Lancet,* **1**, 186–192.

Chen, I. H. Vasavada, A. and Panjabi, M. M. (1994b). Kinematics of the cervical spine canal. *Journal of Spinal Disorders,* **7**, 93–101.

Chen, J. C. and Au, A. W. (1994). Infantile torticollis: a review of 624 cases. *Journal of Pediatric Orthopedics,* **14**, 802–808.

Chen, Q., Baba, H., Kamitani, K. et al. (1994a). Postoperative bone re-growth in lumbar spinal stenosis. A multivariate analysis of 48 patients. *Spine*, **19**, 2144–2149.

Chester, J. B. (1991). Whiplash, postural control and the inner ear. *Spine*, **16**, 716–720.

Chestnut, R. M., Abitbol, J.-J. and Garfin, S. R. (1992). Surgical management of cervical radiculopathy. Indication, techniques, and results. *Orthopedic Clinics of North America*, **23**, 461–474.

Chirls, M. (1975). Retrospective study of cervical spondylosis treatment by anterior interbody fusion in 505 patients performed by the Cloward technique. *Bulletin New York Hospital for Joint Disease*, **39**, 74–82.

Chisin, R., Milgrom, C., Marguilies, J. et al. (1984). Unilateral sacroiliac overuse syndrome in military recruits. *British Medical Journal*, **289**, 590–591.

Cholewicki, J. and McGill, S. M. (1996). Mechanical stability of the in vivo lumbar spine: implications for injury and chronic low back pain. *Clinical Biomechanics*, **11**, 1–15.

Choudury, A. R. and Taylor, J. C. (1980). Cauda equina syndrome in lumbar disc disease. *Orthopaedica Scandinavica*, **51**, 493–499.

Chua, W. H. and Bogduk, N. (1995). The surgical anatomy of thoracic facet denervation. *Acta Neurochirurgica*, **136**, 140–144.

Cibulka, M. T. (1992). The treatment of the sacroiliac joint component to low back pain: a case report. *Physical Therapy*, **72**, 917–922.

Cibulka, M. T. and Koldehoff, R. M. (1986). Leg length disparity and its effect on sacroiliac joint dysfunction. *Clinical Management*, **6**, 10–11.

Cibulka, M. T. Delitto, A. and Koldehoff, R. M. (1988). Changes in innominate tilt after manipulation of the sacroiliac joint in patients with low back pain. An experimental study. *Physical Therapy*, **68**, 1359–1363.

Ciocon, J. O., Galindociocon, D., Amaranath, L. M. and Galindo, D. (1994). Caudal epidural blocks for elderly patients with lumbar canal stenosis. *Journal of the American Geriatrics Society*, **42**, 593–596.

Ciric, I., Mikhael, M. A., Tarkington, J. A. and Vick, N. A. (1980). The lateral recess syndrome. A variant of spinal stenosis. *Journal of Neurosurgery*, **53**, 433–443.

Ciriello, V. M. and Snook, S. H. (1995). The effect of back belt on lumbar muscle fatigue. *Spine*, **20**, 1271–1278.

Ciullo, J. V. and Jackson, D. (1985). Pars interarticularis stress reaction, spondylolysis, and spondylolisthesis in gymnasts. *Clinics in Sports Medicine*, **4**, 95–110.

Civitelli, R., Gonnelli, S., Zacchei, F. et al. (1988). Bone turnover in postmenopausal osteoporosis: effects of calcitonin treatment. *Journal of Clinical Investigation*, **82**, 1268–1274.

Clark, C. R. (1994). Rheumatoid involvement of cervical spine. An overview. *Spine*, **19**, 2257–2258.

Clark, C. R., Goetz, D. D. and Menezes, A. H. (1989). Arthrodesis of the cervical spine in rheumatoid arthritis. *Journal of Bone and Joint Surgery*, **71A**, 381–392.

Clark, S., Campbell, S. M., Forehand, M. E. et al. (1985). Clinical characteristics of fibrositis: II. A blinded controlled study using standard psychological tests. *Arthritis and Rheumatism*, **28**, 132–137.

Clarke, D. P., Higgins, J. N., Valentine, A. R. and Black, C. (1994). Magnetic resonance imaging of osteitis condensans ilii. *British Journal of Rheumatology*, **33**, 599–600.

Clarke, G. R. (1972). Unequal leg length: an accurate method of detection and clinical results. *Rheum. Phys. Med.* **1**, 385–390.

Clarke, N. M. P. and Cleak, D. K. (1983). Intervertebral lumbar disc prolapse in children and adolescents. *Journal of Pediatric Orthopedics*, **3**, 202–206.

Claussen, C. F. and Claussen, E. (1995). Neurootological contributions to the diagnostic follow-up after whiplash injuries. *Acta Oto-Laryngolocica. Supplement*, **520**, 53–56.

Cloward, R. B. (1958). Cervical diskography: technique, indications, and use in cervical of ruptured cervical discs. *Annals of Surgery*, **79**, 690–705.

Cloward, R. B. (1959). Cervical diskography. A contribution to the etiology and mechanism of neck, shoulder and arm pain. *Annals of Surgery*, **150**, 1052–1064.

Cohen, M. J., Ezekiel, J. and Persellin, R. H. (1978). Costovertebral and costotransverse joint involvement in rheumatoid arthritis. *Annals of the Rheumatic Diseases*, **37**, 473–475.

Cohen, M. L. and Quintner, J. L. (1993). Fibromyalgia syndrome, a problem of tautology. *Lancet*, **342**, 906–909.

Colachis, S. C., Strohm, B. R. and Ganter, E. L. (1973). Cervical spine motion in normal women: radiographic study of the effect of cervical collars. *Archives of Physical Medicine and Rehabilitation*, **54**, 161–169.

Colditz, G. A., Hankinson, S. E., Hunter, D. J. et al. (1995). The use of estrogens and progestins and the risk of breast cancer in post-menopausal women. *New England Journal of Medicine*, **332**, 1589–1593.

Collins, D. H. (1940). Fibrositis and infection. *Annals of the Rheumatic Diseases*, **2**, 114–126.

Connell, M. D. and Wiesel, S. W. (1992). Natural history and pathogenesis of cervical disk disease. *Orthopedic Clinics of North America*, **23**, 369–380.

Cooper, R. G., Freemont, A. J., Hoyland, J. A. et al. (1995). Herniated intervertebral disc-associated periradicular fibrosis and vascular abnormalities occur without inflammatory cell infiltration. *Spine*, **20**, 591–598.

Cope, R. (1988). Acute traumatic spondylolysis. *Clinical Orthopaedics and Related Research*, **230**, 162–165.

Cope, S. and Ryan, G. M. S. (1959). Cervical and otolith vertigo *Journal of Laryngology and Otology*, **73**, 113–119.

Copeland, G, P., Machin, D. G. and Shennan, J. M. (1984). Surgical treatment of the 'slipping rib syndrome'. *British Journal of Surgery*, **71**, 522–523.

Coppes, M. H., Marani, E., Thomeer, R. T. W. et al. (1990). Innervation of annulus fibrosis in low back pain. *Lancet*, **336**, 189–190.

Corrigan, A. B. and Maitand, G. D. (1994). *Musculoskeletal and Sports Injuries*. pp. 123–124, Butterworth Heinemann.

Cox, J. M. and Trier, K. K. (1987). Exercise and smoking habits in patients with and without low back and leg pain. *Journal of Manipulative and Physiologial Thrapeutics*, **10**, 239–245.

Coxhead, C. E., Inskip, H., Meade, T. W. et al. (1981). Multicentre trial of physiotherapy in the management of sciatic symptoms. *Lancet*, **1**, 1065–1068.

Craufurd, D. I. O., Creed, F. and Jayson, M. I. V. (1990). Life events and psychological disturbance in patients with low back pain. *Spine*, **15**, 490–494.

Cresswell, A. G., Blake, P. L. and Thorstensson, A. (1994). The effect of an abdominal muscle training program on intra-abdominal pressure. *Scandinavian Journal of Rehabilitation Medicine*, **26**, 79–86.

Crisco, J. J., Panjabi, M. M. and Dvorak, J. (1991). A model of the alar ligaments of the upper cervical spine in axial rotation. *Journal of Biomechanics*, **24**, 607–614.

Crock, H. (1986). Internal disc disruption. A challenge to disc prolapse fifty years on. *Spine*, **11**, 650–653.

Crockard, H. A. (1995). Spine update. Surgical management of cervical rheumatoid problems. *Spine*, **20**, 2584–2590.

Crowe, H. E. (1928). Injuries to the cervical spine. Paper presented to the Western Orthopedic Association, San Francisco. Unpublished.

Cuckler, J., Bernini, P., Wiesel, S. et al. (1985). The use of epidural steroids in the treatment of lumbar radicular pain. A prospective, randomised, double blind study. *Journal of Bone and Joint Surgery*, **67A**, 63–66.

Cummings, G. S. and Crowell, R. S. (1988). Source of error in clinical assessment of innominate rotation. A special communication. *Physical Therapy*, **68**, 77–78.

Cummings, S. R., Nevitt, M. C., Browner, W. S. et al. (1995). Risk factors for hip fractures in white women. *New England Journal of Medicine*, **332**, 767–773.

Curd, J. G. and Thorne, R. P. (1989). Diagnosis and management of the patient with acute back pain. *Hospital Practice*, **15**, 135–148.

Cusick, J. F. (1991). Pathophysiology and treatment of cervical spondylotic myelopathy. *Clinical Neurosurgery*, **37**, 661–681.

Cyron, B. M. and Hutton, W. C. (1978). The fatigue strength of the lumbar neural arch in spondylolysis. *Journal of Bone and Joint Surgery*, **60B**, 234–238.

Cyron, B. M. and Hutton, W.C. (1980). Articular tropism and stability of the lumbar spine. *Spine*, **5**, 168–172.

Cyron, B. M., Hutton, W. C. and Troup, J. D. G. (1976). Spondylolytic fractures. *Journal of Bone and Joint Surgery*, **58B**, 462–466.

Daly, J. M., Frame, P. S. and Rapoza, P. A. (1991). Sacroiliac subluxation: a common cause of low back pain in pregnancy. *Family Practice Research Journal*, **11**, 149–159.

Dan, N. G. and Saccasan, P. A. (1983). Serious complications of lumbar spinal manipulation. *Medical Journal of Australia*, **2**, 672–673.

Danek, V. (1989). Haemodynamic disorders within the vertebrobasilar arterial system following extreme positions of the head. *Manual Medicine*, **4**, 127–129.

Daniel, J. N., Polly, D. W. and van Dam, B. E. (1995). A study of the efficacy of nonoperative treatment of presumed traumatic spondylolysis in a young patient population. *Military Medicine*, **160**, 553–555.

Daragon, A., Mejjad, O., Czernichow, P. et al. (1995). Vertebral hyperostosis and diabetes mellitus: a case-control study. *Annals of the Rheumatic Diseases*, **54**, 375–378.

Daum, W. J. (1995). The sacroiliac joint: an underappreciated pain generator. *American Journal of Orthopedics*, **24**, 475–478.

Dauser, R. C. and Chandler, W. F. (1982). Symptomatic congenital spinal stenosis in a child. *Neurosurery*, **11**, 61–63.

Davies, J. E., Gibson, T. and Tester, L. (1979). The value of exercises in the treatment of low back pain. *Rheumatology and Rehabilitation*, **38**, 243–247.

Davis, J. W., Phreaner, D. L., Hoyt, D. B. and Mackersie, R. C. (1993). The etiology of missed cervical spine injuries. *Journal of Trauma*, **34**, 342–346.

Davis, P. and Lentle, B. C. (1978). Evidence for sacroiliac disease as a common cause of low backache in women. *Lancet*, **1**, 496–497.

Davis, S. J., Teresi, L. M., Bradley, W. G. et al. (1991). Cervical spine hyperextension injuries. MR findings. *Radiology*, **180**, 245–251.

Dawson-Hughes, B., Dallal, G. E., Krall, E. A. et al. (1990). A controlled trial of the effect of calcium supplementation on bone density in postmenopausal women. *New England Journal of Medicine*, **323**, 878–883.

de Jong, P. T. V. M., de Jong, J. M. B. V., Cohen, B. and Jonkees, L. B. W. (1977). Ataxia and nystagmus induced by injection of local anaesthetic in the neck. *Annals of Neurology*, **1**, 240–246.

de Klyn, A. and Nieuwenhuyse, A. (1927). Shewindlelanfalle und nystagmus bei einer bestimmten stellung des kopfes. *Acta Otolaryngology*, **11**, 155–177.

de Orio, J. K. and Bianco, A. (1982). Lumbar disc excision in children and adolescents. *Journal of Bone and Joint Surgery*, **64A**, 991–996.

de Ruiter, M. (1990). Back to basics with Proflex. *Ergonomics*, **33**, 383–385.

Deans, G.T., Magalliard, J. N., Kerr, M. and Rutherford, W. H. (1987). Neck sprain. A common cause of disability following car accidents. *Injury*, **18**, 10–12.

Delamarter, R. B. and Bohlman, H. H. (1994). Postmortem osseous and neuropathologic analysis of the rheumatoid cervical spine. *Spine*, **19**, 2267–2274.

DeLauche-Cavellier, M-C., Budet, C., Laredo, J-D. et al. (1992). Lumbar disc herniation. Computed tomography scan changes after conservative treatment of nerve root compression. *Spine*, **17**, 927–933.

Delitto, A., Cibulka, M. T., Erhard, R. E. et al. (1993). Evidence for use of an extension – mobilization category in acute low back syndrome: a prescriptive validation pilot study. *Physical Therapy*, **73**, 216–228.

Destouet, J. M., Gilula, M. A., Murphy, W. A. and Monsees, B. (1982). Lumbar facet joint injection: indication, technique, clinical correlation and preliminary results. *Radiology*, **145**, 321–325.

Dettori, J. R., Bullock, S. H., Sutlive, T. G. et al. (1995). The effects of spinal flexion and extension exercises and their associated postures in patients with acute low back pain. *Spine*, **20**, 2303–2312.

Deyo, R. A. (1994). Magnetic resonance imaging of the lumbar spine – terrific test or tar baby? *New England Journal of Medicine*, **331**,115–116.

Deyo, R. A. and Bass, J. E. (1989). Lifestyle and low back pain: the influence of smoking and obesity. *Spine*, **14**, 501–506.

Deyo, R. A., Diehl, A. K. and Rosenthal, M. (1986). How many days bed rest for acute low back pain? *New England Journal of Medicine*, **315**, 1064–1070.

Deyo, R. A., Loeser, J. D. and Bigos, S. J. (1990a). Herniated lumbar intervertebral disc. *Annals of Internal Medicine*, **112**, 598–603.

Deyo, R. A., Walsh, N. E., Martin, D. C. et al. (1990b). A controlled trial of transcutaneous electrical nerve stimulation (TENS) and execise for chronic low back pain. *New England Journal of Medicine*, **322**, 1627–1634.

Deyo, R. A., Rainvillle, J. and Kent, D. (1992a). What can the history and physical examination tell us about low back pain. *Journal of the American Medical Association*, **268**, 760–766.

Deyo, R. A., Cherkin, D. C., Loeser, J. D. et al. (1992b). Morbidity and mortality in association with operations on the lumbar spine. *Journal of Bone and Joint Surgery*, **74A**, 536–543.

Di Fabio, R. P. (1992). Efficacy of manual therapy. *Physical Therapy*, **72**, 853–864.

Di Fabio, R. P. (1995). Efficacy of comprehensive rehabilitation programs and back school for patients with low back pain: a meta-analysis. *Physical Therapy*, **75**, 865–878.

Dieck, G. S., Kelsey, J. L., Goel, V. K. et al. (1985). An epidemiologic study of the relationship between postural asymmetry in the teen years and subsequent back and neck pain. *Spine*, **10**, 872–877.

Dietrich, M. and Kurowski, P. (1985). The importance of mechanical factors in the etiology of spondylolysis. *Spine*, **10**, 532–542.

Dietrichs, E. (1991). Anatomy of the pelvic joints – a review. *Scandinavian Journal of Rheumatology Supplement*, **88**, 4–6.

Dihlmann, W. (1991). Osteitis condensans ilii and sacroiliitis. *Journal of Rheumatology*, **18**, 1430–1432.

Dilke, T. F. W., Burry, H. C. and Grahame, R. (1973). Extradural corticosteroid injection in the management of lumbar nerve root compression. *British Medical Journal*, **2**, 635–637.

Disla, E., Rhim, H. R., Reddy, A. et al. (1994). A prospective analysis in an emergency department setting. *Archives of Internal Medicine*, **14**, 2466–2469.

Dodge, L. D., Bohlman, R. H. and Rhodes, R. S. (1988). Concurrrent lumbar spinal stenosis and peripheral vascular disease. *Clinical Orthopaedics and Related Research*, 230, 141–148.

Doita, M., Kanatani, T., Harada, T. and Kosaku, M. (1996). Immunohistologic study of the ruptured intervertebral disc of the lumbar spine. *Spine*, **21**, 235–241.

Dommisse, G. F. (1990). The vulnerable, rapidly growing thoracic spine of the adolescent. *South African Medical Journal*, **78**, 211–213.

Dommisse, G.F. (1975). Morphological aspects of the lumbar spine and lumbosacral region. *Orthopedic Clinics of North America*, **6**, 163–175.

Donat, W. E. (1987). Chest pain; cardiac and noncardiac causes. *Clinics in Chest Medicine*, **8**, 241–252.

Doneison, R., Aprill, C., Medcalf, R. and Grant, W. (1997). A prospective study of centralization of lumbar and referred pain. A predictor of symptomatic discs and anular competence. *Spine*, **22**, 1115–1122.

Donovan, M. J., Bowen, B.C. and Sze, G. (1991). Magnetic resonance imaging of spinal infection. *Rheumatic Diseases Clinics of North America*, **17**, 773–794.

Don'Tigny, R. L. (1985). Function and pathomechanics of the sacroiliac joint. A review. *Physical Therapy*, **65**, 35–44.

DonTigny, R. L. (1990). Anterior dysfunction of the sacroiliac joint as a major factor in the etiology of idiopathic low back pain syndrome. *Physical Therapy*, **70**, 250–265.

Dory, M. A. (1981). Arthrography of the lumbar facet joints. *Radiology*, **140**, 23–27.

Dory, M. A. (1983). Arthrography of the cervical facet joints. *Radiology*, **148**, 379–382.

Dorwart, R. H., Vogler, J. B. and Helms, C.A. (1983). Spinal stenosis. *Radiological Clinics of North America*, **21**, 301–325.

Drewes, A. M., Neilsen, K. D., Taagholt, S. J. et al. (1994). Quantification of alpha-EEG activity during sleep in fibromyalgia: a study based on ambulatory sleep monitoring. *Journal Musculoskeletal Pain*, **2**, 33–53.

Drewes, A. M., Gade, J., Nielsen, K. D. et al. (1995a). Clustering of sleep electroencephalographic patterns in patients with the fibromyalgia syndrome. *British Journal of Rheumatology*, **34**, 1151–1156.

Drewes, A. M., Nielsen, K. D., Taagholt, S. J. et al. (1995b). Sleep intensity in fibromyalgia: focus on the microstructure of the sleep process. *British Journal of Rheumatology*, **34**, 629–635.

Dreyfuss, P., Dryer, S., Griffin, J. et al. (1994a). Positive sacroiliac screening tests in asymptomatic adults. *Spine*, **19**, 1138–1143.

Dreyfuss, P., Michaelsen, M. and Fletcher, D. (1994b). Atlanto-occipital and lateral atlantoaxial joint pain patterns. *Spine*, **19**, 1125–1131.

Dreyfuss, P., Rogers, J., Dreyer, S. and Fletcher, D.

(1994c). Atlanto-occipital joint pain – a report of three cases and description of an intraarticular joint block technique. *Regional Anesthesia*, **19**, 344–351.

Dreyfuss, P., Tibiletti, C. and Dreyer. S. J. (1994d). Thoracic zygapophyseal joint pain patterns – a study in normal volunteers. *Spine*, **19**, 807–811.

Dreyzin, V. and Esses, S. I. (1994). A comparative analysis of spondylolysis repair. *Spine*, **19**, 1909–1914.

Dublin, A. B., McGahan, J. P. and Reid, M. H. (1983). The value of computed tomographic metrizamide myelography in the neuroradiological evaluation of the spine. *Radiology*, **146**, 79–86.

Dubuisson, D. (1995). Treatment of occipital neuralgia by partial posterior rhizotomy at C1–3. *Journal of Neurosurgery*, **82**, 581–586.

Dullerud, R. and Nakstad, P. H. (1994). CT changes after conservative treatment for lumbar disk herniation. *Acta Radiologica*, **35**, 415–419.

Dullerud, R., Amundsen, T., Lie, H. et al. (1995). Clinical results after percutaneous automated lumbar nucleotomy. A follow-up study. *Acta Radiologica*, **36**, 418–424.

Dunlop, R. B., Adams, M. A., and Hutton, W. C. (1984). Disc space narrowing and the lumbar facet joints. *Journal of Bone and Joint Surgery*, **66B**, 706–710.

Dupuis, P. R., Yong-Hong, K., Cassidy, J. D., and Kirkaldy-Willis, W. H. (1985). Radiological diagnosis of degenerative lumbar spine instability. *Spine*, **10**, 262–276.

Dura, P. A., Daniel, T. M., Frierson, H. F. and Brunner, C. M. (1993). Chest wall mass in rheumatoid arthritis. *Journal of Rheumatology*, **20**, 910–912.

Dussault, R. G. and Nicolet, V. M. (1985). Cervical facet joint arthrography. *Journal of the Canadian Association of Radiology*, **36**, 79–80.

Dutton, C. D. and Riley, L. H. (1969). Cervical migraine. Not merely a pain in the neck. *American Journal of Medicine*, **47**, 141–148.

Dvorak, J. and Orelli, F. (1985). How dangerous is manipulation to the cervical spine: case report and results of a survey. *Manual Medicine*, **2**, 1–4.

Dvorak, J., Penning, L., Hayek, J. et al. (1988a). Functional diagnostics of the cervical spine using computer tomography. *Neuroradiology*, **30**, 132–137.

Dvorak, J., Froehlich, D., Penning, L. et al. (1988b). Functional radiographic diagnosis of the cervical spine: flexion/extension. *Spine*, **13**, 748–755.

Dvorak, J., Valach, L. and Schmid, S. (1989). Cervical spine injuries in Switzerland. *Journal of Manual Medicine*, **4**, 7–16.

Dvorak, J., Antinnes, J. A., Panjabi, M. et al. (1992). Age and gender related motion of the cervical spine. *Spine*, **17**(10S), 393–398.

Dwyer, A., Aprill, C. and Bogduk, N. (1990). Cervical zygapophyseal joint pain patterns. 1. A study in normal volunteers. *Spine*, **15**, 453–457.

Dyck, P. and Doyle, J. B. (1977). 'Bicycle test' of van Gelderen in diagnosis of intermittent cauda equina compressive syndrome. *Journal of Neurosurgery*, **46**, 667–670.

Ebara, S., Iatridis, J. C., Setton, L. A. et al. (1996). Tensile properties of non-degenerate human lumbar annulus fibrosus. *Spine*, **21**, 452–461.

Edelmann, R. R. and Warach, S. (1993). Medical progress: magnetic resonance imaging. *New England Journal of Medicine*, **328**, 708–716.

Edgar, M. A. and Park, W. M. (1974). Induced pain patterns on passive straight leg raising in lower lumbar disc protrusion. *Journal of Bone and Joint Surgery*, **56B**, 658–667.

Editorial. (1992). Fibromyalgia: the Copenhagen declaration. *Lancet*, **340**, 663–664.

Edmeads, J. (1988). The cervical spine and headache. *Neurology*, **38**, 1874–1878.

Edwards, W. C. and LaRocca, S. H. (1985). The developmental segmental sagittal diameter in combined cervical and lumbar spondylosis. *Spine*, **10**, 42–49.

Egund, N., Olson, T. H., Schmid, H. and Selvik, G. (1978). Movements of the sacroiliac joints demonstrated with roentgen stereophotogrammetry. *Acta Radiologica Diagnostica*, **19**, 833–846.

Ehni, G. and Benner, B. (1984). Occipital neuralgia and the C1-2 arthrosis syndrome. *Journal of Neurosurgery*, **61**, 961–965.

Eisenstein, S. (1977). The morphometry and pathological anatomy of the lumbar spine in South African negroes and caucasoids with specific reference to spinal stenosis. *Journal of Bone and Joint Surgery*, **59B**, 173–180.

Eisenstein, S. (1978). Spondylolysis – a skeletal

investigation of two population groups. *Journal of Bone and Joint Surgery*, **60B**, 488–494.

Eisenstein, S. (1983). Lumbar vertebral canal morphometry for computerized tomography in spinal stenosis. *Spine*, **8**, 187–191.

Eisenstein, S. M. and Parry, C. R. (1987). The lumbar facet arthrosis syndrome – clinical presentation and articular surface changes. *Journal of Bone and Joint Surgery*, **69B**, 3–7.

Eisenstein, S. M., Ashton, I. K., Roberts, S. et al. (1994). Innervation of the spondylolysis 'ligament'. *Spine*, **19**, 912–916.

Eismont, F. J., Clifford, S., Goldberg, M. and Green, B. (1984). Cervical saggital spinal canal size in spine injury. *Spine*, **9**, 663–666.

Ekberg, K., Bjorkqvist, B., Malm, P. et al. (1994). Controlled two year follow up of rehabilitation for disorders in the neck and shoulders. *Occupational and Environmental Medicine*, **51**, 833–838.

Elders, P. J. M., Lips, P. and Netelenbos, J. C. (1994). Long-term effect of calcium supplementation on bone loss in perimenopausal women. *Journal of Bone and Mineral Research*, **9**, 963–970.

el Garf, A. and Khater, R. (1984). Diffuse idiopathic skeletal hyperostosis (DISH) a clinico-radiological study of the disease pattern in Middle Eastern populations. *Journal of Rheumatology*, **11**, 804–807.

Ellenberger, C. (1994). MR imaging of the low back syndrome. *Neurology*, **44**, 594–600.

Elliott, B. C. and Foster, D. H. (1984). A biomechanical analysis of the front-on and side-on fast bowling techniques. *Journal of Human Movement Studies*, **10**, 83–94.

Elliott, B., Hardcastle, P., Burnett, A. and Foster, D. (1992). The influence of fast bowling and physical factors on radiological features in high performance young fast bowlers. *Sports Medicine Training and Rehabilitation*, **3**, 113–130.

Elliott, B., Davis, J., Khangure, J. E. et al. (1993). Disc degeneration and the young fast bowler in cricket. *Clinical Biomechanics*, **8**, 227–234.

Elliott, B., Burnett, A., Stockill, N. and Bartlett, R. (1995). The fast bowler in cricket: a sports medicine perspective. *Sports, Exercise and Injury*, **1**, 201–206.

Elnaggar, I. M., Nordin, M., Sheikhzadeh, A. et al. (1991). Effects of spinal flexion and extension exercises on low back pain and spinal mobility in chronic mechanical low back pain patients. *Spine*, **16**, 967–972.

el-Shahaly, H. A., and el-Sherif, A. K. (1991). Is the benign joint hypermobility syndrome benign? *Clinical Rheumatology*, **10**, 302–307.

Elster, A. (1989). Bertolotti's syndrome revisited. Transitional vertebrae of the lumbar spine. *Spine*, **14**, 1373–1377.

Elster, A. D. and Jensen, K. M. (1985). Computered tomography of spondylolisthesis: patterns of associated pathology. *Journal of Computer Assisted Tomography*, **9**, 867–874.

Elvey, R. L. (1986). The investigation of arm pain. In *Modern Manual Therapy of the Vertebral Column*. (G. P. Grieve, ed.) pp. 530–535, Churchill Livingstone.

Engel, R. and Bogduk, N. (1982). The menisci of the lumbar zygapophyseal joints. *Journal of Anatomy*, **135**, 795–809.

Enzmann, D. R. (1994). Special report on low back pain. *American Journal of Neuroradiology*, **15**, 109–113.

Epstein, J. B. (1992). Temporomandibular disorders, facial pain and headache following motor vehicle accidents. *Journal of the Canadian Dental Association*, **58**, 488–496.

Epstein, S. E. (1979). Chest wall syndrome. *Journal of the American Medical Association*, **241**, 2793–2797.

Erkintalo, M. O., Salminen, J. J, Alanen, A. M. et al. (1995). Development of degenerative changes in the lumbar intervertebral disc: results of a prospective MR imaging study in adolescents with and without low-back pain. *Radiology*, **196**, 529–533.

Errico, T. J., Fardon, D. F. and Lowell, T. D. (1995). Contemporary concepts in spine care. Open discectomy as treatment for herniated nucleus pulposus of the lumbar spine. *Spine*, **20**, 1829–1833.

Ettlin, T. M., Kishka, U., Reichmann, S. et al. (1992). Cerebral symptoms after whiplash injury of the neck: a prospective clinical and neuropsychological study of whiplash injury. *Journal of Neurology, Neurosurgery and Psychiatry*, **55**, 943–948.

Evans, D. P. (1982). *Backache: Its Evolution and Conservative Treatment*. MTP Press.

Evans, R. W. (1992). Some observations on

whiplash injuries. *Neurologic Clinics*, **10**, 975–997.

Evans, W., Jobe, W. and Seibert, C. (1989). A cross-sectional prevalence study of lumbar disc degeneration in a working population. *Spine*, **14**, 60–64.

Faciszewski, T., Winter, R. B., Lonstein, J. E. et al. (1995). The surgical and medical perioperative complications of anterior spinal fusion surgery in the thoracic and lumbar spine in adults. A review of 1223 procedures. *Spine*, **20**, 1592–1599.

Fairbank, J. C., Park, W. M., McCall, I. W. and O'Brien, J. P. (1981). Apophyseal injection of local anesthetic as a diagnostic aid in primary low back syndrome. S*pine*, **6**, 598–605.

Farfan, H. F. (1980a). The pathological anatomy of degenerative spondylolisthesis: a cadaver study. *Spine*, **5**, 412–418.

Farfan, H. F. (1980b). The scientific basis of manipulative procedures. *Clinics in Rheumatic Diseases*, **6**, 159–177.

Farfan, H. F. (1984). The torsional injury of the lumbar spine. *Spine*, **9**, 53.

Farfan, H. F. and Gracovetsky, S. (1984). The nature of instability . *Spine*, **9**, 714–719.

Farfan, H. F., Cossette, U. W., Robertson, G. H. et al. (1970). The effects of torsion on the lumbar intervertebral joints. The role of torsion in the production of disc degeneration. *Journal of Bone and Joint Surgery*, **52A**, 468–497.

Farfan, H. F., Huberdeau, R. M. and Dubow, H. I. (1972). Lumbar intervertebral disc degeneration. The influence of geometrical features on the pattern of disc degeneration – a post-mortem study. *Journal of Bone and Joint Surgery*, **54A**, 492–510.

Farfan, H. F., Osteria, V. and Lamy, C. (1976). The mechanical etiology of spondylolysis and spondylolisthesis. *Clinical Orthopaedics and Related Research*, **117**, 40–55.

Farina, S., Granella, F., Malferrari, G. and Manzoni, G. (1986). Headache and cervical spine disorders classification and treatment with transcutaneous electrical nerve stimulation. *Headache*, **26**, 431–433.

Farmer, J. C. and Wisenski, R. J. (1994). Cervical nerve root compression. An analysis of neuroforaminal pressures with varying head and arm positions. *Spine*, **19**, 1850–1855.

Farrell, J. P. and Twomey, L. T. (1982). Acute low back pain. Comparison of two conservative approaches. *Medical Journal of Australia*, **1**, 160–164.

Fass, A., van Eijk, J. Th. M., Chavannes, A. W. and Gubbels, J. W. (1995). A randomized trial of exercise therapy in patients with acute low back pain. Efficacy on sickness absence. *Spine*, **20**, 941–947.

Fast, A., Robin, G. C. and Floman, Y. (1985). Surgical treatment of lumbar canal stenosis in the elderly. *Archives of Physical Medicine and Rehabilitation*, **66**, 149–151.

Fehlandt, A. F. and Micheli, L. J. (1993) Lumbar facet stress fracture in a ballet dancer. *Spine*, **18**, 2537–2539.

Feinstein, B., Langton, N. J. K., Jameson, R. M. and Schiller, F. (1954). Experiments on pain referred from deep somatic tissues. *Journal of Bone and Joint Surgery*, **36A**, 981–987.

Felson, D. T. and Goldenberg, D. L. (1986). The natural history of fibromyalgia. *Arthritis and Rheumatism*, **29**, 1522–1526.

Ferguson, R. J. L. and Caplan, L. (1985). Cervical spondylotic myelopathy. *Neurologic Clinics*, **3**, 373–382.

Ferguson, R. J., McMaster, J. H. and Stanitski, C. L. (1974). Low back pain in college football linemen. *Journal of Sports Medicine*, **2**, 63–69.

Ferreira-Alves, A., Resina, J. and Palma-Rodrigues, R. (1995). Scheuermann's kyphosis. The Portuguese technique of surgical treatment. *Journal of Bone and Joint Surgery*, **77B**, 943–950.

Fewins, H. E., Whitehouse, G. H. and Bucknall, R. C. (1990). Role of computed tomography in the evaluation of suspected sacroiliac joint disease. *Journal of the Royal Society of Medicine,.* **83**, 430–432.

Finch, P. and Taylor, J. (1996). Functional anatomy of the spine. In *Interventional Pain Management*. (H. Waldeman and R. Winnie, eds.) pp. 39–64, Saunders.

Finkenberg, J. G. (1993). Pyogenic and nonpyogenic infections of the spine: indications and treatment. In *Current Opinion in Orthopedics*. (J. P. Kostuik and J. P. W. Errico, eds.) pp. 4,11, 177–185.

Fisher, S. V. Bowar, J. F. and Awad, E. A. (1977). Cervical orthoses' effect on cervical spine motion: roentgenographic and goniometric methods of study. *Archives of Physical Medicine and Rehabilitation*, **58**, 109–115.

Fishman, E. K. and Magid, D. (1992). Cervical fracture in ankylosing spondylitis: value of multidimensional imaging. *Clinical Imaging*, **16**, 31–33.

Fishman, L. M. and Zybert, P. A. (1992). Electrophysiologic evidence of piriformis syndrome. *Archives of Physical Medicine and Rehabilitation*, **73**, 359–364.

Fleisch, H. (1993). Prospective use of bisphosphonates in osteoporosis (editorial). *Journal of Clinical Endocrinology and Metabolism*, **76**, 1397–1398.

Floman, Y, Wiesel, S. W. and Rothman, R. H. (1980). Cauda equina syndrome presenting as a herniated lumbar disc. *Clinical Orthopaedics and Related Research*, **147**, 234–237.

Flynn, K. T. (1981). Musculoskeletal chest wall pain. *Nurse Practitioner*, **18**, 407–412.

Foley-Nolan, D., Moore, K., Codd, M. et al. (1992). Low energy high frequency pulsed electromagnetic therapy for acute whiplash injuries. *Scandinavian Journal of Rehabilitation Medicine*, **24**, 51–59.

Fortin, J. D., Aprill, C., Ponthieux, B. and Pier, J. (1994a). Sacroiliac joint: pain referral maps upon applying a new injection arthrography technique. Part II. Clinical evaluation. *Spine*, **19**, 1475–1482.

Fortin, J. D., Dwyer, A. P., West, S. and Pier, J (1994b). Sacroiliac joint: pain referral maps upon applying a new injection technique. Part I. Asymptomatic volunteers. *Spine*, **19**, 1483–1489.

Foster, D., John, D., Elliot, B. et al. (1989). Back injuries to young fast bowlers in cricket: a prospective study. *British Journal of Sports Medicine*. **23**, 150–154.

Foster, D. N. and Fulton, M. N. (1991). Back pain and the exercise prescription. *Clinics in Sports Medicine*, **10**, 197–209.

Fox, M. W., Onofrio, B. M. and Kilgore, J. E. (1993). Neurological complications of ankylosing spondylitis. *Journal of Neurosurgery*, **78**, 871–878.

Francois, R. J., Eulderink, F. and Bywaters, E. G. L. (1995). Commented glossary for rheumatic spinal diseases, based on pathology. *Annals of the Rheumatic Diseases*, **54**, 615–625.

Franson, R., Saal, J. S. and Saal, J. A. (1992). Human disc phospholipase A2 is inflammatory. *Spine*, **17**, S129–S132.

Fredrickson, B. E., Baker, D., McHolick, W. J. et al. (1984). The natural history of spondylolysis and spondylolisthesis. *Journal of Bone and Joint Surgery*, **66A**, 699–707.

Fredriksen, T. A., Hovdal, H. and Sjaastad, O. (1987). Cervicogenic headache: clinical manifestations. *Cephalalgia*, **7**, 147–160.

Frennered, K. (1994). Isthmic spondylolisthesis among patients receiving disability pension under the diagnosis of chronic low back pain syndromes. *Spine*, **19**, 2766–2769.

Friberg, O. (1983). Clinical symptoms and biomechanics of lumbar spine and hip joint in leg length inequality. *Spine*, **8**, 643–651.

Friberg, O. (1991). Instability in spondylolisthesis. *Orthopedics*, **14**, 463–466.

Fricton, J. R., Auvinen, M. D., Dykstra, D. and Schiffman, E. (1985). Myofascial pain syndromes: electromyographic changes associated with local twitch response. *Archives of Physical Medicine and Rehabilitation*, **66**, 314–317.

Frigerio, N., Stowe, R. and Howe, J. (1974). Movements of the sacroiliac joint. *Clinical Orthopaedics and Related Research*, **100**, 370–377.

Frisoni, G. B. and Anzola, G. P. (1991). Vertebrobasilar ischemia after neck motion. *Stroke*, **22**, 1452–1460.

Frumkin, L. R. and Baloh, R. W. (1990). Wallenberg's syndrome following neck manipulation. *Neurology*, **40**, 611–615.

Frymoyer, J. W. (1992). Predicting disability from low back pain. *Clinical Orthopaedics and Related Research*, **279**, 101–109.

Frymoyer, J. W. (1988). Back pain and sciatica. *New England Journal of Medicine*, **318**, 291–300.

Frymoyer, J. W. and Selby, D. K. (1985). Segmental instability . Rationale for treatment. *Spine*, **10**, 280–296.

Frymoyer, J. W., Pope, M. H., Clements, F. H. et al. (1983). Risk factors in low back pain: an epidemiological survey. *Journal of Bone and Joint Surgery*, **65A**, 213–218.

Fujita, K., Nakagawa, T., Hirabayashi, K. and Nagai, Y. (1993). Neutral proteinases in human intervertebral disc. Role in degeneration and probable origin. *Spine*, **18**, 1766–1773.

Fukushima, T., Ikata, T., Taoka, Y. and Takata, S. (1991). Magnetic resonance imaging study on spinal cord plasticity in patients with cervical compression myelopathy. *Spine*, **16**, S534–S538.

Fukuyama S., Nakamura, T., Ikeda, T. and Takagi, K. (1995). The effect of mechanical stress on hypertrophy of the lumbar ligamentum flavum. *Journal of Spinal Disorders*, **8**, 126–130.

Fyler, G. W. (1980). Pain in the xiphisternal joint. Letter. *Journal of the American Medical Association*, **243**, 1896.

Gainor, B. J., Hagen, R. J. and Allen, W. C. (1983). Biomechanics of the spine in the pole-vaulter as related to spondylolysis. *American Journal of Sports Medicine*, **11**, 53–57.

Gallinaro, P. and Cartesegna, M. (1983). Three cases of lumbar disc rupture and one of cauda equina associated with spinal manipulation (chiropraxis) (letter). *Lancet*, **2**, 986–987.

Gamble, J. G., Simmons, S. C. and Freedman, M. (1986). The symphysis pubis: anatomic and pathologic considerations. *Clinical Orthopaedics and Related Research*, **203**, 261–272.

Garfin, S. R. (1995). A 50-year old woman with disabling spinal stenosis. *Journal of the American Medical Association*, **274**, 1949–1954.

Garfin, S. R., Rydevik, B., Lind, B. and Massie, J. (1995). Spinal nerve root compression. *Spine*, **20**, 1810–1820.

Gargan, M. F. and Bannister, G. C. (1990). Long-term prognosis of soft-tissue injuries of the neck. *Journal of Bone and Joint Surgery*, **72B**, 901–903.

Gargan, M. F. and Bannister, G. C. (1994). The rate of recovery following whiplash injury. *European Spine Journal*, **3**, 162–164.

Gelb, D.E., Lenke, L.G., Bridwell, K.H. et al. (1995). An analysis of sagittal spinal alignment in 100 asymptomatic middle and older aged volunteers. *Spine*, **20**, 1351–1358.

Gemmell, H. A. and Jacobson, B. H. (1990). Incidence of sacroiliac dysfunction and low back pain in fit college students. *Journal of Manipulative and Physiological Therapeutics*, **13**, 63–67.

Genaidy, A. M., Simmons, R. J. and Christensen, D. M. (1995). Can back supports relieve the load on the lumbar spine for employees engaged in industrial operations? *Ergonomics*, **38**, 996–1010.

Ghabrial, Y. A. and Tarrant, M. J. (1989). Adolescent lumbar disc prolapse. *Acta Orthopaedica Scandinavica*, **60**, 174–176.

Ghelman, B., Lospinuso, M. F., Levine, D. B. et al. (1991). Percutaneous computed tomography guided biopsy of the thoracic and lumbar spine. *Spine*, **16**, 736–739.

Ghormley, R. K. (1933). Low back pain with special reference to the articular facets, with presentation of an operative procedure. *Journal of the American Medical Association*, **101**, 1773–1777.

Ghosh, P. (1990a). Basic biochemistry of intervertebral disc and its variation with ageing and degeneration. *Journal of Manual Medicine*, **5**, 48–51.

Ghosh, P. (1990b). The role of mechanical and genetic factors in degeneration of the disc. *Journal of Manual Medicine*, **5**, 62–65.

Gibson, T., Grahame, R., Harkness, J. et al. (1985). Controlled comparison of short-wave diathermy with osteopathic treatment in non-specific low back pain. *Lancet*, **2**, 1258–1261.

Giles, L. G. F. and Taylor, J. R. (1981). Low back pain associated with leg length inequality. *Spine*, **6**, 510–521.

Giles, L. G. F. and Taylor, J. R. (1982). Lumbar spine structural changes associated with leg length inequality. *Spine*, **7**, 159–162.

Giles, L. G. F. and Taylor, J. R. (1987). Innervation of lumbar zygapophyseal joint synovial folds. *Acta Orthopaedica Scandinavica*, **58**, 43–46.

Giroux, J. C. and Leclercq, T. A. (1982). Lumbar disc excision in the second decade. *Spine*, **7**, 168–170.

Glover, M. G., Hargens, A. R., Mahmood, M. M. et al. (1991). A new technique for the in vitro measurement of nucleus pulposus swelling pressure. *Journal of Orthopaedic Research*, **9**, 61–67.

Godfrey, C. M., Morgan, P. P. and Schatzker, J. (1984). A randomized trial of manipulation for low-back pain in a medical setting. *Spine*, **9**, 301–304.

Goeken, L. N. and Hof, A. L. (1994). Instrumental straight leg raising: results in patients. *Archives of Physical Medicine and Rehabilitation*, **75**, 470–477.

Goel, V. K., Kong, W., Hans, J. S. et al. (1993). A combined finite element and optimization investigation of lumbar spine mechanics with and without muscles. *Spine*, **18**, 1531–1541.

Goldberg, A. L., Rothfus, W. E., Deeb, Z. L. et al. (1988). The impact of magnetic resonance on the diagnostic evaluation of acute cervico-thoracic trauma. *Skeletal Radiology*, **17**, 89–95.

Goldberg, A. L., Soo, M. S. C., Deeb, Z. L. and Rothfus, W. E. (1991). Degenerative disease of the lumbar spine: role of CT-Myelography in the M.R. era. *Clinical Imaging*, **15**, 47–55.

Goldenberg, D. L. (1987). Fibromyalgia syndrome. An emerging but controversial condition. *Journal of the American Medical Association*, **257**, 2782–2787.

Goldenberg, D. L. (1995). Fibromyalgia: why such controversy? *Annals of the Rheumatic Diseases*, **54**, 3–5.

Goldthwait, J. E. (1911). The lumbosacral articulation: an explanation of many cases of 'lumbago', sciatica and paraplegia. *Boston Medical and Surgical Journal*, **164**, 365–372.

Good, D. C., Couch, J. R. and Wacaser, L. (1984). 'Numb, clumsy hands' and high cervical spondylosis. *Surgical Neurology*, **22**, 285–291.

Gordon, S. J., Yang, K. H., Mayer, P. J. et al. (1991). Mechanisms of disk rupture, preliminary report. *Spine*, **16**, 450–456.

Gordon, T. P., Sage, M. R., Bertouch, J. V. and Brooks, P. M. (1984). Computed tomography of paraspinal musculature in ankylosing spondylitis. *Journal of Rheumatology*, **11**, 794–797.

Gore, D. R., Sepic, S. B. and Gardner, G. M. (1986). Roentgenographic finding of the cervical spine in asymptomatic people. *Spine*, **6**, 521–524.

Gore, D. R., Sepic, S. B. and Gardner, G. M. (1987). Neck pain: a long-term follow-up of 205 patients. *Spine*, **12**, 1–5.

Gottten, N. (1956). Survey of one hundred cases of whiplash injury after settlement of litigation. *Journal of the American Medical Association*, **162**, 865–867.

Goupille, P., Fitoussi, V., Cotty, B. et al. (1993). Lumbar facet joint injections with corticosteroids for chronic low back pain – results in 206 patients. *Revue du Rhumatisme*, **60**, 797–801.

Gower, W. R. (1904). A lecture on lumbago: its lessons and analogues. *British Medical Journal*, **1**, 117–121.

Grabias, S. (1980). Current concepts review. The treatment of spinal stenosis. *Journal of Bone and Joint Surgery*, **62A**, 308–313.

Gracovetsky, S., Farfan, H. F. and Helleur, C. (1985). The abdominal mechanism. *Spine*, **10**, 317–324.

Grahame, R. (1993). Joint hypermobility and the performing musician (editorial). *New England Journal of Medicine*, **329**, 1120–1121.

Granges, G., Zilko, P. and Littlejohn, G. (1994). Fibromyalgia syndrome: assessment of the severity of the condition 2 years after diagnosis. *Journal of Rheumatology*, **21**, 523–529.

Granhed, H. and Morelli, B. (1988). Low back pain among retired wrestlers and heavyweight lifters. *American Journal of Sports Medicine*, **16**, 530–533.

Green, T. P., Allvey, J. C. and Adams, M. A. (1994). Spondylolysis. Bending of the inferior articular processes of lumbar vertebrae during simulated spinal movements. *Spine*, **19**, 2683–2691.

Greenbarg, P. E., Brown, M. D., Pallares, V. S. et al. (1988). Epidural anesthesia for lumbar spine surgery. *Journal of Spinal Disorders*, **1**, 139–143.

Greenberg, J. O. and Schell, R. G. (1991). Magnetic resonance imaging of the lumbar spine in asymptomatic adults. *Journal of Neuroimaging*, **1**, 2–9.

Greene, P., Kang, U. J. and Fahn, S. (1995). Spread of symptoms in idiopathic torsion dystonia. *Movement Disorders*, **10**, 143–152.

Greenman, P. E. and Tait, B. (1988). Structural diagnosis in chronic low back pain. *Journal of Manual Medicine*, **3**, 114–117.

Gregg, R. (1994). Chronic pain management and lumbar stenosis. *Seminars in Spine Surgery*, **6**, 156–161.

Grieve, E. F. M. (1983). Mechanical dysfunction of the sacroiliac joint. *International Rehabilitation Medicine*, **5**, 46–52.

Grieve, G. P. (1976). The sacroiliac joint. *Physiotherapist*, **62**, 383–400.

Grob, D., Dvorak, J., Panjabi, M. M., and Antinnes, J. A. (1994). The role of plate and screw fixation in occipitocervical fusion in rheumatoid arthritis. *Spine*, **19**, 2545–2551.

Grob, D., Humke, T., and Dvorak, J. (1995). Degenerative lumbar spinal stenosis. Decompression with and without arthrodesis. *Journal of Bone and Joint Surgery*, **77A**, 1036–1041.

Grobler, L., Novotny, J .E., Wilder, D. G. et al. (1994). L4–5 isthmic spondylolisthesis. A biomechanical analysis comparing stability in L4-5 and L5-S1 isthmic spondylolisthesis. *Spine*, **19**, 222–227.

Grobler, L. J., Robertson, P. A., Novotny, J. E. and Pope, M. H. (1993). Etiology of spondylolisthesis. Assessment of the role played by lumbar facet joint morphology. *Spine*, **18**, 80–91.

Grogaard, B., Dullerud, R. and Magnaes, B. (1993). Acute torticollis in children due to atlanto-axial rotary fixation. *Archives of Orthopaedic and Trauma Surgery*, **112**, 185–188.

Grogan, J. P., Hemminghytt, S., Williams, A. L. et al. (1982). Spondylolysis studied with computered tomography. *Radiology*, **145**, 737–742.

Gross, A. R., Aker, P. D. and Quartly, C. (1996). Manual therapy in the treatment of neck pain. *Rheumatic Diseases Clinics of North America*, **22**, 579–598.

Gunzberg, R., Parkinson, R., Moore, R. et al. (1992). A cadaveric study comparing discography, magnetic resonance imaging, histology, and mechanical behavior of the human lumbar disc. *Spine*, **17**, 417–426.

Guyer, R. D. and Ohnmeiss, D. D. (1995). Contemporary concepts in spine care. Lumbar discography. Position statement from the North American spine society diagnostic and therapeutic committee. *Spine*, **20**, 2048–2059.

Hadler, N. M. (1986). A critical reappraisal of the fibrositis concept. *American Journal of Medicine*, **81**, suppl 3A, 26–30.

Hadler, N. M., Curtis, P., Gillings, D. B. and Stinnett, S. (1987). A benefit of spinal manipulation as adjunctive therapy for acute low back pain: a stratified controlled trial. *Spine*, **12**, 702–706.

Hagg, O. and Wallner, A. (1990). Facet joint asymmetry and protrusion of the intervertebral disc. *Spine*, **15**, 356–359.

Haher, T. R., O'Brien, M., Kauffman, C. et al. (1993). Biomechanics of the spine in sports. *Clinics in Sports Medicine*, **12**, 449–464.

Haher, T. R., O'Brien, M., Dryer, J. W. et al. (1994). The role of the lumbar facet joint in spinal stability. Identification of alternative paths of loading. *Spine*, **19**, 2667–2670.

Hainline, B. (1995). Low back injury. *Clinics in Sports Medicine*, **14**, 241–265.

Hakelius, A. and Hindmarsh, J. (1972). The significance of neurological signs and myelographic finding in the diagnosis on lumbar root compression. *Acta Orthopaedica Scandinavica*, **43**, 234–238.

Halal, F., Gledhill, R. B. and Fraser, F. C. (1978). Dominant inheritance of Scheuermman's juvenile kyphosis. *American Journal of Diseases of Children*, **132**, 1105–1107.

Haldeman, S. (1983). Spinal manipulative therapy. A status report. *Clinical Orthopaedics and Related Research*, **179**, 62–70.

Haldeman, S. and Rubinstein, S. M. (1992). Cauda equina syndrome in patients undergoing manipulation of the lumbar spine. *Spine*, **17**, 1469–1473.

Hales, T. A., Yunus, M. B. and Masi, A. T. (1987). Is chronic pain a variant of depressive disease? *Pain*, **29**, 105–111.

Halilgolu, M., Kleiman, M. B., Siddiqui, A. R. and Cohen, M. D. (1994). Osteomyelitis and pyogenic infection of the sacroiliac joint. MRI findings and review. *Pediatric Radiology*, **24**, 333–335.

Hall, H. and Hadler, N. M. (1995). Low back school. Education or exercise? *Spine*, **20**, 1097–1098.

Hall, S., Barelson, J. D., Onfrio, B. M. et al. (1985). Lumbar spinal stenosis: clinical features, diagnostic procedures, and results of surgical treatment in 68 patients. *Annals of Internal Medicine*, **103**, 271–275.

Halliday, J. L. (1941). Concepts of psychosomatic rheumatism. *Annals of Internal Medicine*, **15**, 666–667.

Halm, H., Metz-Stavenhagen, P. and Zielke, K. (1995). Results of surgical correction of kyphotic deformities of the spine in ankylosing spondylitis on the basis of the modified arthritis impact measurement scales. *Spine*, **20**, 1612–1619.

Hanly, J. G., Mitchell, M. J., Barnes, D. C. and Macmillan, L. (1994). Early recognition of sacroiliitis by magnetic resonance imaging and single photon emission computed tomography. *Journal of Rheumatology*, **21**, 2088–2095.

Hansson, T. and Holm, S. (1991). Clinical implications of vibration-induced changes in the lumbar spine. *Orthopedic Clinics of North America*, **22**, 247–253.

Hardcastle, P. (1993). Repair of spondylolysis in young fast bowlers. *Journal of Bone and Joint Surgery*, **75B**, 398–402.

Hardcastle, P., Annear, P., Foster, D. H. et al. (1992). Spinal abnormalities in young fast bowlers. *Journal of Bone and Joint Surgery*, **74B**, 421–425.

Harreby, M., Neergaard, K., Hesselsoe, G. and Kjer, J. (1995). Are radiologic changes in the thoracic and lumbar spine of adolescents risk factors for low back pain in adults? A 25-year prospective cohort study of 640 school children. *Spine*, **20**, 2298–2302.

Harris, S. T., Watts, N. B., Jackson, R. D. et al. (1993). Four-year study of intermittent cyclic etidronate treatment of postmenopausal osteoporosis: three years of blind therapy followed by one year of open therapy. *American Journal of Medicine*, **95**, 557–567.

Hart, R. G. and Easton J. D. (1983). Dissections of cervical and cerebral arteries. *Neurologic Clinics*, **1**, 155–182.

Hartman, J. T., Palumbo, F. and Hill, B. J. (1975). Cineradiography of the braced normal cervical spine. A comparative study of five commonly used cervical orthoses. *Clinical Orthopaedics and Related Research*, **109**, 97–102.

Harvey, J. and Tanner, S. (1991). Low back pain in young athletes. A practical approach. *Sports Medicine*, **12**, 394–406.

Hassall, J. (1992). The psyche and the soma in rheumatic disease. *Modern Medicine of Australia*, **Aug.**, 58–69.

Hasue, M. (1993). Pain and the nerve root. An interdisciplinary approach. *Spine*, **18**, 2053–2058.

Hasvold, T. and Johnsen, R. (1993). Headache and neck or shoulder pain – frequent and disabling complaints in the general population. *Scandinavian Journal of Primary Health Care*, **11**, 219–224.

Heggeness, M. H. and Doherty, B. J. (1993). Discography causes end plate deflection. *Spine*, **18**, 1050–1053.

Hehne, H. J., Zielke, K. and Bohm, H. (1990). Polysegmental lumbar osteotomies and transpedicled fixation for correction of long-curved kyphotic deformities in ankylosing spondylitis. *Clinical Orthopaedics and Related Research*, **258**, 49–55.

Heinz, G. J. and Zavala, D. C. (1977). Slipping rib syndrome. *Journal of the American Medical Association*, **237**, 794–795.

Heise, A. P., Laskin, D. M. and Gervin, A. S. (1992). Incidence of temporomandibular joint symptoms following whiplash injury. *Journal of Oral and Maxillofacial Surgery*, **50**, 825–828.

Helbig, T. and Lee, C. K. (1988). The lumbar facet syndrome. *Spine*, **13**, 61–64.

Heliovaara, M. (1989). Risk factors for low back pain and sciatica. *Annals of Medicine*, **21**, 257–264.

Heliovaara, M., Makela, M., Knekt, P. et al. (1991). Determinants of sciatica and low back pain. *Spine*, **16**, 608–614.

Heller, C. A., Stanley, P., Lewis-Jones, B. and Heller, R. F. (1983). Value of x-ray examination on the cervical spine. *British Medical Journal*, **287**, 1276–1278.

Heller, J. G. (1992). The syndromes of degenerative cervical disease. *Orthopaedic Clinics of North America*, **23**, 381–394.

Helliwell, P. S. (1995). Osteoarthritis and Paget's disease. *British Journal of Rheumatology*, **34**, 1061–1063.

Hellstrom, M., Jacobsson, B., Sward, L. and Peterson, L. (1990). Radiological abnormalities in the spine of top athletes. *Acta Radiologica*, **31**, 127–132.

Hench, P. K. (1977). Nonarticular rheumatism. In 22nd Rheumatism Review: review of the American and English literature for the years 1973 and 1974. *Arthritis and Rheumatism Supplement*, **19**, 1081–1089.

Hendrix, P. W., Melany, M., Miller, F. and Rogers, L. F. (1994). Fracture of the spine in patients with ankylosis due to diffuse skeletal hyperostosis: clinical and imaging findings. *American Journal of Roentgenology*, **162**, 899–904.

Hendrix, R. W., Lin, P. J. and Kane, W. J. (1982). Simplified aspiration or injection technique for the sacroiliac joint. *Journal of Bone and Joint Surgery*, **64A**, 1249–1252.

Henry, D., Lim, L. L. Y., Rodriguez, L. A. G. et al.

(1996). Variability in risk of gastrointestinal complications with individual non-steroidal anti-inflammatory drugs: results of a collaborative meta-analysis. *British Medical Journal*, **312**, 1563–1566.

Hensinger, R. N. (1989). Current concepts review. Spondylolysis and spondylolisthesis in children and adolescents. *Journal of Bone and Joint Surgery*, **71A**, 1098–1107.

Herkowitz, H. N. (1995). Spine update. Degenerative lumbar spondylolisthesis. *Spine*, **20**, 1084–1090.

Herkowitz, H. N. and Kurz, L. T. (1991). Degenerative lumbar spondylolisthesis with spinal stenosis: a prospective study comparing decompression with decompression and intertransverse process arthrodesis. *Journal of Bone and Joint Surgery*, **73A**, 802–808.

Hermanus, N., de Becker, D., Baleriaux, D. and Hauzer, J. P. (1983). The use of CT scanning for the study of posterior lumbar intervertebral articulations. *Neuroradiology*, **24**, 159–161.

Herno, A., Airaksinen, O. and Saari, T. (1994a). Computed tomography after laminectomy for lumbar spinal stenosis. Patients' pain patterns, walking capacity, and subjective disability had no correlation with computed tomography findings. *Spine*, **19**, 1975–1978.

Herno, A., Airaksinen, O., Saari, T. and Miettinen, H. (1994b). The predictive value of preoperative myelography in lumbar spinal stenosis. *Spine*, **19**, 1335–1338.

Herno, A., Airaksinen, O., Saari, T. and Sihvonen, T. (1995). Surgical results of lumbar spinal stenosis – a comparison of patients with or without previous back surgery. *Spine*, **20**, 964–969.

Herron, L. D. and Mangelsdorf, C. (1991). Lumbar spine stenosis: results of surgical treatment. *Journal of Spinal Disease*, **4**, 26–33.

Herzog, J. M., Guyer, R. D., Graham-Smith, A. and Simmons, E. D. (1995). Contemporary concepts in spine care. Magnetic resonance imaging use in patients with low back or radicular pain. *Spine*, **20**, 1834–1838.

Herzog, W., Read, L. J., Conway, P. J. W. et al. (1989). Reliability of motion palpation procedures to detect sacroiliac joint fixations. *Journal of Manipulative and Physiological Therapy*, **12**, 86–92.

Herzog, W., Conway, P. J., Kawchuk, G. N. et al. (1993). Forces exerted during spinal manipulative therapy. *Spine*, 18, 1206–1212.

Hidding, A. and Vanderlinden, S. (1995). Factors related to change in global health after group physical therapy in ankylosing spondylitis. *Clinical Rheumatology*, **14**, 347–351.

Hidding, A., Vanderlinden, S. and de Witte, L. (1993). Therapeutic effects of individual physical therapy in ankylosing spondylitis related to duration of disease. *Clinical Rheumatology*, **12**, 334–340.

Hijikata, S. (1989). Percutaneous nucleotomy – a new concept and 12 years' experience. *Clinical Orthopaedics and Related Research*, **238**, 9–23.

Hildingsson, C., Wenngren, B.-I., Bring, G. and Toolanen, G. (1989). Oculomotor problems after cervical spine injury. *Acta Orthopaedica Scandinavica*, **60**, 513–516.

Hirsch, C., Inglemark, B. and Miller, M. (1963). The anatomical basis for low back pain. *Acta Orthopaedica Scandinavica*, **33**, 1–17.

Hirsch, S. A., Hirsch, P. J., Hiramoto, H. and Weiss, A. (1988). Whiplash syndrome – fact or fiction? *Orthopaedic Clinics of North America*, **19**, 791–795.

Hitselberger, W. E. and Witten, R. M. (1968). Abnormal myelograms in asymptomatic patients. *Journal of Neurosurgery*, **28**, 204–206.

Hodgkinson, A. (1979). Neck pain localisation by cervical disc stimulation and treatment by anterior interbody fusion (abstract). *Journal of Bone and Joint Surgery*, **52B**, 789.

Hoehler, F. K. and Tobis, J. S. (1983). Psychological factors in the treatment of back pain by spinal manipulation. *British Journal of Rheumatology*, **22**, 206–212.

Hoehler, F. K., Tobis, J. S. and Beurger, A. A. (1981). Spinal manipulation for low back pain. *Journal of the American Medical Association*, **245**, 1835–1838.

Hoffman, R. M., Wheeler, K. J. and Deyo, R. A. (1993). Surgery for herniated lumbar discs: a literature synthesis. *Journal of General Internal Medicine*, **8**, 487–496.

Hohl, M. (1974). Soft-tissue injuries of the neck in automobile accidents. Factors influencing prognosis. *Journal of Bone and Joint Surgery*, **56A**, 1675–1682.

Hohl, M. (1989). Soft-tissue neck injuries. In *The*

Cervical Spine. 2nd ed. Cervical Spine Research Society, pp. 436–439, Lipincott.

Holder, L. E. (1990). Clinical radionuclide bone imaging. *Radiology*, **176**, 607–614.

Holm, S. and Nachemson, A. (1988). Nutrition of the intervertebral disc: acute effects of cigarette smoking. An experimental animal study. Upsala. *Journal of Medical Sciences*, **93**, 91–99.

Holmes, A., Wang, C., Han, Z. H. and Dang, G. T. (1994). The range and nature of flexion-extension motion in the cervical spine. *Spine*, **19**, 2505–2510.

Holmstrom, E. B., Lindell, J. and Moritz, U. (1992). Low back and neck shoulder pain in construction workers: occupational workload and psychosocial risk factors. Part 1: relationship to low back pain. *Spine*, **17**, 663–671.

Holt, E. P. (1968). The question of lumbar discography. *Journal of Bone and Joint Surgery*, **50A**, 720–726.

Holt, S. and Yates, P. O. (1966). Cervical spondylosis and nerve root lesions. *Journal of Bone and Joint Surgery*, **48B**, 407–423.

Honan, M., White, G. W. and Eisenberg, G. M. (1996). Spontaneous infectious discitis in adults. *American Journal of Medicine*, **100**, 85–89.

Hopp, E. and Tsu, P. M. (1988). Postdecompression lumbar instability. *Clinical Orthopaedics and Related Research*, **227**, 143–151.

Horne, J., Cockshott, P. and Shannon, H. (1987). Spinal column damage from water ski jumping. *Skeletal Radiology*, **16**, 612–616.

Horowitz, M. B. and Yonas, H. (1993). Occipital neuralgia treated by intradural dorsal nerve root sectioning. *Cephalalgia*, **13**, 354–360.

Hoshina, H. (1980). Spondylolysis in athletes. *Physician and Sports Medicine*, **8**, 75–79.

Howe, D. H., Newcombe, R. G. and Wade, M. T. (1983). Manipulation of the cervical spine: a pilot study. *Journal of the Royal College of General Practitioners*, **33**, 564–579.

Howell, D. W. (1984). Musculoskeletal profile and incidence of musculoskeletal injuries in lightweight women rowers. *American Journal of Sports Medicine*, **12**, 278–282.

Howell, J. M. (1992). Xiphoidynia: a report of three cases. *Journal of Emergency Medicine*, **10**, 435–438.

Howes, R. G. and Isdale, I. C. (1971). The loose back: an unrecognised syndrome. *Rheumatology and Physical Medicine*, **11**, 72–77.

Hsieh, C. Y., Walker, J. M. and Gillis, K. (1983). Straight leg raising test: comparison of three instruments. *Physical Therapy*, **63**, 1429–1432.

Hsu, K., Zucherman, J., Shea, W. et al. (1990). High lumbar disc degeneration. Incidence and etiology. *Spine*, **15**, 679–682.

Hsu, K. Y., Zucherman, J. F., Shea, W. J. and Jeffrey, R. A. (1995). Lumbar intraspinal synovial and ganglion cysts (facet cysts). Ten-year experience in evaluation and treatment. *Spine*, **20**, 80–89.

Hudgins, R. W. (1979). The crossed straight leg raising test: a diagnostic sign of herniated disc. *Journal of Occupational Medicine*, **21**, 407–408.

Hudson, J. L. and Pope, H. G. (1989). Fibromyalgia and psychopathology: is fibromyalgia a form of 'affective spectrum disorder'? *Journal of Rheumatology* suppl 19, **16**, 15–22.

Hudson, J. L., Hudson, M. S., Pliner, L. F. et al. (1985). Fibromyalgia and major affective disorders: a controlled phenomenology and family history study. *American Journal of Psychiatry*, **142**, 441–446.

Hughes, A. J. (1994). Botulinum toxin in clinical practice. *Drugs*, **48**, 888–893.

Hughes, R. A. and Keats, A. C. (1994). Reiter's syndrome and reactive arthritis: a current view. *Seminars in Arthritis and Rheumatism*, **24**, 190–210.

Hult, L. (1954). Cervical, dorsal, and lumbar spinal syndromes: a field investigation of a non-selected material of 1200 workers in different occupations with special reference to disc degeneration and so-called muscular rheumatism. *Acta Orthopaedica Scandinavica Supplementum*, **17**, 1–102.

Humphrey, S. M. and Inman, R. D. (1995). Metastatic adenocarcinoma mimicking unilateral sacroiliitis. *Journal of Rheumatology*, **22**, 970–982.

Hunter, C. R. and Mayfield, F. H. (1949). Role of the upper cervical roots in the production of pain in the head. *American Journal of Surgery*, **78**, 743–749.

Hurwitz, E. L., Aker, P. D., Adams, A. H. et al. (1996). Manipulation and mobilization of the cervical spine: a systematic review of the literature. *Spine*, **21**, 1746–1760.

Husni, E. A. and Storer, J. (1967). The syndrome of mechanical occlusion of the vertebral artery: further observations. *Angiology*, **18**, 106–116.

Huston, G. J. (1988). Collars and corsets. *British Medical Journal*, **296**, 276.

Hutchinson, E. C. and Yates, P. O. (1956). The cervical portion of the vertebral artery; a clinicopathological study. *Brain*, **79**, 319–331.

Hutton, W. and Cyron, B. (1978). Spondylolysis: the role of the posterior elements in resisting the intervertebral compressive force. *Acta Orthopaedica Scandinavica*, **49**, 604–609.

Ichikawa, N., Ohara, Y., Morishita, T. et al. (1982). An aetiological study on spondylolysis from a biomechanical aspect. *British Journal of Sports Medicine*, **16**, 135–141.

Ignelzi, R. and Cummings, T. W. (1980). A statistical analysis of percutaneous radiofrequency lesions in the treatment of chronic low back pain and sciatica. *Pain*, **8**, 181–187.

Ikata, T., Morita, T., Katoh, S. and Miyake, R. (1996). Pathomechanism of sports-related spondylolisthesis in adolescents: radiographic and MRI study. *American Journal of Sports Medicine*, **24**, 94–98.

Inman, R. D. and Schofield, R. H. (1994). Etiopathogenesis of ankylosing spondylitis and reactive arthritis. *Current Opinion in Rheumatology*, **6**, 360–370.

International Headache Society. (1988). Headache classification. *Cephalalgia*, **8**, suppl 7, 1–96.

Ippolito, E., and Ponsetti, I. V. (1981). Juvenile kyphosis: histological and histochemical studies. *Journal of Bone and Joint Surgery*, **63A**, 175–182.

Ireland, M. L. and Micheli, L. J. (1987). Bilateral stress fracture of the lumbar pedicles in a ballet dancer. *Journal of Bone and Joint Surgery*, **69A**, 140–142.

Ishikawa, S., Kumar, J. and Torres, B. C. (1994). Surgical treatment of dysplastic spondylolisthesis. Results after in situ fusion. *Spine*, **19**, 1691–1696.

Ito, T., Yamada, M., Ikuta, F. et al. (1996a). Histologic evidence of absorption of sequestration-type herniated disc. *Spine*, **21**, 230–234.

Ito, T., Shirado. O., Suzuki, H. et al. (1996b). Lumbar trunk muscles endurance testing: an inexpensive alternative to a machine for evaluation. *Archives of Physical Medicine and Rehabilitation*, **77**, 75–79.

Ito, T., Oyanagi, K., Takahashi, H. et al. (1996c). Cervical spondylotic myelopathy. Clinicopathological study on the progression pattern and thin myelinated fibers of the lesions of seven patients examined during complete autopsy. *Spine*, **21**, 827–833.

Itoi, E. and Sinaki, M. (1994). Effect of back-strengthening exercises on posture in healthy women 49 to 65 years of age. *Mayo Clinical Proceedings*, **69**, 1054–1059.

Jackson, D., Wiltse, L. and Cirincione, R. (1976). Spondylolysis in the female gymnast. *Clinical Orthopaedics and Related Research*, **117**, 68–73.

Jackson, R. P., Jacobs, R. R. and Montesaro, P. X. (1988). Facet joint injection in low back pain – a prospective statistical study. *Spine*, **13**, 966–971.

Jacob, H. A. C. and Kissling, R. O. (1995). The mobility of the sacroiliac joints in healthy volunteers between 20 and 50 years of age. *Clinical Biomechanics*, **10**, 352–361.

Jaffray, D. and O'Brien, J. P. (1986). Isolated intervertebral disc resorption. A source of mechanical and inflammatory back pain? *Spine*, **11**, 397–401.

Jaffray, D., Becker, V. and Eisenstein, S. (1992). Closing wedge osteotomy with transpedicular fixation in ankylosing spondylitis. *Clinical Orthopaedics and Related Research*, **279**, 122–126.

Jankiewicz, J. J., Hennrikus, W. L. and Houkom, J. A. (1991). The appearance of the piriformis muscle syndrome in CT and magnetic resonance imaging: a case report and review of the literature. *Clinical Orthopaedics and Related Research*, **262**, 205–209.

Jayson, M. I. V., Keegan, A., Million, R. and Tomlinson, I. (1984). A fibrinolytic defect in chronic back pain syndromes. *Lancet*, **2**, 1186–1187.

Jenkinson, T., Armas, J., Evison, G. et al. (1994). The cervical spine in psoriatic arthritis: a clinical and radiological study. *Annals of the Rheumatic Diseases*, **33**, 255–259.

Jensen, M. C., Brantzawadzki, M., Obuchowski, N. et al. (1994a). Magnetic resonance imaging of the lumbar spine in people without back pain. *New England Journal of Medicine*, **331**, 115–116.

Jensen, M. C., Kelly, A. P. and Brant-Zawadzki, M. N. (1994b). MRI of degenerative disease of the lumbar spine. *Magnetic Resonance Quarterly*, **10**, 173–190.

Jensen, O. K., Nielsen, F. F. and Vosmar, L. (1990). An open study comparing manual therapy with the use of cold packs in the treatment of post-traumatic headache. *Cephalalgia*, **10**, 243–250.

Johanning, E. (1991). Back disorders and health problems among subway train operators exposed to whole body vibration. *Scandinavian Journal of Work, Environment and Health*, **17**, 414–419.

Johnson, D. W., and Thompson, A. G. (1992). The Scott wiring technique for direct repair of lumbar spondylolysis. *Journal of Bone and Joint Surgery*, **74B**, 426–430.

Johnson, R. M., Hart, J. R., Simmons, E. F. et al. (1977). Cervical orthoses: a study comparing their effectiveness in restricting cervical motion in normal subjects. *Journal of Bone and Joint Surgery*, **59A**, 332–339.

Johnson, R. M., Owen, R. R., Hart, D. L. et al. (1981). Cervical orthoses: a guide to their selection and use. *Clinical Orthopaedics and Related Research*, **154**, 34–42.

Johnsson, B. and Stromqvist, B. (1994). Decompression for lateral lumbar spinal stenosis. *Spine*, **19**, 2381–2386.

Johnsson, K., Willner, S. and Johnsson, K. (1986). Postoperative instability after decompression for lumbar spinal stenosis. *Spine*, **11**, 107–110.

Johnsson, K. E., Johnell, I., Udena, A. et al. (1989). Pre-operative and post-operative instability in lumbar spinal stenosis. *Spine*, **14**, 591–593.

Johnsson, K. E., Rosen, I. and Uden, A. (1992). A natural course of lumbar spinal stenosis. *Clinical Orthopaedics and Related Research*, **279**, 82–86.

Johnston, C. C., Miller, J. Z., Slemenda, C. W. et al. (1992). Calcium supplementation and increases in bone mineral density in children. *New England Journal of Medicine*, **327**, 82–87.

Johnston, R. A. and Kelly, I. G. (1990). Surgery of the rheumatoid cervical spine. *Annals of the Rheumatic Diseases*, **49**, 845–850.

Johnstone, B. and Bayliss, M. T. (1995). The large proteoglycans of the human intervertebral disc. *Spine*, **20**, 674–684.

Jonathan, D. and Baer, S. (1990). Cervical osteophytes: their significance in ENT practice (ankylosing vertebral hyperostosis – Forestier's disease). *Journal of Laryngology and Otology*, **104**, 236–238.

Jones, G., Nguyen, T., Sambrook, P. N. et al. (1994a). Progressive femoral neck bone loss in the elderly: longitudinal findings from the Dubbo osteoporosis epidemiology study. *British Medical Journal*, **309**, 691–695.

Jones, G., Nguyen, T., Sambrook, P. N. et al. (1994b). Symptomatic fracture incidence in elderly men and women: the Dubbo osteoporosis epidemiology study. *Osteoporosis International*, **4**, 277–282.

Jones, T. R., James, J. E., Adams, J. W. et al. (1989). Lumbar zygapophyseal joint meniscoids: evidence of their role in chronic intersegmental hypomobility. *Journal of Manipulative and Physiological Therapeutics*, **12**, 374–385.

Jonsson, B. and Stromqvist, B. (1994). Decompression for lateral lumbar stenosis – results and impact on sick leave and working conditions. *Spine*, **19**, 2381–2386.

Jonsson, B. and Stromqvist, B. (1995). The straight leg raising test and the severity of symptoms in lumbar disc herniation. A preoperative evaluation. *Spine*, **20**, 27–30.

Jonsson, H., Bring, G., Rauschning, W. and Sahlstedt, B. (1991). Hidden cervical spine injuries in traffic accident victims with skull fractures. *Journal of Spinal Disorders*, **4**, 251–263.

Jonsson, H., Cesarini, K., Sahlstedt, B. and Rauschning, W. (1994). Finding and outcome in whiplash-type neck distortions. *Spine*, **19**, 2733–2743.

Jougon, J. B., Lepront, D. J. and Dromer, C. E. (1996). Posterior dislocation of the sternoclavicular joint leading to mediastinal compression. *Annals of Thoracic Surgery*, **61**, 711–733.

Jull, G. A., Bogduk, N. and Marsland, A. (1988). The accuracy of manual diagnosis for cervical zygapophyseal joint pain syndromes. *Medical Journal of Australia*, **148**, 233–236.

Jurik, A. G. (1992). Seronegative anterior chest wall syndromes: a study of the findings and course at radiology. *Acta Radiologica*, **32**, suppl 381, 1–42.

Jurik, A. G., Justesen, T. and Graudal, H. (1987). Radiographic findings in patients with clinical Tietze syndrome. *Skeletal Radiology*, **16**, 517–523.

Kaapa, E., Holm, S., Han, X. et al. (1994). Collagens in the injured porcine intervertebral disc. *Journal of Orthopaedic Research*, **12**, 92–103.

Kahanovitz, M. (1993). Surgical disc excision. *Clinical Sports Medicine*, **12**, 579–585.

Kahmann, R D., Buttermann, G. R., Lewis, J. L. and Bradford, D. S. (1990). Facet loads in the canine lumbar spine before and after disc alteration. *Spine*, **15**, 971–978.

Kaigle, A. M., Holm, S. H., Holm, S. H. and Hansson, T. H. (1995). Experimental instability in the lumbar spine. *Spine*, **20**, 421–430.

Kallina, C. (1985). Degenerative lumbar stenosis. *Clinical in Geriatric Medicine*, **1**, 391–400.

Kalyan-Raman, U. P., Kalyan-Raman, K., Yunus, M. B. and Masi, A. T. (1984). Muscle pathology in primary fibromyalgia syndrome: a light microscopic, histochemical and ultrastructural study. *Journal of Rheumatology*, **11**, 808–813.

Kambin, P. and Cohen, L. F. (1993). Arthroscopic microdiscectomy versus nucleotomy techniques. *Clinics in Sports Medicine*, **12**, 587–598.

Kamel, M. and Rosman, M. (1984). Disc protrusion in the growing child. *Clinical Orthopaedics and Releaed Research*, **185**, 46–52.

Kamiyama, T., Hashizuma, Y., Ando, T. and Takahashi, A. (1994). Morphometry of the normal cadaveric cervical spine cord. *Spine*, **18**, 2077–2081.

Kana, S. M. and Wiesel, S. W. (1994). Conservative therapy for spinal stenosis. *Semininars in Spine Surgery*, **6**, 109–115.

Kanner, R. (1994). Low back pain. *Seminars in Neurology*, **14**, 272–280.

Kapandji, I. A. (1983). *The Physiology of the Joints*, Vol. 3. pp. 63–71, Churchill Livingstone.

Karbowski, K. and Dvorak, J. (1995). Historical perspective. Description of variations of the sciatica stretch phenomenon. *Spine*, **20**, 1525–1527.

Karlson, B. W., Herlitz, J., Pettersson, P. et al. (1991). Patients admitted to the emergency room with symptoms indicative of acute myocardial infarction. *Journal of Internal Medicine*, **230**, 251–258.

Karppinen, J., Inkinen, R. I., Kaapa, E. et al.

(1995). Effects of tiaprofenic acid and indomethacin on proteoglycans in the degenerating porcine intervertebral disc. *Spine*, **20**, 1170–1177.

Katz, J. N., Lipson, S. J., Larson, M. G. et al. (1991). The outcome of decompressive laminectomy for degenerative lumbar stenosis. *Journal of Bone and Joint Surgery*, **73A**, 809–816.

Katz, J. N., Dalgas, M., Stucki, G. and Lipson, S. J. (1994) The diagnosis of lumbar spinal stenosis. *Rheumatic Diseases Clinics of North America*, **20**, 471–483.

Katz, J. N., Dalgas, M., Stucki, G. et al. (1995a). Degenerative lumbar spinal stenosis: Diagnostic value of the history and physical examination. *Arthritis and Rheumatism*, **38**, 1236–1241.

Katz, J. N., Lipson, S. J., Brick G. W. et al. (1995b). Clinical correlates of patient satisfaction after laminectomy for degenerative lumbar spinal stenosis. *Spine*, **20**, 1155–1160.

Katz, M. E., Shier, C. K., Ellis, B. I. et al. (1989). A unified approach to symptomatic juxtasternal arthritis and enthesitis. *American Journal of Roentgenology*, ***153***, 327–333.

Katz, S. S. and Savitz, M. H. (1986). Percutaneous radio frequency rhizotomy of the lumbar facets. *Mt. Sinai Journal of Medicine (NY)*, **53**, 523–525.

Kauppi, M. and Anttila, P.(1995). A stiff collar can restrict atlantoaxial instability in rheumatoid cervical spine in selected cases. *Annals of the Rheumatic Diseases*, **54**, 305–307.

Kawakami, M., Weinstein, J. N., Chatani, K. et al. (1994a). Experimental lumbar radiculopathy. Behavioural and histologic changes in a model of radicular pain after spinal nerve root irritation with chromic gut ligatures in the rat. *Spine*, **19**, 1795–1802.

Kawakami, M., Weinstein, J. N., Spratt, K. F. et al. (1994b). Experimental lumbar radiculopathy. Immunohistochemical and quantitative demonstrations of pain induced by lumbar nerve root irritation of the rat. *Spine*, **19**, 1780–1794.

Keats, A. (1994). HIV and overlap with Reiterís syndrome. *Clinical Rheumatology*, **8**, 363–377.

Keim, H. A., Hadjdu, M., Gonalez, E. G. et al. (1985). Somatosensory evoked potentials as an aid in the diagnosis and intraoperative management of spinal stenosis. *Spine*, **10**, 338–344.

Keith, W. S. (1986). 'Whiplash' – injury to the 2nd cervical ganglion and nerve. *Canadian Journal of Neurological Sciences*, **13**, 133–137.

Keller, T. S., Holm, S., Hansson, T. H. and Spengler, D. M. (1990). The dependence of intervertebral disc mechanical properties on physiologic conditions. *Spine*, **15**, 751–761.

Kelscy, J. L. (1975). An epidemiological study of acute herniated lumbar intervertebral discs. *Rheumatology and Rehabilitation*, **14**, 144–159.

Kelsey, J. L. and Ostfield, A. M. (1975). Demographic characteristics of persons with acute herniated lumbar intervertebral disc. *Journal of Chronic Diseases*, **28**, 37–50.

Kelsey, J. L., Gittens, P. B., O'Connor, T. et al. (1984a). Acute prolapsed lumbar intervertebral disc: an epidemiologic study with special reference to driving automobiles and cigarette smoking. *Spine*, **9**, 608–613.

Kelsey, J., Gittens, P. B., White, A. A. et al. (1984 b). An epidemiologic study of lifting and twisting on the job and risk for acute prolapsed lumbar intervertebral disk. *Journal of Orthopaedic Research*, **2**, 61–66.

Kelsey, J., Golden, A. and Mundt, D. (1990). Low back pain in prolapsed intervertebral disc. *Epidemiology Rheumatic Disease*, **16**, 699–716.

Kendall, P. H. and Jenkins, J. M. (1968). Exercises for backache: a double-blind controlled trial. *Physiotherapist*, **54**, 154–157.

Kenneally, M., Rubenach, H. and Elvey, R. L. (1988). The upper limb tension test: the SLR test to the arm: physical therapy of the cervical and thoracic spine. In *Clinics in Physical Therapy*. (R. Grant ed.) pp. 167–194, Churchill Livingstone.

Kent, D. L., Haynor, D. R., Larson, E. B. et al. (1994). Diagnosis of lumbar spinal stenosis in adults: a meta-analysis of the accuracy of CT, MRI, and myelography. *American Journal of Roentgenology*, **158**, 1135–1144.

Kepes, E. R. and Duncalf, D. (1985). Treatment of backache with spinal injection of local anaesthetics, spinal and systemic steroids. A review. *Pain*, **22**, 33–47.

Kerr, F. W. L. (1972). Central relationships of trigeminal and cervical primary afferents in the spinal cord and medulla. *Brain Research*, **43**, 561–572.

Kerr, F. W. L. and Olafson, R. A. (1961). Trigeminal and cervical vollleys. *Archives of Neurology*, **5**, 171–178.

Kesuib, F., Thomas, C. E., Lozes, G. et al. (1985). Has the safety belt replaced the hangman's noose (letter)? *Lancet*, **1**, 1341.

Khalil, T. M., Asfour, S. S., Martinez, L. M. et al. (1991). Stretching in the rehabilitation of low back pain patients. *Spine*, **17**, 311–317.

Khan, M. A. (1992). An overview of clinical spectrum and heterogeneity of spondyloarthropathies. *Rheumatic Diseases Clinics of North America*, **18**, 1–10.

Kiely, M. J. (1993). Neuroradiology case of the day: lumbar synovial cyst. *American Journal of Roentgenology*, **160**, 1336–1337.

Kikuchi, S. and Macnab, I. (1981). Localisation of the level of symptomatic cervical disc degeneration. *Journal of Bone and Joint Surgery*, **63B**, 272–277.

Kinalski, R., Kuwik, W. and Pietrzak, D. (1989). The comparison of the results of manual therapy versus physiotherapy methods used in treatment of patients with low back pain syndromes. *Journal of Manual Medicine*, **4**, 44–46.

King, J. S. and Lagger, R. (1976). Sciatica viewed as a referred pain syndrome. *Surgical Neurology*, **5**, 46–50.

King, W. (1992). Clinical biomechanics of the sacroiliac joint. *Australian Assocociation of Manual Medicine Bulletin*, **8**, 50–54.

Kip, P. C., Esses, S. I., Doherty, B. I. et al. (1994). Biomechanical testing of pars defect repairs. *Spine*, **19**, 2692–2697.

Kirkaldy-Willis, W. H. and Farfan, H. F. (1982). Instability of the lumbar spine. *Clinical Orthopaedics and Related Research*, **165**, 110–123.

Kirkaldy-Willis, W. H., Wedge, J. H., Yong-Hing, K. and Reilly, J. (1978). Pathology and pathogenesis of lumbar spondylosis and stenosis. *Spine*, **3**, 319–328.

Kischka, U., Ettlin, T. M., Heim, S. et al. (1991). Cerebral symptoms following whiplash injury. *European Neurology*, **31**, 136–140.

Klein, D. M., Weiss, R. L. and Allen, J. E. (1986). Scheuermann's dorsal kyphosis and spinal cord compression: case report. *Neurosurgery*, **18**, 628–631.

Klenerman, L., Greenwood, R., Davenport, H. T. et al. (1984). Lumbar epidural injections in the treatment of sciatica. *British Journal of Rheumatology*, **23**, 35–38.

Koes, B. W., Assendelft, W. J. J., van der Heijden, G. J. M. G. et al. (1991a). Spinal manipulation and mobilization for back and neck pain: a blinded review. *British Medical Journal*, **303**, 1298–1303.

Koes, B. W., Bouter, L. M., Beckerman, H. et al. (1991b). Physiotherapy exercises and back pain: a blinded review. *British Medical Journal*, **302**, 1572–1576.

Koes, B. W., Bouter, L. M. and van Mameren, H. (1992). Randomised clinical trial of manipulative therapy and physiotherapy for persistent back and neck complaints: results of one year follow up. *British Medical Journal*, **304**, 601–605.

Koes, B. W., Bouter, L. M., van Mameren, H. and Essers, A. H. M. (1993). The effectiveness of manual therapy, physiotherapy and treatment by the general practitioner for nonspecific back and neck complaints: a randomized clinical trial. *Spine*, **17**, 28–35.

Koes, B. W., Vantulder, M. W., Vanderwindt, D. A. W. M. and Bouter, L. M. (1994). The efficacy of back schools: a review of randomized clinical trials. *Journal of Clinical Epidemiology*, **47**, 851–862.

Koes, B. W., Scholten, R. I., Mens, J. M. A. and Bouter, L. M. (1995). Efficacy of epidural steroid injections for low-back pain and sciatica: a systematic review of randomized clinical trials. *Pain*, **63**, 279–288.

Kokubun, S., Sakurai, N. and Tanaka, Y. (1996). Cartilage end-plate in cervical disc herniation. *Spine*, **21**, 190–195.

Komori, H., Shinomiya, K., Nakai, O. et al. (1996). The natural history of herniated nucleus pulposus with radiculopathy. *Spine*, **21**, 225–229.

Konno, S., Olmarker, K., Byrod, G. et al. (1995). Intermittent cauda equina compression. An experimental study of the porcine cauda equina with analyses of nerve impulse conduction properties. *Spine*, **20**, 1223–1226.

Kornberg, M. (1995). Nerve root compression by a ganglion cyst of the lumbar anulus fibrosus. *Spine*, **20**, 1633–1635.

Kortelainen, P., Puranen, J., Koivisto, E. and Lahde, S. (1985). Symptoms and signs of sciatica and their relation to the localization of the lumbar disc herniation. *Spine*, **10**, 88–92.

Kosteljanetz, M., Bang, F. and Schmidt-Olsen, S. (1988). The clinical significance of straight leg raising (Lasegue's sign) in the diagnosis of prolapsed lumbar disc. *Spine*, **13**, 393–395.

Kostuik, J. P. (1993a). Controversies in cauda equina syndrome and lumbar disc herniation. *Current Opinion in Orthopedics*, **4**,11,125–128.

Kostuik, J. P. (1993b). Metastatic disease of the spine. *Current Opinion in Orthopedics*, **4**,11, 169–176.

Kostuik, J., Harringon, I., Alexander, D. et al. (1986). Cauda equina syndrome and lumbar disc herniation. *Journal of Bone and Joint Surgery*, **68A**, 382–391.

Kotani, P. T., Ichikawa, N., Wakabayashi, W. et al. (1971). Studies of spondylolysis found among weight-lifters. *British Journal of Sports Medicine*, **6**, 4–12.

Kraemer, J. (1995). Natural course and prognosis of intervertebral disc disease. *Spine*, **20**, 635–639.

Kraft, G. H., Johnson, E. W. and LaBan, M. M. (1968). The fibrositis syndrome. *Archives of Physical Medicine and Rehabilitation*, **49**, 155–161.

Krag, M. H., Cohen, M. C., Haugh, L. D. and Pope, M. H. (1990). Body height change during upright and recumbent posture. *Spine*, **15**, 202–207.

Kramer, J., Rivera, C. A. and Kleefield, J. (1991). Degenerative disorders of the cervical spine. *Rheumatic Diseases Clinics of North America*, **17**, 741–756.

Kraus, H. (1976). Effect of lordosis on the stress in the lumbar spine. *Clinical Orthopaedics and Related Research*, **117**, 56–58.

Kreuger, B. R. and Okazaki, H. (1980). Vertebral-basilar distribution infarction following chiropractic cervical manipulation. *Mayo Clinic Proceedings*, **55**, 322–332.

Kronn, E. (1993). The incidence of TMJ dysfunction in patients who have suffered a cervical whiplash injury following a traffic accident. *Journal of Orofacial Pain*, **7**, 209–213.

Kummel, B. M. (1996). Nonorganic signs of significance in low back pain. *Spine*, **21**, 1077–1081.

Kunnasmaa, K. T. T. and Thiel, H. W. (1994).

Vertebral artery syndrome: a review of the literature. *Journal of Orthopaedic Medicine*, **16**, 17–20.

Kurihara, A. and Katoka, O. (1980). Lumbar disc herniation in children and adolescents. A review of 70 operated cases and their minimum 5-year follow-up studies. *Spine*, **5**, 443–451.

Kumar, S. (1990). Cumulative load as a risk factor for back pain. *Spine*, **15**, 1311–1316.

Kurz, L. T. and Herkowitz, H. (1992). Surgical management of cervical myelopathy. *Clinical Orthopedic Clinics of North America*, **23**, 495–504.

Kuslich, S. D., Ulstrom, C. L. and Michael, C. J. (1991). The tissue origin of low back pain and sciatica; a report of pain response to tissue stimulation during operation on the lumbar spine using local anesthesia. *Orthopedic Clinics of North America*, **22**, 181–187.

LaBan, M. M. and Taylor, R. S. (1992). Manipulation: an objective analysis of the literature. *Orthopedic Clinics of North America*, **23**, 451–459.

Lacroix, J. M., Powell, J., Lloyd, G. J. et al. (1990). Low back pain. Factors of value in predicting outcome. *Spine*, **15**, 495–499.

Lahad, A., Malter, A. D., Berg, A. O. and Deyo, R. A. (1994). The effectiveness of four interventions for the prevention of low back pain. *Journal of the American Medical Association*, **272**, 1286–1291.

Lamy, C., Bazergui, A., Kraus, H. and Farfan, H. F. (1975). The strength of the neural arch and the etiology of spondylolysis. *Orthopedic Clinics of North America*, **6**, 215–231.

Lance, J. W. (1982). *Mechanism and Management of Headache*, 4th Edition. Butterworth.

Lander, J. E., Hundley, J. R. and Simonton, R. L. (1992). The effectiveness of weight belts during multiple repetitions of the squat exercise. *Medicine and Science in Sports and Exercise*, **24**, 603–609.

La Rocca, H. and Macnab, I. (1970). Value of preemployment radiographic assessment of the lumbar spine. *Industrial Medicine*, **39**, 253–258.

Larouche, M., Delisle, M. B., Aziza, R. et al. (1995). Is camptocormia a primary muscular disease? *Spine*, **20**, 1011–1016.

LaRoy, L. L., Cormier, P. J., Matalon, T. A. S. et al. (1989). Imaging of abdominal aortic aneurysms. *American Journal of Roentgenology*, **152**, 785–792.

Larsson, E. M., Holtas, S. and Zygmunt, S. (1989). Pre- and postoperative MR imaging of the craniocervical junction in rheumatoid arthritis. *American Journal of Roentgenology*, **152**, 561–566.

Larsson, L-G., Mudholkar, G. S., Baum, J. and Srivastava, D. K. (1995). Benefits and liabilities of hypermobility in the back pain disorders of industrial workers. *Journal of Internal Medicine*, **238**, 461–467.

Laslett, M. and Williams, M. (1994). The reliability of selected pain provocation tests for sacroiliac joint pathology. *Spine*, **19**, 1243–1249.

Laslett, M., Crothers, C., Beattie, P. et al. (1991). The frequency and incidence of low back pain and sciatica in an urban population. *New Zealand Medical Journal*, **104**, 424–426.

Latham, J. M., Pearcy, M. J., Costi, J. J. et al. (1994). Mechanical consequences of annular tears and subsequent intervertebral disc degeneration. *Clinical Biomechanics*, **9**, 211–219.

Lau, L. S. W., Littlejohn, G. O. and Miller, M. H. (1985). Clinical evaluation of intra-articular injections for lumbar facet joint pain. *Medical Journal of Australia*, **143**, 563–565.

Lavignolle, B., Vital, J. M., Senegas, J. et al. (1983). An approach to the functional anatomy of the sacroiliac joints in vivo. *Anatomia Clinica*, **5**, 169–176.

Lavyne, M. H. (1994). Cauda equina syndrome secondary to lumbar disc herniation (correspondence). *Neurosurgery*, **34**, 591.

Law, M. D., Bernhardt, M. and White, A. A. (1993). Cervical spondylotic myelopathy: a review of surgical indications and decision making. *Yale Journal of Biology and Medicine*, **66**, 165–167.

Lawrence, J. S., Bremner, J. M., and Bier, F. (1966). Osteoarthritis: prevalence in the population and relationship between symptoms and x-ray changes. *Annals of the Rheumatic Diseases*, **25**, 1–24.

Leak, A. M., Cooper, J., Dyer, S. et al. (1994). The Northwick Park neck pain questionnaire, devised to measure neck pain and disability. *British Journal of Rheumatology*, **33**, 469–474.

Leavitt, F., Garron, D. C., McNeill, T. W. and Whisler, W. W. (1982). Organic status, psychological disturbance, and pain report characteristics in low back pain patients on compensation. *Spine*, **7**, 398–402.

Lee, C. K. (1983). Lumbar spinal instability after extensive posterior spinal decompression. *Spine*, **8**, 429–433.

Lee, C. K., Rauschning, W. and Glenn, W. (1988). Lateral lumbar spinal canal stenosis: classification, pathologic anatomy and surgical decompression. *Spine*, **13**, 313–320.

Lee, C. K., Vessa, P. and Lee, J. K. (1995a). Chronic disabling low back pain syndrome caused by internal disc derangements. The result of disc excision and posterior lumbar interbody fusion. *Spine*, **20**, 356–361.

Lee, J., Giles, G. and Drummond, P. D. (1993b). Psychological disturbances and an exaggerated response to pain in patients with whiplash injury. *Journal of Psychosomatic Research*, **37**, 105–110.

Lee, K. P., Carlini, W. G., McCormick, G. F. and Albers, G. W. (1995b). Neurologic complications following chiropractic manipulation: a survey of California neurologists. *Neurology*, **45**, 1213–1215.

Lee, M., Latimer, J. and Maher, C. (1993a). Manipulation: investigation of a proposed mechanism. *Clinial Biomechanics*, **8**, 302–306.

Leino, P. (1993). Does leisure time physical activity prevent low back disorders? *Spine*, **18**, 863–871.

Lenz, G. P., Assheuer, J., Lenz, W. and Gottschlich, K. W. (1990). New aspects of lumbar disc disease. MR imaging and histological findings. *Archives of Orthopaedic and Trauma Surgery*, **109**, 75–82.

Levine, P. R. and Mascette, A. M. (1989). Musculoskeletal chest pain in patients with 'angina': a prospective study. *Southern Medical Journal*, **82**, 580–585.

Lewinnek, G. E. and Warfield, C. A. (1986). Facet joint degeneration as a cause of low back pain. *Clinical Orthopaedics and Related Research*, **213**, 216–222.

Lewit, K. (1985). Examination of locomotor function and its disturbance. In: *Manipulative Therapy in Rehabilitation of the Motor System*. pp. 109–114.

Liberman, U. A., Weiss, S. R., Broll, J. et al. (1995). Effect of oral alendronate on bone mineral density and fracture incidence in postmenopausal osteoporosis. *New England Journal of Medicine*, **333**, 1437–1443.

Lillius, G., Laasonen, E. M., Myllynen, P. et al. (1989). Lumbar facet joint syndrome: a randomised clinical trial. *Journal of Bone and Joint Surgery*, **68B**, 681–684.

Lillius, G., Harilainen, A., Laasonen, E. M. and Myllynen, P. (1990). Chronic unilateral low back pain. Predictors of outcome of facet joint injections. *Spine*, **15**, 780–782.

Lindsay, D. M., Meeuwisse, W. H., Vyse, A. et al. (1993). Lumbosacral dysfunction in elite cross-country skiers. *Journal of Orthopedic and Sports Physical Therapy*, **18**, 580–585.

Lindstrom, I., Ohlund, C., Eek, C. et al. (1992a). The effect of graded activity on patients with subacute low back pain: a randomized prospective, clinical study with an operant-condition behavioral approach. *Physical Therapy*, **72**, 279–290.

Lindstrom, I., Ohlund, C., Eek, C. et al. (1992b). Mobility, strength, and fitness after a graded activity program for patients with subacute low back pain: a randomized prospective clinical study with a behavioral therapy approach. *Spine*, **17**, 641–652.

Linson, M. A. and Crowe, C. H. (1990). Comparison of magnetic resonance imaging and lumbar discography in the diagnosis of disc degeneration. *Clinical Orthopaedics and Related Research*, **250**, 160–163.

Lippit, A .B. (1984). The facet joint and its role in spinal pain: management with facet joint injections. *Spine*, **9**, 746–750.

Lipson, S. (1989a). Clinical diagnosis of spinal stenosis. *Seminars in Spine Surgery*, **1**, 143–144.

Lipson, S. J. (1989b). Rheumatoid arthritis in the cervical spine. *Clinical Orthopaedics and Related Research*, **239**, 121–127.

Livingston, M. (1994). Back exercises. What patients are taught and what they do. *Journal of Orthopaedic Medicine*, **16**, 9–11.

Lora, J. and Long, D. (1976). So-called facet denervation in the management of intractable back pain. *Spine*, **1**, 121–126.

Lord, S. M., Barnsley, L. and Bogduk, N. (1993). The utility of comparative local anaesthetic blocks versus placebo-controlled blocks for the diagnosis of cervical zygapophyseal joint pain. *Clinical Journal of Pain*, **11**, 208–213.

Lord, S. M., Barnsley, L. and Bogduk, N. (1995a). Percutaneous radiofrequency neurotomy in the treatment of cervical zygapophyseal joint pain: a caution. *Neurosurgery*, **36**, 732–739.

Lord, S. M., Barnsley, L. Wallis, B. J. and Bogduk, N. (1995b). Third occipital nerve headache: a prevalence study. *Journal of Neurology, Neurosurgery and Psychiatry*, **57**, 1187–1190.

Lord, S. M., Barnsley, L., Wallis, B. J. and Bogduk, N. (1996). Chronic cervical zygapophyseal joint pain after whiplash. *Spine*, **21**, 1737–1745.

Lorenz, M. and McCulloch, J. (1985). Chemonucleolysis for herniated nucleus pulposus in adolescents. *Journal of Bone and Joint Surgery*, **67A**, 1402–1404.

Lorenz, M., Patwardhan, A. and Vanderby, R. (1983). Load-bearing characteristics of lumbar facets in normal and surgically altered spinal segments. *Spine*, **8**, 122–130.

Louw, J. A., Dommissee, G. F. and Roos, M. F. (1988). Spinal stenosis following anterior spinal fusion. *Spine*, **13**, 952–953.

Lowe, T. G. (1990). Scheuermann's disease. *Journal of Bone and Joint Surgery*, **72A**, 940–945.

Lowell, T. D., Errico, T. J., Fehlings, M. G. et al. (1995). Microdiskectomy for lumbar disc herniation: a review of 100 cases. *Orthopedics*, **18**, 985–990.

Luk, K. D. K. and Leong, J. C. Y. (1986). The iliolumbar ligament: a study of its anatomy, development and clinical significance. *Journal of Bone and Joint Surgery*, **68B**, 197–200.

Lund, N., Bengtsson, A. and Thorburg, P. (1986). Muscle tissue oxygen pressure in primary fibromyalgia. *Scandinavian Journal of Rheumatology*, **15**, 165–173.

Lusins, J. O., Elting, J. J., Cicoria, A. D. and Goldsmith, S. J. (1994). SPECT evaluation of unilateral spondylolysis. *Clinical Nuclear Medicine*, **19**, 1–5.

Lynch, M. C. and Taylor, J. F. (1986). Facet joint injection for low back pain: a clinical study. *Journal of Bone and Joint Surgery*, **68B**, 138–141.

Lyritis, G. P., Tsakatakos, N., Maglasis, B. et al. (1991). Analgesic effect of salmon calcitonin in osteoporotic vertebral fractures: a double-blind placebo-controlled clinical study. *Calcified Tissue International*, **49**, 369–372.

MacLennan, A. H. (1991). The role of the hormone relaxin in human reproduction and pelvic girdle relaxation. *Scandinavian Journal of Rheumatology Supplement*, **88**, 7–15.

Macnab, I. (1971a). The traction spur. *Journal of Bone and Joint Surgery*, **53A**, 663–670.

Macnab, I. (1971b). The whiplash syndrome. *Orthopedic Clinics of North America*, **2**, 389–403.

Magnaes, B. (1982). Clinical recording of pressure on the spinal cord and cauda equina: Part I: The spinal block infusion test methods and clinical studies. Part II. Position changes in pressure on the cauda equina in central lumbar stenosis. *Journal of Neurosurgery*, **57**, 48–63.

Magni, G., Marchetti, M., Moreschi, C. et al. (1993). Chronic musculoskeletal pain and depressive symptoms in the national health and nutrition examination. I. Epidemiologic follow-up study. *Pain*, **53**, 163–168.

Magni, G., Moreschi, C., Rigatti-Luchini, S. and Merskey, H. (1994). Prospective study on the relationship between depressive symptoms and chronic musculoskeletal pain. *Pain*, **56**, 289–297.

Magnusson, T. (1994). Extra-cervical symptoms after whiplash trauma. *Cephalalgia*, **14**, 223–227.

Magora, A., and Schwarz, A. (1976). Relation between the low back pain syndrome and x-ray findings. I. Degenerative osteoarthritis. *Scandinavian Journal of Rehabilitation Medicine*, **8**, 115–125.

Maheshwaran, S., Davies, A. M., Evans, N. et al. (1995). Sciatica in degenerative spondylolisthesis of the lumbar spine. *Annals of the Rheumatic Diseases*, **54**, 539–543.

Maigne, J.-Y., Rime, B. and Deligne, B. (1992). Computed tomographic follow-up studies of forty-eight cases of nonoperatively treated lumbar intervertebral disc herniation. *Spine*, **17**, 1071–1074.

Maigne, J.-Y., Aivaliklis, A. and Pfefer, F. (1996). Results of sacroiliac joint double block and value of sacroiliac pain provocation tests in 54 patients with low back pain. *Spine*, **21**, 1889–1892.

Maigne, R. (1980). Low back pain of thoracolumbar origin. *Archives of Physical Medicine and Rehabilitation*, **61**, 389–395.

Maimaris, C., Barnes, M. R. and Allen, M. J. (1988). Whiplash injuries of the neck: a retrospective study. *Injury*, **19**, 393–396.

Maitland, G. D. (1979). Negative disc exploration: positive canal signs. *Australian Journal of Physiotherapy*, **25**, 129–134.

Maitland, G. D. (1985). The slump test: exercise and treatment. *Australian Journal of Physiotherapy*, **31**, 215–219.

Maitland, G. D. (1986). *Vertebral Manipulation*, 5th edn. Butterworth.

Makela, M., Heilovaara, M., Sievers K. et al. (1993). Musculoskeletal disorders as determinants of disability in Finns aged 30 years or more. *Journal of Clinical Epidemiology*, **46**, 549–559.

Malawski, S. K. and Lukawski, S. (1991). Pyogenic infection of the spine. *Clinical Orthopaedics and Related Research*, **272**, 58–66.

Malchaire, J. B. and Masset, D. F. (1995). Isometric and dynamic performances of the trunk and associated factors. *Spine*, **20**, 1649–1656.

Maldague, B., Mathurin, P. and Malghem, J. (1981). Facet joint arthrography in lumbar spondylolysis. *Radiology*, **140**, 29–36.

Malmivaara, A. and Pohjola, R. (1982). Cauda equina syndrome caused by chiropraxic on a patient previously free of lumbar spine symptoms (letter). *Lancet*, **1**, 411.

Malmivaara, A., Videman, T., Kuosma, E. and Troup, J. D. G. (1987). Facet joint orientation, facet and costovertebral joint osteoarthrosis, disc degeneration, vertebral body osteophytosis and Schmorl's nodes in the thoracolumbar region of cadaveric spines. *Spine*, **12**, 458–463.

Malter, A. D., Larson, E. B., Urban, N. and Deyo, R. A. (1996). Cost-effectiveness of lumbar discectomy for the treatment of herniated intervertebral disc. *Spine*, **21**, 1048–1055.

Mandell, G. A., Morales, R. W., Harcke, H. T. and Bowen, J. R. (1993). Bone scintigraphy in patients with atypical lumbar Scheuermann's disease. *Journal of Pediatric Orthopedics*, **13**, 622–627.

Mann, N. H., Brown, M. D., Hertz, D. B. et al. (1993). Initial-impression diagnosis using low-back pain patient pain drawings. *Spine*, **18**, 41–53.

Maravilla, K. R., Lesh, P., Weinreb, J. C. et al. (1985). Magnetic resonance imaging of the lumbar spine with CT correlation. *American Journal of Neuroradiology*, **6**, 237–245.

Marchand, F. and Ahmed, A. M. (1990). Investigation of the laminate structure of lumbar disc annulus fibrosus. *Spine*, **15**, 402–410.

Marchand, S., Charest, J., Li, J. et al. (1993). Is TENS purely a placebo effect? A controlled study on chronic low back pain. *Pain*, **54**, 99–106.

Marcus, R. (1995). Cyclical etidronate: has the rose lost its bloom (editorial)? *American Journal of Medicine*, **95**, 555–556.

Marder, W. D., Meenan, R. F., Felson, D. T. et al. (1991). The present and future adequacy of rheumatology manpower: a study of health care needs and physician supply. *Arthritis and Rheumatism*, **34**, 1209–1217.

Marks, R. (1989). Distribution of pain provoked from lumbar facet joints and related structures during diagnostic spinal infiltration. *Pain*, **39**, 37–40.

Marks, R. C., Houston, T. and Thulbourne, T. (1992). Facet joint injection and facet nerve block: a randomised comparison in 86 patients with chronic low back pain. *Pain*, **49**, 325–328.

Markwalder, Th-M. and Merat, M. (1994). The lumbar and lumbosacral facet-syndrome. Diagnostic measures, surgical treatment and results in 119 patients. *Acta Neurochirurgica*, **128**, 40—46.

Marras, W. S. and Mirka, G. A. (1996). Intra-abdominal pressure during trunk extension motions. *Clinical Biomechanics*, **11**, 267–274.

Marshall, L. L, Trethewie, E. R. and Curtain, C. C. (1977). Chemical radiculitis. A clinical, physiological and immunological study. *Clinical Orthopaedics and Related Research*, **129**, 61–67.

Martin, A. (1995). Osteoporosis: a geriatric public health issue. *Topics in Geriatric Rehabilitation*, **10**, 1–11.

Martin, J. C., Harvey, J. and Dixey, J. (1996). Chest pain in patients with rheumatoid arthritis. *Annals of Rheumatic Disease*, **55**, 152–153.

Martino, F., D'Amore, M., Angelelli, G. et al. (1991). Echographic study of Tietze's syndrome. *Clinics in Rheumatology*, **10**, 2–4.

Masaryk, T. J. (1991). Neoplastic disease of the spine. *Radiologic Clinics of North America*, **29**, 829–845.

Matsunaga, S., Sakou, T., Morizono, Y. et al. (1990). Natural history of degenerative spondylolisthesis. *Spine*, **15**, 1204–1210.

Matsuyama, Y., Kawakami, N. and Mimatsu, K. (1995). Spinal cord expansion after decompression in cervical myelopathy. Investigation by myelography and ultrasonography. *Spine*, **20**, 1657–1663.

Mathews, J. A., Mills, S. B., Jenkins, V. M. et al. (1987). Back pain and sciatica: controlled trials on manipulation, traction, sclerosant and epidural injection. *British Journal of Rheumatology*, **26**, 416–423.

Mau, W., Zeidler, H., Mau, R. et al. (1988). Clinical features and prognosis of patients with possible ankylosing spondylitis: results of a 10-year follow up. *Journal of Rheumatology*, **15**, 1109–1114.

Maugars, Y., Mathis, C., Vilon, P. and Prost, A. (1992). Corticosteroid injection of the sacroiliac joint in patients with seronegative spondyloarthropathy. *Arthritis and Rheumatism*, **35**, 564–568.

Mayer, H. M. (1994). Percutaneous lumbar disc surgery. *Spine*, **19**, 2719–2723.

Mayer, H. M. and Brock, M. (1993). Percutaneous endoscopic discectomy. Surgical technique and preliminary results compared to micrsurgical discectomy. *Journal of Neurosurgery*, **78**, 216–225.

McAfree, P. C., Regan, J. R., Zdeblick, T. et al. (1995). The incidence of complications in endoscopic anterior thoracolumbar spinal surgery. *Spine*, **20**, 1624–1632.

McCain, G. A. (1989. Nonmedical treatment in primary fibromyalgia. *Rheumatic Diseases Clinics of North America*, **15**, 73 90.

McCall, I. W., Park, W. M. and OiBrien, J. P. (1979). Induced pain referral from posterior lumbar elements in normal subjects. *Spine*, **4**, 441–446.

McCarroll, J. R., Miller, J. M. and Ritter, M. A. (1986). Lumbar spondylolysis and spondylolisthesis in college football players. *American Journal of Sports Medicine*, **14**, 404–406.

McCarron, R. F., Wimpee, M. W., Hudkins, P. and Laros, G. S. (1987). The inflammatory effect if nucleus pulposus. A possible element in the pathogenesis of low back pain. *Spine*, **12**, 760–764.

McCombe, P. F., Fairbank, J. C. T., Cockersole, B. C. and Pynsent, P. B. (1989). Reproducibility of physical signs in low back. *Spine*, **14**, 908–918.

McCulloch, J. H. and Organ, L. W. (1977). Percutaneous radiofrequency lumbar rhizolysis (rhizotomy). *Canadian Medical Association Journal*, **116**, 30–32.

McDonald, R. S. and Bell, C. M. (1990). An open controlled assessment of osteopathic manipulation in nonspecific low back pain. *Spine*, **15**, 364–370.

McGaughey, I. (1994). Pyogenic infection of the sacroiliac joint. *Australian and New Zealand Journal of Surgery*, **66**, 282–286.

McGill, S. M. (1987). A biomechanical perspective of sacroiliac pain. *Clinical Biomechanics*, **2**, 145–151.

McGill, S., Seguin, J. and Bennett, G. (1994). Passive stiffness of the upper torso in flexion, extension, lateral bending and axial rotation: effect of belt wearing and breath holding. *Spine*, **19**, 696–704.

McGuire, R. A. and Amundson, G. M. (1993). The use of primary internal fixation in spondylolisthesis. *Spine*, **18**, 1662–1672.

McKenzie, L. and Sillence, D. (1992). Familial Scheuermann's disease: a genetic and lingkage study. *Journal of Medical Genetics*, **29**, 41–45.

McKinney, L. A. (1989). Early mobilization and outcome in acute sprains of the neck. *British Medical Journal*, **299**, 1006–1008.

McKinney, L. A., Dornan, J. O. and Ryan, M. (1989). The role of physiotherapy in the management of acute neck sprains following road-traffic events. *Archives of Emergency Medicine*, **6**, 27–33.

McNally, D. S., Adams, M. A., and Goodship, A. E. (1993). Can intervertebral disc prolapse be predicted by disc mechanics? *Spine*, **18**, 1525–1530.

McRae. D. L. (1956). Asymptomatic intervertebral disc protrusions. *Acta Radiologica*, **46**, 9–27.

McRorie, E. R., McLoughlin, P., Russell, T. et al. (1996). Cervical spine surgery in patients with rheumatoid arthritis: an appraisal. *Annals of the Rheumatic Diseases*, **55**, 99–104.

Meade, T. W., Dyer, S., Browne, W. et al. (1990). Low back pain of mechanical origin: randomised comparison of chiropractic and outpatient treatment. *British Medical Journal*, **300**, 1431–1437.

Mealy, K., Brennan, H. and Fenelon, G. C. C. (1986). Early mobilization to acute whiplash injuries. *British Medical Journal*, **292**, 656–657.

Mehta, M. and Sluijter, M. E. (1979). The treatment of chronic back pain: a preliminary survey of the effect of radiofrequency denervation of the posterior vertebral joints. *Anaesthesia*, **34**, 768–775.

Mehta, M. and Wynn Parry, C. B. (1994). Mechanical back pain and the facet joint syndrome. *Disability and Rehabilitation*, **16**, 2–12.

Meloche, J. P., Bergeron, Y., Bellavance, A. et al. (1993). Painful intervertebral dysfunction: Robert Maigne's original contribution to headache of cervical origin. The Quebec headache study group. *Headache*, **33**, 328–334.

Mendelson, G. (1982). Not 'cured by a verdict'. Effect of legal settlements on compensation claimants. *Medical Journal of Australia*, **2**, 132–134.

Mendelson, G. (1984). Follow-up studies of personal injury litigants. *International Journal of Law and Psychiatry*, **7**, 179–188.

Mendelson, G. (1992). Compensation and chronic pain. *Pain*, **48**, 121–123.

Merbs, C. F. (1995). Incomplete spondylolysis and healing. A study of ancient Canadian Eskimo skeletons. *Spine*, **21**, 2328–2334.

Merskey, H. (1984). Psychiatry and the cervical sprain syndrome. *Canadian Medical Association Journal*, **130**, 1119–1121.

Merskey, H. (1993). Psychological consequences of whiplash. *Spine: State of the Art Reviews*, **7**, 471–480.

Micheli, L. (1983). Back injuries in dancers. *Clinics in Sports Medicine*, **2**, 473–484.

Micheli, L. (1985). Back injuries in gymnasts. *Clinics in Sports Medicine*, **4**, 85–93.

Micheli, L. and Wood, R. (1995). Back pain in young athletes. Significant differences from adults in causes and patterns. *Archives of Paediatrics and Adolescent Medicine*, **149**, 15–18.

Micheli, L., Hall, J. E. and Miller, M. E. (1980). Use of modified Boston brace for back injuries in athletes. *American Journal of Sports Medicine*, **8**, 351–355.

Michler, R. P., Bovim, G. and Sjaastad, O. (1991). Disorders in the lower cervical spine: a cause of unilateral headache. *Headache*, **31**, 550–551.

Miles, K. A., Maimaris, C., Finlay, D. and Barnes, M. R. (1988). The incidence and prognostic significance of radiological abnormalities in soft tissue injuries to the cervical spine. *Skeletal Radiology*, **17**, 493–496.

Milgrom, C., Finestone, A. and Lev, B. (1993). Overexertional lumbar and thoracic back pain among recruits: a prospective study of risk factors and treatment regimens. *Journal of Spinal Disorders*, **6**, 187–193.

Miller, J. A., Schmatz, C. and Schult, A. B. (1988). Lumbar disc degeneration: correlation with age, sex, and spine level in 600 autopsy specimens. *Spine*, **13**, 173–178.

Miller, J. A. A., Shultz, A. B. and Andersson, G. B. (1987). Load-displacement behaviour of sacroiliac joints. *Journal of Orthopaedic Research*, **5**, 92–100.

Miller, R. G. and Burton, R. (1974). Stroke following chiropractic manipulation of the spine. *Journal of the American Medical Association*, **229**, 189–190.

Mimura, M., Panjabi, M. M., Oxland, T. R. et al. (1994). Disc degeneration affects the multidirectional flexibility of the lumbar spine. *Spine*, **19**, 1371–1380.

Miniaci, A. and Johnson, P. Q. (1993). Spondylolysis of the lumbar vertebrae with associated reactive sclerosis of the pedicle of the contralateral side: report of a case. *Clinical Journal of Sports Medicine*, **3**, 189–191.

Mixter, W. J. and Barr, J. S. (1934). Rupture of the intervertebral disc with involvement of the spinal canal. *New England Journal of Medicine*, **11**, 210–215.

Miyake, R., Ikata, T., Katoh, S. and Morita, T. (1996). Morphologic analysis of the facet joint in the immature lumbosacral spine with special reference to spondylolysis. *Spine*, **21**, 783–789.

Modic, M. (1994). Degenerative disorders of the spine. In *Magnetic Resonance Imaging of the Spine*. (M. Modic, T. Masaryk and J. Ross eds) pp. 80–150, Mosby.

Modic, M. T. and Herzog, R. J. (1994). Spinal imaging modalities what's available and who should order them? *Spine*, **19**, 1764–1765.

Modic, M. T. and Ross, J. S. (1991). MRI in the evaluation of low back pain. *Orthopedic Clinics of North America*, **22**, 283–301.

Modic, M. T., Masaryk, T., Bundschuh, C. et al. (1986). Cervical radiculopathy: prospective evaluation with surface coil MR imaging, CT with metrizamide, and metrizamide myelography. *Radiology*, **161**, 753–759.

Modic, M. T., Masaryk, T. J., Ross, J. S. and Carter, J. R. (1988a). Imaging of degenerative disc disease. *Radiology*, **168**, 177–186.

Modic, M.T, Steinberg, P. M., Ross, J. S. et al. (1988b). Degenerative disk disease: assessment of changes in vertebral body marrow with MR imaging. *Radiology*, **166**, 193–199.

Moldofsky, H., Scarisbrick, P., England, R. and Smythe, H. A. (1975). Musculoskeletal symptoms and non-REM sleep disturbances in patients with fibrositic syndromes and healthy subjects. *Psychosomatic Medicine*, **38**, 35–44.

Moneta, G. B., Videman, T., Kaivanto, K. et al. (1994). Reported pain during lumbar discography as a function of annular ruptures and disc degeneration. A re-analysis of 833 discograms. *Spine*, **19**, 1968–1974.

Montgomery, D. M. and Brower, R. S. (1992). Cervical spondylotic myelopathy. Clinical syndrome and natural history. *Orthopedic Clinics of North America*, **23**, 487–493.

Mooney, V. (1987). Where is the pain coming from? *Spine*, **12**, 754–759.

Mooney, V. and Andersson, G. B. (1994). Trunk strength testing in patient evaluation and treatment. *Spine*, **19**, 2483–2485.

Mooney, V. and Robertson, J. (1976). The facet syndrome. *Clinical Orthopaedics and Related Research*, **115**, 149–156.

Moore, R. J., Vernon-Roberts, B., Osti, O. L. and Fraser, R. D. (1996). Remodelling of vertebral bone after outer anular injury in sheep. *Spine*, **21**, 936–940.

Moran, R., O'Connell, D. and Walsh, M. G. (1988). The diagnostic value of facet joint injections. *Spine*, **13**, 1407–1410.

Morand, E. F., Leech, M., Cooley, H. and Littlejohn, G. O. (1996). Advances in the understanding of neuroendocrine function in rheumatic disease. *Australian and New Zealand Journal of Medicine*, **26**, 543–551.

Moreland, L. W., Lopez-Mendez, A. and Alarcon, G. S. (1989). Spinal stenosis: a comprehensive review of the literature. *Seminars in Arthritis and Rheumatism*, **19**, 127–149.

Morita, T., Ikata, T., Katoh, S. and Miyake, R. (1995). Lumbar spondylolysis in children and adolescents. *Journal of Bone and Joint Surgery*, **77B**, 620–625.

Morris, F. (1989). Do head restraints protect the neck from whiplash injuries? *Archives of Emergency Medicine*, **6**, 17–21.

Mundt, D., Kelsey, J., Golden, A. et al. (1983). An epidemiological study of lifting and twisting on the job and risk for prolapsed lumbar intervertebral disc. *Spine*, **18**, 595–599.

Murata, M., Morio, Y. and Kuranobu, K. (1994). Lumbar disc degeneration and segmental instability: a comparison of magnetic resonance images and plain radiographs of patients with low back pain. *Archives of Orthopaedic and Trauma Surgery*, **113**, 297–301.

Murphey, M. D., Wetzel, L. H., Bramble, J. M. et al. (1991). Sacroiliitis: magnetic resonance imaging findings. *Radiology*, **180**, 239–244.

Murphy, W. A. (1984). The facet syndrome. Opinions. *Radiology*, **151**, 533.

Murtagh, F. R. (1988). Computered tomography and fluoroscopy guided anesthesia and steroid injection in facet syndrome. *Spine*, **13**, 686–689.

Nachemson, A. (1969). Intradiscal measurements of pH in patients with lumbar rhizopathics. *Acta Orthopaedica Scandinavica*, **40**, 23–42.

Nachemson, A. (1985). Lumbar spine instability: a critical update and symposium summary. *Spine*, **10**, 290–291.

Nachemson, A. (1989). Lumbar discography – Where are we today? *Spine*, **14**, 555–557

Nachemson, A. L. (1992). Newest knowledge of low back pain: a critical look. *Clinical Orthopaedics and Related Research*, **279**, 8–20.

Nachemson, A. and Elfstrom, G. (1970). Intravital dynamic pressure measurements in lumbar disc. *Scandinavian Journal of Rehabilitation Medicine Supplement*, 2, 1–40.

Nachemson, A. and Morris, J. M. (1964). In vivo measurements of intradiscal pressure. *Journal of Bone and Joint Surgery*, **46A**, 1077–1092.

Nagler, W. (1973). Vertebral artery obstruction by hyperextension of the neck: report of three cases. *Archives of Physical Medicine and Rehabilitation*, **54**, 237–240.

Nakai, O., Ookawa, A. and Yamaura, I. (1991). Long-term roentgenographic and functional changes in patients who were treated with wide fenestration for central lumbar stenosis.

Journal of Bone and Joint Surgery, **73A**, 1184–1191.

Nasca, R. J. (1987). Surgical management of lumbar spinal stenosis. *Spine,* **12**, 809–816.

Nathan, H., Weinberg, H., Robin, G. C. and Aviad, I. (1964). The costovertebral joints: anatomical–clinical observations in arthritis. *Arthritis and Rheumatism,* **7**, 228–240.

Naylor, J. R. and Mulley, G. P. (1991). Surgical collars: a survey of their prescription and use. *British Journal of Rheumatology,* **30**, 282–284.

Nelson, C. L., Janecki, C. J., Gildenberg, P. L. and Sava, G. (1972). Disc protrusions in the young. *Clinical Orthopaedics and Related Research,* **88**, 142–150.

Nelson, J. M., Walmsley, R. P. and Stevenson, J. M. (1995). Relative lumbar and pelvic motion during loaded spinal flexion/extension. *Spine,* **20**, 199–204.

Newell, R. L. M. (1995). Spondylolysis. An historic review. *Spine,* **20**, 1950–1956.

Newman, P. H. (1976). Stenosis of the lumbar spine in spondylolisthesis. *Clinical Orthopaedics and Related Research,* **115**, 116–121.

Newman, P. K. (1990). Whiplash injury. Long term prospective studies are needed, and, meanwhile, pragmatic treatment (editorial). *British Medical Journal,* **301**, 395–396.

Nicholas, J. J., Smith, W. F. and Andersson, G. B. (1996). Bacterial discitis caused by limb gangrene requiring below-knee amputation. *Archives of Physical Medicine and Rehabilitation,* **77**, 301–304.

Nilsson, N. (1995). The prevalence of cervicogenic headache in a random population sample of 20-59 year olds. *Spine,* **20**, 1884–1888.

Nissila, M., Lahesmaa, R., Leirisalo-Repo, M. et al. (1994). Antibodies to *Klebsiella pneumoniae, Escherichia coli, Proteus mirabilis* in ankylosing spondylitis: effect of sulfasalazine treatment. *Journal of Rheumatology,* **21**, 2082–2087.

Nordemar, R. and Thorner, C. (1981). Treatment of acute cervical pain: a comparative group study. *Pain,* **10**, 93–101.

Nordstrom, D., Santavirta, S., Seitsalo, S. et al. (1994). Symptomatic lumbar spondylolysis. Neuroimmunologic studies. *Spine,* **19**, 2752–2758.

Noren, R., Trafimow, J., Andersson, G. B. and Huckman, M. S. (1991). The role of facet joint tropism and facet angle in disc degeneration. *Spine,* **16**, 530–532.

Normelli, H. C., Svensson, O. and Aaro, S. I. (1991). Cord compression in Scheuermann's kyphosis. A case report. *Acta Orthopaedica Scandinavica,* **62**, 70–72.

Norris, S. H. and Watt, I. (1983). The prognosis of neck injuries resulting from rear-end vehicle collisions. *Journal of Bone and Joint Surgery,* **65B**, 608–611.

North, R. B., Han, M., Zahurak, M. and Kidd, D. H. (1994). Radiofrequency lumbar facet denervation: analysis of prognostic factors. *Pain,* **57**, 77–83.

Nugent, P. J. and Kostuik, J. P. (1993). Degenerative spondylolisthesis. *Current Opinion in Orthopedics,* **4**, 11, 125–128.

Nwuga, G. and Nwuga, V. (1985). Relative therapeutic efficacy of the Williams and McKenzie protocols in back pain management. *Physiotherapy Practice,* **1**, 99–105.

Nwuga, V. C. (1982). Relative therapeutic efficacy of vertebral manipulation and conventional treatment in back pain management. *American Journal of Physical Medicine,* **61**, 273–278.

O'Brien, C. P. (1996). 'Rugby neck': cervical degeneration in two front row rugby union players. *Clinical Journal of Sports Medicine,* **6**, 56–59.

Oda, T., Fujiwara, K., Yonenobu, K. et al. (1995). Natural course of cervical spine lesions in rheumatoid arthritis. *Spine,* **20**, 1128–1135.

Oegema, T. R. (1993). Biochemistry of the intervertebral disc. *Clinics in Sports Medicine,* **12**, 419–438.

Ogsbury, J. A., Simon, R. H. and Lehman, R. A. W. (1977). Facet denervation in the treatment of low back syndrome. *Pain,* **3**, 257–263.

Ohlund, C., Eek, C., Palmblad, S. et al. (1996). Quantified pain drawing in subacute low back pain. Validation in a nonselected outpatient industrial sample. *Spine,* **21**, 1021–1031.

Ohnmeiss, D. D., Guyer, R. D. and Hochschuler, S. H. (1994). Laser disc decompression. The importance of proper patient selection. *Spine,* **19**, 2054–2059.

Ohshima, H., Hirano, N., Osada, R. et al. (1993). Morphologic variation of lumbar posterior longitudinal ligament and the modality of disc herniation. *Spine,* **18**, 2408–2411.

Ohshima, H. and Urban, J. P. G. (1992). The effect of lactate and pH on proteoglycans and protein synthesis rates in the intervertebral disc. *Spine*, **17**, 1079–1082.

Okada, Y., Ikata, T., Katoh, S. and Yamada, H. (1994). Morphologic analysis of the cervical spinal cord, dural tube, and spinal canal by magnetic resonance imaging in normal adults and patients with cervical spondylotic myelopathy. *Spine*, **19**, 2331–2335.

O'Leary, P. F., Camino, M. B., Polifroni, N. V. et al. (1984). Thoracic disc disease: clinical manifestations and surgical treatment. *Bulletin of the Hospital for Joint Diseases*, **44**, 27–40.

Olivieri, I., Gemignani, G., Camerini, E. et al. (1990). Differential diagnosis between osteitis condensans ilii and sacroiliitis. *Journal of Rheumatology*, **17**, 1504–1512.

Olivieri, I., Ferri, S. and Barozzi, L. (1994). Osteitis condensans ilii. *British Journal of Rheumatology*, **35**, 295–297.

Olmarker, K. and Rydevik, B. (1991). Pathophysiology of sciatica. *Orthopedic Clinics of North America*, **22**, 223–234.

Olmarker, K., Rydevik, B. and Nordborg, C. (1993). Autologous nucleus pulposus induces neurophysiologic and histologic changes in porcine cauda equina nerve roots. *Spine*, **18**, 1425–1432.

Olmarker, K., Byrod, G., Cornefjord, M. et al. (1994). Effects of methylprednisolone on nucleus pulposus – induced nerve root injury. *Spine*, **10**, 1803–1808.

Olmarker, K., Blomquist, J., Stromberg, J. et al. (1995) Inflammatogenic properties of nucleus pulposus. *Spine*, **20**, 665–669.

Olsnes, B. T. (1989). Neurobehavioral findings in whiplash patients with long lasting symptoms. *Acta Neurologica Scandinavica*, **80**, 584–588.

Onel, D., Sari, H. and Donmez, C. (1993). Lumbar spinal stenosis: clinical/radiologic therapeutic evaluation in 145 patients. Conservative treatment or surgical intervention? *Spine*, **18**, 291–298

Ongley, M. J., Klein, R. G., Dorman, T. A. et al. (1987). A new approach to the treatment of chronic low back pain. *Lancet*, **2**, 143–146.

Onik, G., Mooney, V., Maroon, J. S. et al. (1990). Automated percutaneous discectomy: a prospective multi-institutional study. *Neurosurgery*, **26**, 228–232.

Oosterveld, W. J., Kortschot, H. W., Kingma, G. G. et al. (1991). Electronystagmographic findings following cervical whiplash injuries. *Acta Oto-Laryngologica*, **111**, 201–205.

Orvieto, R., Achiron, A., Ben Ralail, Z. et al. (1994). Low back pain of pregnancy. *Acta Obstetrica et Gynecologica Scandinavica*, **73**, 209–214.

Osman, A. A. and Govender, S. (1995). Septic sacroiliitis. *Clinical Orthopaedics and Related Research*, **313**, 214–219.

Osman, A. A.-H., Bassiouni, H., Koutri, R. et al. (1994). Aging of the thoracic spine: distinction between wedging in osteoarthritis and fracture in osteoporosis. A cross-sectional and longitudinal study. *Bone*, **15**, 437–442.

Ostgaard, H. C., Andersson, G. B. J. and Karlsson, K. (1991). Prevalence of back pain in pregnancy. *Spine*, **16**, 549–542.

Ostgaard, H. C., Andersson, G. B., Schultz, A. B. and Miller, J. A. (1993). Influence of some biomechanical factors on low back pain in pregnancy. *Spine*, **18**, 61–65.

Ostgaard, H. C, Zetherstrom. G., Roos-Hansson, E. and Svanberg, B. (1994). Reduction of back and posterior pelvic pain in pregnancy. *Spine*, 19, 894–900.

Osti, O. L. and Fraser, R. D. (1992). MRI and discography of annular tears and intervertebral disc degeneration. A prospective clinical comparison. *Journal of Bone and Joint Surgery*, **74B**, 431–435.

Osti, O. L., Vernon-Roberts, B. and Fraser, R. D. (1990). Anulus tears and intervertebral disc degeneration. An experimental study using an animal model. *Spine*, **15**, 762–767.

Otani, A., Yoshida, M. Fujii, E. et al. (1988). Thoracic disk herniation. Surgical treatment in 23 patients. *Spine*, **13**, 1262–1267.

Ottenbacher, K. and Di Fabio, R. P. (1985). Efficacy of spinal manipulation mobilization therapy. A meta-analysis. *Spine*, **10**, 833–837.

Oudenhoven, R. C. (1979). The role of laminectomy, facet rhizotomy and epidural steroids. *Spine*, **4**, 145–147.

Overgaard, K., Hansen, M. A., Jensen, S. B. and Christiansen, C. (1992). Effect of calcitonin given intranasally on bone mass and fracture rates in established osteoporosis: a dose-response study. *British Medical Journal*, **305**, 556–561.

Paajanen, H., Erkintalo, M., Kuusela, T. et al. (1989). Magnetic resonance study of disc degeneration in young low-back pain patients. *Spine*, **14**, 982–985.

Paajanen, H., Lehto, I., Alenen, A. et al. (1994). Diurnal fluid changes of lumbar discs measured indirectly by magnetic resonance imaging. *Journal of Orthopaedic Research*, **12**, 509–514.

Pal, B., Mangion, P., Hossain, M. A. and Diffey, B. L. (1986). A controlled trial of continuous lumbar traction in the treatment of back pain and sciatica. *British Journal of Rheumatology*, **25**, 181–183.

Pang, L. Q. (1971). The otological aspects of whiplash injuries. *Laryngoscope*, 81, 1381–1387.

Panjabi, M. M., Abumi, K., Duranceau, J. and Oxland, T. (1989). Spinal stability and intersegmental muscle forces. A biomechanical model. *Spine*, **14**, 194–199.

Parfenchuck, T. A. and Janssen, M. E. (1994). A correlation of cervical magnetic resonance imaging and discography/computed tomographic discograms. *Spine*, **19**, 2819–2825.

Parke, W. W. (1988). Correlative anatomy of cervical spondylotic myelopathy. *Spine*, **13**, 831–837.

Parke, W. W. and Watanabe, R. (1985). The intrinsic vasculature of the lumbosacral spinal nerve roots. *Spine*, **10**, 508–515.

Parker, G. B., Tupling, H. and Pryor, D. S. (1978). A controlled trial of cervical manipulation for migraine. *Australian and New Zealand Journal of Medicine*, **8**, 598–593.

Pascual, E., Castelanno, J. A. and Lopez, E. (1992). Costovertebral joint changes in ankylosing spondylitis with thoracic pain. *British Journal of Rheumatology*, **31**, 413–415.

Patijn, J. (1991). Complications in manual medicine: a review of the literature. *Journal of Manual Medicine*, **6**, 89–92.

Patwardhan, A. G. (1994). The role of the lumbar facet joints in spinal stability: identification of alternative paths of loading (point of view). *Spine*, **19**, 2671.

Pawl, R. P. (1977). Headache, cervical spondylosis and anterior cervical fusion. *Surgery Annals*, **9**, 391–408.

Payne, T. C., Leavitt, F., Garron, D. C. et al. (1982). Fibrositis and psychological disturbance. *Arthritis and Rheumatism*, **25**, 213–217.

Pearce, J. M. (1989). Whiplash injury: a reappraisal. *Journal of Neurology, Neurosurgery and Psychiatry*, **52**, 1329–1331.

Pearce, J. M. (1994). Polemics of chronic whiplash injury (editorial). *Neurology*, **44**, 1993–1997.

Pech, P., Daniels, D. L., Williams, A. L. and Haughton, V. M. (1985). The cervical neural foramina: correlation of microtomy and CT anatomy. *Radiology*, **155**, 143–146.

Pellecchia, G. L. (1994). Lumbar traction: a review of the literature. *Journal of Orthopedic and Sports Physical Therapy*, **20**, 262–267.

Pennell, R. G., Maurer, A. H. and Bonakdarpour, A. (1985). Stress injuries of the pars interarticularis: radiologic classification and indications for scintigraphy. *American Journal of Roentgenology*, **145**, 763–766.

Pennie, B. and Agambar, L. J. (1990). Whiplash injuries. A trial of early management. *Journal of Bone and Joint Surgery*, **72B**, 277–279.

Pennie, B. and Agambar, L. J. (1991). Patterns of injury and recovery in whiplash. *Injury*, **22**, 57–59.

Penning, L. (1991). Differences in anatomy, motion development and aging in the upper and lower cervical disk segments. *Clinical Biomechanics*, **3**, 37–41.

Penning, L. and Wilmink, J. T. (1987). Rotation of the cervical spine. A CT study in normal subjects. *Spine*, **12**, 732–738.

Penning, L., Wilmink, J. T., Van Woerden, H. H. et al. (1986). CT myelography findings in degenerative disorders of the cervical spine: clinical significance. *American Journal of Neuroradiology*, **7**, 793–801.

Peterson, D. I., Austin, G. M. and Dayes, L. A. (1975). Headache associated with discogenic disease of the cervical spine. *Bulletin of the Los Angeles Neurological Society*, **40**, 96–100.

Pettersson, H., Larsson, E. M., Holtas, S. et al. (1988). MR imaging of the cervical spine in rheumatoid arthritis. *American Journal of Neuroradiology*, **9**, 573–577.

Pettersson, K., Karrholm, J., Toolanen, G and

Hildingsson, C. (1995). Decreased width of the spinal canal in patients with chronic symptoms after whiplash injury. *Spine*, **20**, 1664–1667.

Pettine, K. A., Salib, R. M. and Walker, S. G. (1993). External electrical stimulation and bracing for treatment of spondylosis. *Spine*, **18**, 436–439.

Pevsener, P. H., Ondra, S., Radcliff, W. et al. (1986). Magnetic resonance imaging of the lumbar spine. A comparison with CT and myelography. *Acta Radiologica Scandinavica*, **369**, 706–707.

Peyton, F. W. (1983). Unexpected frequency of idiopathic costochondral pain. *Obstetrics and Gynecology*, **62**, 605–608.

Pfaffenrath, V. and Kaube, H. (1990). Diagnositics of cervicogenic headache. *Functional Neurology*, **5**, 157–164.

Pfaffenrath, V., Dandekar, R. and Pollman, W. (1987). Cervicogenic headache – the clinical picture, radiological findings and hypothesis on its pathophysiology. *Headache*, **27**, 495–499.

Pfaffenrath, V., Dandekar, R., Mayer, E. T. et al. (1988). Cervicogenic headache: results of computer-based measurements of cervical spine mobility in 15 patients. *Cephalalgia*, **8**, 45–48.

Pierrynowski, M., Schroeder, B. C, and Garrity, C. B. (1988). Three-dimensional sacroiliac motion during locomotion in asymptomatic male and female subjects. In *Proceedings of the Fifth Biennial Conference and Human Locomotion Symposium of the Canadian Society for Biomechanics*. (Cotton, LaMontagne, Robertson, and Strothart eds.) pp. 132–133.

Pietri, F., Lecierc, A., Boitel, L. et al. (1992). Low back pain in commercial travellers. *Scandinavian Journal of Work, Environment and Health*, 18, 52-58.

Pintar, F. A., Cusick, J. F., Yoganandan, R. J. et al. (1992). The biomechanics of lumbar facetectomy under compression-flexion. *Spine*, **17**, 804–810.

Pitkanen, M. and Manninen, H. (1994). Sidebending versus flexion-extension radiographs in lumbar spinal instability. *Clinical Radiology*, **49**, 109–114.

Ponte, A., Gebbia, F. and Eliseo, F. (1985). Non-operative treatment of adolescent hyperkyphosis. *Orthopaedic Transactions*, **9**, 108

Ponte, J. D., Jensen, G. J. and Kent, B. E. (1984). A preliminary report on the use of the McKenzie protocol versus Williams protocol in the treatment of low back pain. *Journal of Orthopedic and Sports Physical Therapy*, **6**, 130-139.

Pope, M. (1989). Risk indicators in low back pain. *Annals of Medicine*, **21**, 387–392.

Pope, M. and Hansson, T. (1992). Vibration and the spine. *Clinical Orthopaedics and Related Research*, **279**, 49–59.

Pope, M. H., Phillips, R. B., Haugh, L. D. et al. (1994) A prospective randomized 3-week trial of spinal manipulation, transcutaneous muscle stimulation, massage and corset in the treatment of subacute low back pain. *Spine*, **19**, 2571–2577.

Porter, G. E. (1985). Slipping rib syndrome. An infrequently recognised entity in children: a report of three cases and review of the literature. *Pediatrics*, **76**, 810–813.

Porter, K. M. (1989). Neck sprains after car accidents (editorial). *British Medical Journal*, **298**, 973–974.

Porter, R. W. (1996). Spinal stenosis and neurogenic claudication. *Spine*, **21**, 2046–2052.

Porter, R. W. and Park, W. (1982). Unilateral spondylolysis. *Journal of Bone and Joint Surgery*, **64B**, 344–347.

Porter, R. W., and Thorp, L. (1986). Familial aspects of disc protrusion. Orthop. Trans. **10**, 524–527.

Porter, R. W. and Ward, D. (1992). Cauda equina dysfunction; the significance of two-level pathology. *Spine*, **17**, 9–15

Porter, R. W., Adams, M. A. and Hutton, W. C. (1989). Physical activity and the strength of the lumbar spine. *Spine*, **14**, 201–203.

Post, M. J., Bowen, B. C. and Sze, G. (1991). Magnetic resonance imaging of spinal infection. *Rheumatic Diseases Clinics of North America*, **17**, 773–794.

Postacchini, F. (1985). Familial lumbar stenosis, case report of three siblings. *Journal of Bone and Joint Surgery*, **67A**, 321–323.

Postacchini, F. (1996). Management of lumbar spinal stenosis. *Journal of Bone and Joint Surgery*, **78B**, 154–164.

Postacchini, F., Lami, R., Pugliese, O. et al. (1988). Familial predispositiion to disco genic low back pain: an epidemologic and immunogenic study. *Spine*, **13**, 1403–1406.

Postacchini, F., Cinotti, G., Perugia, D. and Gumina, S. (1993). The surgical treatment of central lumbar stenosis. *Journal of Bone and Joint Surgery*, **75B**, 386–392.

Postacchini, F., Gumina, S., Cinotti, G. et al. (1994). Ligamenta flava in lumbar disc herniation and spinal stenosis. Light and electron microscopic morphology. *Spine*, **19**, 917–922.

Potter, N. A. and Rothstein, J. M. (1985). Intertester reliability for selected clinical tests of the sacroiliac joint. *Physical Therapy*, **65**, 1671–1675.

Powell, F. C., Hanigan, W. C. and Olivero, W. C. (1993). A risk/benefit analysis of spinal manipulation therapy for relief of lumbar or cervical pain. *Neurosurgery*, **33**, 73–79.

Powell, M. C., Wilson, M., Szypryt, P. et al. (1986). Prevalence of lumbar disc degeneration observed by magnetic resonance in symptomless women. *Lancet*, **2**, 1366–1367.

Pratt-Thomas, H. R. and Berger, K. E. (1947). Cerebellar and spinal injuries after chiropractic manipulation. *Journal of the American Medical Association*, **133**, 600–603.

Preisinger, E., Alacamliogllu, Y., Pil, K. et al. (1995). Therapeutic exercise in the prevention of bone loss: a controlled trial with women after menopause. *American Journal of Physical Medicine and Rehabilitation*, **74**, 120–123.

Prince, R., Devine, A., Dick, I. et al. (1995). The effects of calcium supplementation (milk powder or tablets) and exercise on bone density in postmenopausal women. *Journal of Bone and Mineral Research*, **10**, 1068–1075.

Professional Development. (1995). Lifting and handling: knowledge for practice. *Nursing Times*, **91** suppl, 1–4.

Pullos, J. (1986). The upper limb tension test. *Australian Journal of Physiotherapy*, **32**, 258–259.

Putz, R. L. and Muller-Gerbl, M. (1996). The vertebra column – a phylogenetic failure? A theory explaining the function and vulnerability of the human spine. *Clinical Anatomy*, **9**, 205–212.

Quebec Task Force on Spinal Disorders (1987). Scientific approach to the assessment and management of activity-related spinal disorders: A monograph for clinicians. Report of the Quebec task force on spinal disorders. *Spine*, **12**, S1–S59.

Quinter, J. L. (1989). A study of upper limb pain paraesthesiae following neck injury in motor vehicle accidents: assessment of the brachial plexus tension test of Elvey. *British Journal of Rheumatology*, **28**, 528–533.

Raby, N. and Mathews, S. (1993). Symptomatic spondylolysis: correlation of CT and SPECT with clinical outcome. *Clinical Radiology*, **48**, 97–99.

Radanov, B. P. and Dvorak, J. (1996). Spine update. Impaired cognitive functioning after whiplash injury of the cervical spine. *Spine*, **21**, 392–397.

Radanov, B. P., Stefano, G., Schnidrig, A. and Balinari, P. (1991). Role of psychosocial stress in recovery from common whiplash. *Lancet*, **338**, 712–715.

Radanov, B. P., Dvorak, J. and Valach, L. (1992). Cognitive deficits in patients after soft tissue injury of the cervical spine. *Spine*, **17**, 127–131.

Radanov, B. P., Sturzenegger, M., DiStephano, G. et al. (1993). Factors influencing recovery from headache after common whiplash. *British Medical Journal*, **307**, 652–655.

Rahim, K. A. and Stambough, J. L. (1992). Radiographic evaluation of the degenerative cervical spine. *Orthopedic Clinics of North America*, **23**, 395–403.

Raininko, R., Manninen, H., Battie, M. C. et al. (1995). Observer variability in the assessment of disc degeneration on MRI of the lumbar and thoracic spine. *Spine*, **20**, 1029–1035.

Ramos, R. C., Gomez, V. A., Guzman, J. L. et al. (1995). Frequency of atlantoaxial subluxation and neurologic involvement in patients with ankylosing spondylitis. *Journal of Rheumatology*, **22**, 2120–2125.

Randell, A., Sambrook, P. N., Nguyen, T. V. et al. (1995). Direct clinical and welfare costs of osteoporotic fracture in elderly men and women. *Osteoporosis International*, **5**, 427–432.

Ranu, H. S. (1990). Measurement of pressures in the nucleus and within the annulus of the human spinal disc: due to extreme loading. *Proceedings of the Institute of Mechanical Engineering*, **204**, 141-146.

Rapp, S. E., Haselkorn, J. K., Elam, J. K. et al. (1994). Epidural steroid injection in the treatment of low back pain: a meta-analysis (abstract). *Anesthesiology*, *81*, 923.

Rashbaum, R. F. (1983). Radiofrequency facet denervation. *Orthopedic Clinics of North America*, **14**, 569–575.

Rasmussen, B. K., Jensen, R., Schroll, M. and Olesen, J. (1991). Epidemiology of headache in a general population – a prevalence study. *Journal of Clinical Epidemiology*, **44**, 1147–1157.

Ray, C. D. (1991). Facet syndrome: pathophysiology, clinical picture and treatment. *International Journal of Pain Therapy*, **1**, 80–93.

Raymond, J. and Dumas, J. M. (1984). Intraarticular facet block: diagnostic test or therapeutic procedure? *Radiology*, **151**, 333–336.

Read, M. T. (1994). Single photon emission computed tomography (SPECT) scanning for adolescent back pain. A sine qua non? *British Journal of Sports Medicine*, **28**, 56–57.

Rees, W. E. S. (1971). Multiple bilateral subcutaneous rhizolysis of segmental nerves in the treatment of the indication syndrome. *Annals of General Practice*, **26**, 126–127.

Refshauge, K. (1994). Rotation: a valid premanipulative dizziness test. Does it predict safe manipulation? *Journal of Manipulative and Physiological Therapeutics*, **17**, 15–19.

Reid, I. R., Ames, R. W., Evans, M. C. and Gamble, G. D. (1995). Long-term effects of calcium supplementation on bone loss and fractures in postmenopausal women: a randomised controlled trial. *American Journal of Medicine*, **98**, 331–335.

Reilly, T. and Chana, D. (1994). Spinal shrinkage in fast bowling. *Ergonomics*, **37**, 127–132.

Resnick, D., Niwayama, G. and Georgen, T. G. (1975). Degenerative disease of the sacroiliac joint. *Investigative Radiology*, **10**, 608–621.

Resnick, D., Shapiro, R. F., Wiesner, K. B. et al. (1978). Diffuse idiopathic skeletal hyperostosis (DISH): ankylosing hyperostosis of Forestier and Rôtes-Querol. *Seminars in Arthritis and Rheumatism*, **7**, 153–187.

Revel, M. E., Listrat, V. M., Chevalier, X. J. et al. (1992). Facet joint block for low back pain: identifying predictors of a good response. *Archives of Physical Medicine and Rehabilitation*, **73**, 824–828.

Rhyne, A. L., Smith, S. E., Wood, K. E. and

Darden, B. V. (1995). Outcome of unoperated discogram-positive low back pain. *Spine*, **20**, 1997–2001.

Ricciardi, J. E., Pflueger, P. C., Isaza, J. and Whitecloud, T. S. (1995). Transpedicular fixation for the treatment of isthmic spondylolisthesis in adults. *Spine*, **20**, 1917–1922.

Rich, B. S. and McKeag, D. (1992). When sciatica is not disk disease. Detecting piriformis syndrome in active patients. *Physician and Sportsmedicine*, **20**, 105–115.

Richardson, C. A. and Jull, G. A (1995). Muscle control-pain control. What exercises would you prescribe? *Manual Therapy*, **1**, 2–10.

Richmond, F. (1988). The sensorium: Receptors of neck muscles and joints. In *Control of Head Movements*, L. Peterson and F. Richmond, eds pp. 49–62, Oxford University Press.

Richter, J. E. (1991). Investigation and management of non-cardiac chest pain. *Clinics in Gasteroenterology*, **5**, 281–306.

Ridenour, T. R., Haddad, S. F., Hitchon, P. W. et al. (1993). Herniated thoracic disks: treatment and outcome. *Journal of Spinal Disorders*, **6**, 218–224.

Ridley, M. G., Kingsley, G. M., Gibson, T. and Grahame, R. (1988). Outpatient lumbar epidural corticosteroid injection in the management of sciatica. *British Journal of Rheumatology*, **27**, 295–299.

Rifat, S. F. and Lombardo, J. A. (1995). Occipital neuralgia in a football player: a case report. *Clinical Journal of Sports Medicine*, **5**, 251–253.

Riihimaki, H., Tola, S., Videman, T. and Hanninen, K. (1989). Low back pain and occupation. *Spine*, **14**, 204–208.

Riihimaki, H., Mattsson, T., Zitting, A. et al. (1990). Radiographically detectable degenerative changes of the lumbar spine among concrete reinforcement workers and house painters. *Spine*, **15**, 114–119.

Roberts, S., Menage, J. and Urban, J. P. G. (1989). Biochemical and structural properties of the cartilage endplate and its relation to the intervertebral disc. *Spine*, 14, 166–174.

Roberts, S., Eisenstein, S. M., menage, J. et al. (1995). Mechanoreceptors in intervertebral discs. Morphology, distribution, and neuropeptides. *Spine*, 20, 2645–2651.

Roberts, S., Urban, J. P. G., Evans, H. and

Eisenstein, S. M. (1996). Transport properties of the human cartilage end-plate in relation to its composition and calcification. *Spine*, **21**, 415–420.

Robertson, J. A. (1978). Facet joints and low back pain. Letter. *British Medical Journal*, **1**, 1238.

Robinson, M. E., Greene, A. F., O'Connor, P. et al. (1993). Reliability of lumbar isometric torque in patients with chronic low back pain. *Physical Therapy*, **72**, 186–190.

Rocco, A., G., Frank, E., Kaul, A. F. et al. (1989). Epidural steroids, epidural morphine and epidural steroids combined with morphine in the treatment of post laminectomy syndrome. *Pain*, **36**, 297–303.

Roche, M. B. and Rowe, G. G. (1952). The incidence of separate neural arch and coincident bone variations: summary. *Journal of Bone and Joint Surgery*, **34A**, 491–494.

Rogers, M. A., Crockford, H. A., Moskovich, R. et al. (1994). Nystagmus and joint position sensation: their importance in posterior occipitocervical fusion in rheumatoid arthritis. *Spine*, **19**, 16–20.

Rosenberg, N. J. (1975). Degenerative spondylolisthesis: predisposing factors. *Journal of Bone and Joint Surgery*, **57A**, 467–474.

Rosenberg, N. J., Barer, W. L. and Friedman, B. (1981). The incidence of spondylolysis and spondylolisthesis in non-ambulatory patients. *Spine*, **6**, 35–42.

Ross, J. S., Modic, M. T. and Masaryk, T. J. (1990). Tears of the annulus fibrosus: assessment with Gd-DTPA-enhanced MR imaging. *American Journal of Roentgenology*, **154**, 159–162.

Rossi, F. (1978). Spondylolysis, spondylolisthesis and sports. *Journal of Sports Medicine and Physical Fitness*, **18**, 317–340.

Rossi, F. and Dragoni, S. (1990). Lumbar spondylolysis: occurrence in competitive athletes. Updated achievements in a series of 390 cases. *Journal of Sports Medicine and Physical Fitness*, **30**, 450–452.

Rothman, S. L. G. (1996). The diagnosis of infections of the spine by modern imaging techniques. *Orthopedic Clinics of North America*, **27**, 15–31.

Rothschild, B. M., Poteat, G. B., Williams, E. and Crawford, W. L. (1994). Inflammatory sacroiliac joint pathology: evaluation of radiologic assessment techniques. *Clinical and Experiemental Rheumatology*, **12**, 267–274.

Rubin, W. (1973). Whiplash with vestibular involvement. *Archives of Otolaryngology*, **97**, 85–87.

Rupp, R. E., Ebraheim, N. A. and Coombs, R. J. (1995). Magnetic resonance imaging differentiation of compression spine fractures or vertebral lesions caused by osteoporosis or tumor. *Spine*, **20**, 2499–2504.

Russell, E. J. (1990). Cervical disk disease. *Radiology*, **177**, 313–325.

Ryan, G. A., Taylor, G. W., Moore, V. M. and Dolinis, J. (1993). Neck strain in car occupants. The influence of crash-related factors on initial severity. *Medical Journal of Australia*, **159**, 651–656.

Ryan, G. M. S. and Cope, S. (1955). Cervical vertigo. *Lancet*, **2**, 1355–1358.

Rydevik, B., Brown, M. and Lundborg, G. (1984). Pathoanatomy and pathophysiology of nerve compression. *Spine*, **9**, 7-15.

Saal, J. S. (1995). The role of inflammation in lumbar pain. *Spine*, **20**,1821–1827.

Saal, J. A. and Saal, J. S. (1989). Nonoperative treatment of herniated lumbar intervertebral disc with radiculopathy: an outcome study. *Spine*, **14**, 431–437.

Saal, J. A., Saal, J. S. and Herzog, R. J. (1990). The natural history of lumbar intervertebral disc extrusion treated nonoperatively. *Spine*, **15**, 683–686.

Saal, J. S., Franson, R., Dobrow, R. et al. (1992). High levels of inflammatory phospholipase A2 activity in lumbar disc hernations. *Spine*, **15**, 674–678.

Saal, J. S., Saal, J. A. and Yurth, E. F. (1996). Nonoperative management of herniated cervical intervertebral disc with radiculopathy. *Spine*, **21**, 1877–1883.

Sadasivan, K. K., Reddy, R. P. and Albright, J. A. (1993). The natural history of cervical spondylotic myelopathy. *Yale Journal of Biology and Medicine*, **66**, 235–242.

Salminen, J. J., Erkintalo, M. O. and Paajanen, H. E. (1993). Magnetic resonance imaging findings of lumbar spine in the young: correlation with leisure time, physical activity, spinal mobility and trunk muscles strength in 15 year old pupils with or without low back pain. *Journal of Spinal Disorders*, **6**, 386–391.

Salminen, J. J., Erkintalo, M., Laine, M. and Pentti, J. (1995). Low back pain in the young. A prospective three-year follow-up study of subjects with and without low back pain. *Spine*, **19**, 2101–2108.

Sambrook, P. N. (1995). The treatment of post-menopausal osteoporosis. *New England Journal of Medicine*, **333**, 1495–1496.

Sambrook, P. N. (1996). Osteoporosis. *Medical Journal of Australia*, **165**, 332–336.

Sambrook, P. N., Birmingham, J., Kelly, P.J. et al. (1993). Prevention of corticosteroid osteoporosis: a comparison of calcium, calcitriol, and calcitonin. *New England Journal of Medicine*, **328**, 1747–1752.

Sambrook, P. N., Kelly, P.J., Morrison, N. A. and Eisman, J. A. (1994). Genetics of osteoporosis. *Journal of Rheumatology*, **33**, 1007–1011.

Sanderson, P. L. and Wood, P. L. R. (1993). Surgery for lumbar stenosis in old people. *Journal of Bone and Joint Surgery*, **75B**, 393–397.

Sandover, J. (1983). Dynamic loading as a possible source of low back disorders. *Spine*, **8**, 652–658.

Sanzhang, C. and Rothschild, B. M. (1993). Zygapophyseal and costovertebral-costotransverse joints: an anatomic assessment of arthritis impact. *British Journal of Rheumatology*, **32**, 1066–1071.

Saraste, H. (1987). Long-term clinical and radiographic follow-up of spondylolysis and spondylolisthesis. *Journal of Pediatric Orthopedics*, **7**, 631–638.

Sato, H. and Kikuchi, S. (1993). The natural history of radiographic instability of the lumbar spine. *Spine*, **18**, 2075–2079.

Savini, R., Martucci, E., Nardi, S. et al. (1991). The herniated lumbar intervertebral disc in children and adolescents. *Italian Journal of Orthopaedics and Traumatology*, **17**, 505–511.

Sayson, S. C., Ducey, J. P., Maybrey, J. B. et al. (1994). Sciatic entrapment neuropathy associated with an anomalous piriformis muscle. *Pain*, **59**, 149–152.

Scapinelli, R. (1994). Three-dimensional computed tomography in infantile atlantoaxial rotatory fixation. *Journal of Bone and Joint Surgery*, **76**, 367–370.

Scheer, S. J., Radack, K. L. and O'Brien, D. R. (1995). Randomized controlled trials in industrial low back pain relating to return to work. Part 1. Acute interventions. *Archives of Physical Medicine and Rehabilitation*, **76**, 966–973.

Schellhas, K. P., Pollei, S. R. and Dorwart, R. H. (1994). Thoracic discography. *Spine*, **19**, 2103–2109.

Schellhas, K. P., Smith, M. D., Gundry, C. R. and Pollei, S. R. (1996). Cervical discogenic pain. Prospective correlation of magnetic resonance imaging and discography in asymptotic subjects and pain sufferers. *Spine*, **21**, 300–312.

Schiebler, M., Grenier, M., Fallon, M. et al. (1991). Normal and degenerated intervertebral disc: in vivo and in vitro MR imaging with histopathologic correlation. *American Journal of Roentgenology*, **157**, 93–97.

Schippel, A. H. and Robinson, G. K. (1986). Radiological and magnetic resonance imaging of cervical spine instability. *Journal of Manipulative and Physiological Therapeutics*, **10**, 316–322.

Schlegel, J. D., Smith, J. A. and Schleusener, R. L. (1996). Lumbar motion segment pathology adjacent to thoracolumbar, lumbar, and lumbosacral fusions. *Spine*, **21**, 970–981.

Schmidt, M., Reddy, V. and Massa, M. C. (1994). Costochondritis presenting as a peculiar skin lesion. *Cutis*, **54**, 187–188.

Schneiderman, G. A., McLain, R. F., Hambly, M. F. and Nielsen, S. L. (1995). The pars defect as a pain source. A histologic study. *Spine*, **20**, 1761–1764.

Schochat, T., Croft, P. and Raspe, H. (1994). The epidemiology of fibromyalgia. *British Journal of Rheumatology*, **33**, 783–786.

Schoensee, S. K., Jensen, G., Nicholson, G. et al. (1995). The effect of mobilization on cervical headaches. *Journal of Orthopedic and Sports Physical Therapy*, **21**, 184–196.

Scholes, P. V., Latimer, B. M., DiGiovanni, F. et al. (1991). Vertebral alterations in Scheuermann's kyphosis. *Spine*, **16**, 509–515.

Scholten, P. J. M., Schultz, A. B., Luchico, C. W. and Miller, J. A. A. (1988). Motions and loads within the human pelvis: a biomechanical model study. *Journal of Orthopaedic Research*, **6**, 840–850.

Schonstrom, N. S., Bolender, N. F. and Spengler,

D. M. (1985). The pathomorphology of spinal stenosis as seen on CT scans of the lumbar spine. *Spine*, **10**, 806–811.

Schonstrom, N., Lindahl, S., Willer, J. et al. (1989). Dynamic changes in the dimensions of the lumbar spinal canal: an experimental study in vitro. *Journal of Orthopaedic Research*, **7**, 115–121.

Schrader, H., Obelieniene, D., Bovim, G. et al. (1996). Natural evolution of late whiplash syndrome outside the medicolegal context. *Lancet*, **347**, 1207–1211.

Schwartz, D. P., Barth, J.T., Dane, J. R. et al. (1987). Cognitive deficits in chronic pain patients with and without history of head neck injury: development of a brief screening battery. *Clinical Journal of Pain*, **3**, 94–101.

Schwarzer, A. C., Wang, S., Laurent, R. et al. (1992). The role of the zygapophyseal joint in chronic low back pain (abstract). *Australian and New Zealand Journal of Medicine*, **22**, 185.

Schwarzer, A. C., Aprill, C. N., Derby, R. et al. (1994a). The false-positive rate of uncontrolled diagnostic blocks of the lumbar zygoapophyseal joints. *Pain*, **58**, 195–200.

Schwarzer, A. C., Aprill, C. N., Derby, R. et al. (1994b). Clinical features of patients with pain stemming from lumbar zygoapophyseal joints. Is the lumbar facet syndrome a clinical entity? *Spine*, **19**, 1132–1137.

Schwarzer, A. C., Aprill, C. N., Derby, R. et al. (1994c). The relative contribution of the disc and zygoapophyseal joint in chronic low back pain. *Spine*, **19**, 801–806.

Schwarzer, A. C., Derby, R., Aprill, C. N. et al. (1994d). The value of provocation response in lumbar zygoapophyseal joint injection *Clinical Journal of Pain*, **10**, 309–313.

Schwarzer, A. C., Derby, R., Aprill, C.N. et al. (1994e) Pain from the lumbar zygoapophyseal joints: a test of two models. *Journal of Spinal Disorders*, **7**, 331–336.

Schwarzer, A. C., Aprill, C. N., Derby, R. et al. (1995a). The prevalence and clinical features of internal disc disruption in patients with chronic low back pain. *Spine*, **20**, 1878–1883.

Schwarzer, A. C., Shih-Chang, W., Bogduk, N. et al. (1995b). Prevalence and clinical features of lumbar zygoapophyseal joint pain: a study in an Australian population with chronic low back

pain. *Annals of the Rheumatic Diseases*, **54**, 100–106.

Schwarzer, A. C., Shih-Chang, W., O'Driscoll, D. et al. (1995c). The ability of computed tomography to identify a painful zygoapophyseal joint in patients with chronic low back pain. *Spine*, **20**, 907–912.

Schwarzer, A. C., Aprill, C. N. and Bogduk, N. (1995d). The sacroiliac joint in chronic low back pain. *Spine*, **20**, 31–37.

Scudds, R. A., McCain, G. A., Rollman, G. B. and Harth, M. (1989). Improvement in pain responsiveness in patients with fibrositis after successful treatment with amitriptyline. *Journal of Rheumatology*, **16**, suppl 19, 98–103.

Seidenwurm, D. and Litt, A. W. (1995). The natural history of lumbar spine disease. *Radiology*, **195**, 323–324.

Selvaratnam, P. J., Matyas, T. A. and Glasgow, E. F. (1994). Noninvasive discrimination of brachial plexus involvement in upper limb pain. *Spine*, **19**, 26–33.

Semble, E. L., Loesser, R. F. and Wise, C. M. (1990). Therapeutic exercise for rheumatoid arthritis and osteoarthritis. *Seminars in Arthritis and rheumatism*, **20**, 32–40.

Semon, R. L. and Spengler, D. (1981). Significance of lumbar spondylolysis in college football players. *Spine*, **6**, 172–174.

Serrao, J. M., Marks, R. J., Morley, S. J. and Goodchild, C. S. (1992). Intrathecal midazolam for the treatment of chronic mechanical low back pain; a controlled comparison with epidural steroid in a pilot study. *Pain*, **48**, 5–12.

Severy, D. M., Mathewson, J. H. and Bectol, C. O. (1955). Controlled automobile rear end collisions, an investigation of related engineering and medical phenomena. *Canadian Services Medical Journal*, **11**, 727–759.

Shahriaree, H., Sajadi, K. and Rooholamini, S. A. (1979). A family with spondylolisthesis. *Journal of Bone and Joint Surgery*, **61A**, 1256–1258.

Shapiro, A. P. and Roth, R. S. (1993). The effect of litigation on recovery from whiplash. *Spine: State of the Art Reviews*, **7**, 531–556.

Sharma, M., Langrana, N. A. and Rodriguez, J. (1995). Role of ligaments and facets in lumbar spinal stability. *Spine*, **20**, 887–900.

Shea, M., Takeuchi, T. Y., Wittenberg, R. H. et al. (1994). A comparison of the effects of automated percutaneous diskectomy and conventional diskectomy on intradiscal pressure, disk geometry, and stiffness. *Journal of Spinal Disorders*, **7**, 317–325.

Shealy, C. N. (1975). Percutaneous radiofrequency denervation of spinal facets: an alternative approach to treatment of chronic back pain and sciatica. *Journal of Neurosurgery*, **43**, 448–451.

Shealy, C. N. (1976). Facet denervation in the management of back and sciatic pain. *Clinical Orthopaedics and Related Research*, **115**, 157–164.

Sheehan, S., Bauer, R. B. and Meyers, J. S. (1960). Vertebral artery compression in cervical spondylosis. *Neurology*, **10**, 968–986.

Shekelle, P. G. (1994). Spine update. Spinal manipulation. *Spine*, **19**, 858–861.

Shekelle, P. G., Adams, A. H., Chassin, M. R. et al. (1992). Spinal manipulation for low back pain. *Annals of Internal Medicine*, **117**, 590–598.

Sherk, H. H., Black, J., Rhodes, A. et al. (1993). Laser Discectomy. *Clinics in Sports Medicine*, **12**, 569–577.

Sherlock, R. A. (1981). A criticism of the article 'movement of the sacroiliac joint' (letter). *Clinical Orthopaedics and Related Research*, **155**, 293–296.

Sherman, C. (1992). Managing fibromyalgia with exercise. *Physician and Sportsmedicine*, **20**, 166–172.

Sherman, F. C., Wilkinson, R. H. and Hall, J. E. (1977). Reactive sclerosis of a pedicle and spondylolysis in the lumbar spine. *Journal of Bone and Joint Surgery*, **59A**, 49–54.

Sherman, J. L., Hart, R. G. and Easton, J. D. (1981). Abrupt change in head position and cerebral infarction. *Stroke*, **12**, 2–6.

Shinomiya, K., Komori, K., Matsuoka, T. et al. (1994). Neuroradiologic and electrophysiologic assessment of cervical spondylotic amyotrophy. *Spine*, **19**, 21–25.

Shiqing, X., Quanzhi, Z. and Dehao, F. (1987). Significance of straight leg raising test in the diagnosis and clinical evaluation of lower lumbar intervertebral disc protrusion. *Journal of Bone and Joint Surgery*, **69A**, 517–522.

Shiraishi, T. and Crock, H. V. (1995). Excision of laminal pseudoarthroses in spondylolytic spondylolisthesis. A review of 13 cases. *European Spine Journal*, **4**, 52–55.

Shvartzman, L., Weingarten, E., Sherry, H. et al. (1992). Cost-effectiveness analysis of extended conservative therapy versus surgical intervention in the management of herniated lumbar intervertebral disc. *Spine*, **17**, 176–181.

Silver, J. (1984). Injuries of the spine sustained in rugby. *British Medical Journal*, **288**, 27–43.

Silvers, H. R., Lewis, P. J. and Asch, H. L. (1993). Decompressive lumbar laminectomy for spinal stenosis. *Journal of Neurosurgery*, **78**, 695–701.

Silvers, H. R., Lewis, P. J., Clabeaux, D. E. and Asch, H. L. (1994). Lumbar disc excisions in patients under the age of 21 years. *Spine*, **19**, 2387–2392.

Simeone, F. A. and Goldberg, H. I. (1968). Thrombosis of the vertebral artery from hyperextension injury to the neck. *Journal of Neurosurgery*, **29**, 540–544.

Simeone, F. A. and Rothman, R. H. (1983). Clinical usefulness of CT scanning in the diagnosis and treatment of lumbar spine disease. *Radiologic Clinics of North America*, **21**, 197–200.

Simkin, P. A. (1982). Simian stance: a sign of spinal stenosis. *Lancet*, **2**, 652–653.

Simmons, E. D., Guyer, R. D., Graham-Smith, A. and Herzog, R. (1995). Contemporary concepts in spine care. Radiographic assessment for patients with low back pain. *Spine*, **20**, 1839–1841.

Simms R. W., Roy, S. H., Hrovat, M. et al. (1994). Lack of association between fibromyalgia syndrome and abnormalities in muscle energy metabolism. *Arthritis and Rheumatism*, **37**, 794–800.

Simons, D. G. (1986). Fibrositis/fibromyalgia: a form of myofascial trigger points? *American Journal of Medicine*, **81** suppl 3A, 93–98.

Simons, D. G. (1988). Myofascial pain syndromes: where are we going? *Archives of Physical Medicine and Rehabilitation*, **69**, 207–212.

Simons, D. G. and Travell, J. G. (1983). Myofascial origins of low back pain. *Postgraduate Medicine*, **73**, 66–108.

Simpson, J. M., Silveri, C. P., Simeone, F. A. et al. (1993). Thoracic disk herniation. Re-evaluation of the posterior approach using a modified costotransversectomy. *Spine*, **18**, 1872–1877.

Sims-Williams, H., Jayson, M. I. V. and Baddeley, H. (1977). Rheumatoid involvement of the lumbar spine. *Annals of the Rheumatic Diseases*, **36**, 524–531.

Singer, C., Green, B. A., Bruce, J. H. et al. (1994). Late presentation of congenital muscle torticollis: use of MR imaging and CT scan in diagnosis. *Movement Disorders*, **9**, 100–103.

Sivakumaran, P. and Wilsher, M. (1995). Diaphragmatic palsy and chiropractic manipulation (letter). *New Zealand Medical Journal*, **108**, 279–280.

Sjaastad, O., Saunte, O., Hovdal, H. et al. (1983). Cervicogenic headache. An hypothesis. *Cephalalgia*, **3**, 249–256.

Sjaastad, O., Fredriksen, T. A. and Stolt-Nielsen, A. (1986). Cervicogenic headache, C2 neurotomy and occipital neuralgia: a connection? *Cephalalgia*, **6**, 189–195.

Sjaastad, O., Fredriksen, T. A. and Pfaffenrath, V. (1990). Cervicogenic headache: diagnostic criteria. *Headache*, **30**, 725–726.

Skaggs, D. L., Weidenbaum, M., Iatridis, J. C. et al. (1994). Regional variation in tensile properties and biochemical composition of the human lumbar annulus fibrosus. *Spine*, **19**, 1310–1319.

Skubic, J. W. (1993). Thoracic disc disease. *Current Opinion in Orthopaedics*, **4**, 96–103.

Sloop, P. R., Smith, D. S., Goldenberg, E. and Dore, C. (1982). Manipulation for chronic neck pain. A double-blind controlled study. *Spine*, **7**, 532–535.

Slotman, G. J. and Stein, S. C. (1996). Laparoscopic L5-S1 diskectomy: a cost-effective, minimally invasive general surgery–neurosurgery team alternative to laminectomy. *American Surgeon*, **62**, 64–68.

Sluijter, M. E. and Mehta. M. (1981). Treatment of chronic back and neck pain by percutaneous thermal lesions. In *Modern Methods of Treatment*, vol. 3. *Persistent Pain*. (S. Lipton and J. Miles, eds.) pp. 141–179, Academic Press.

Smidt, G. L., McQuade, K., Wei, S. and Barakatt, F. (1995). Sacroiliac kinematics for reciprocal straddle positions. *Spine*, **20**, 1047–1054.

Smith, A. S. and Blaser, S. I. (1991). Infectious and inflammatory process of the spine. *Radiologic Clinics of North America*, **29**, 809–827.

Smith, E. B., Rasmussen, A. A., Lechner, D. E. et al. (1996). The effects of lumbosacral support belts and abdominal muscle strength on functional lifting ability in healthy women. *Spine*, **21**, 356–366.

Smith, S. A., Massie, J. B., Chestnut, R. and Garfin, S. R. (1993). Straight leg raising – anatomical effects on the spinal nerve root without and with fusion. *Spine*, **18**, 992–999.

Smyth, M. J. and Wright, V. (1958). Sciatica and the intervertebral disc. An experimental study. *Journal of Bone and Joint Surgery*, **40A**, 1401–1418.

Smythe, H. A. (1979). Nonarticular rheumatism and psychogenic musculoskeletal syndromes. In *Arthritis and Allied Conditions*. 9th edn. D. J. McCarthy ed.) pp. 881–891, Lea and Febiger.

Smythe, H. A. (1986). Referred pain and tender points. *American Journal of Medicine*, **81** suppl 3A, 90–92.

Smythe, H. A. (1992). Links between fibromyalgia and myofascial pain syndromes (editorial). *Journal of Rheumatology*, **19**, 842–843.

Smythe, H. A. (1995). Studies of sleep in fibromyalgia; techniques, clinical significance, and future directions. *British Journal of Rheumatology*, **34**, 897–899.

Smythe, H. A. and Moldofsky, H. (1977). Two contributions to understanding of 'fibrositis' syndrome. *Bulletin of the Rheumatic Diseases*, **28**, 928–931.

Snoek, W., Weber, H. and Jorgensen, B. (1977). Double blind evaluation of extradural methyl prednisolone for herniated lumbar discs. *Acta Orthopaedica Scandinavica*, **48**, 635–661.

Solheim, L. F., Siewers, P. and Paus, B. (1981). The piriformis muscle syndrome: sciatic nerve entrapment treated with section of the piriformis muscle. *Acta Orthopaedica Scandinavica*, **52**, 73–75.

Somhegyi, A. and Ratko, I. (1993). Hamstring tightness and Scheuermann's disease (commentary). *American Journal of Physical Medicine and Rehabilitation*, **72**, 44.

Sortland, O., Magnaes, B. and Hauge, T. (1977). Functional myelography with metrizamide in the diagnosis of lumbar spinal stenosis. *Acta Radiologica*, **355**, 42–54.

Spaccarelli, K. C. (1996). Lumbar and caudal epidural corticosteroid injections. *Mayo Clinic Proceedings*, **71**, 169–178.

Spence, E. K. and Rosato, E. F. (1983). The slipping rib syndrome. *Archives of Surgery*, **118**, 1330–1332.

Spengler, D. M. (1987). Degenerative stenosis of the lumbar spine. *Journal of Bone and Joint Surgery*, **69A**, 305–308.

Spitzer, W. O., Skovron, M. L., Salmi, L. R. et al. (1995). Scientific monograph of the Quebec task force on whiplash-associated disorders: redefining 'whiplash' and its management. *Spine*, **20**, S1–S73.

Star, M. J., Curd, J. G. and Thorne, R. P. (1992). Atlantoaxial lateral mass osteoarthritis: a frequently overlooked cause of severe occipito-cervical pain. *Spine*, **17S**, S71–S76.

Sternbach, R. A. (1986). Survey of pain in the US: the Nuprin Pain Report. *Clinical Journal of Pain*, **2**, 49–53.

Stevens, A. J. (1991). Functional Doppler sonography of the vertebral artery and some considerations about manual techniques. *Journal of Manual Medicine*, **6**, 102–105.

Stewart, T. D. (1953). The age incidence of neural arch defects in Alaskan natives considered from the standpoint of aetiology. *Journal of Bone and Joint Surgery*, **35A**, 937–950.

Stewart, T. D. (1984). Pathologic changes in aging sacroiliac joints: a study of dissecting room skeletons. *Clinical Orthopaedics and Related Research*, **183**, 188–196.

Stinson, J. T. (1993). Spondylolysis and spondylolisthesis in the athlete. *Clinics in Sports Medicine*, **12**, 517–528.

Stockman, R. (1904). The causes, pathology and treatment of chronic rheumatism. *Edinburgh Medical Journal*, **15**, 107–116.

Stoddard, A. and Osborn, J. F. (1979). Scheuermanní s disease or spinal osteochondrosis. Its frequency and relationship with spondylosis. *Journal of Bone and Joint Surgery*, **61B**, 56–58.

Stokes, I. A. F. (1988). Mechanical function of facet joints in the lumbar spine. *Clinical Biomechanics*, **3**, 101–105.

Stokes, I. A. F. and Frymoyer, J. W. (1987). Segmental motion and instability. *Spine*, **12**, 688–691.

Stokes, I. A. F., Counts, D. F. and Frymoyer, J. W. (1989). Experimental instability in the rabbit lumbar spine. *Spine*, **14**, 68–72.

Stolker, R. J., Vervest, A. C. M. and Groen, G. J. (1994). The management of chronic spinal pain by blockades: a review. *Pain*, **58**, 1–20.

Stucki, G., Daltroy, L., Liang, M. et al. (1996). Measurement properties of a self-administered outcome measure in lumbar spinal stenosis. *Spine*, **21**, 796–803.

Sturesson, B., Selvik, G. and Uden, A. (1989). Movements of the sacroiliac joints: a roentgen stereophotogrammetric analysis. *Spine*, **14**, 162–165.

Sturm, P. F., Dobson, J. C. and Armstrong, G. W. (1993). The surgical management of Scheuermann's disease. *Spine*, **18**, 685–691.

Sturzenegger, M., Radanov, B. P. and Di Stefano, G. (1995). The effect of accident mechanisms and initial findings on the long-term course of whiplash injury. *Journal of Neurology*, **242**, 443–449.

Subotnick, S. I. (1981). Limb length discrepancies of the lower extremity (the short leg syndrome). *Journal of Orthopedic and Sports Physical Therapy*, **3**, 11–16.

Sumchai, A., Eliastam, M. and Werner, P. (1988). Seatbelt cervical injury in an intersection type vehicular collision. *Journal of Trauma*, **28**, 1384–1388.

Supik, L. F. and Broom, M. J. (1994). Sciatic tension signs and lumbar disc herniation. *Spine*, **19**, 1066–1069.

Svensson, H. and Andersson, G. (1989). The relationship of low back pain, work environment, and stress. *Spine*, **14**, 517–520.

Svensson, H., Vedin, A., Whilchellmsson, C. and Andersson, G. (1983). Low back pain in relation to other diseases and cardiovascular risk factors. *Spine*, **8**, 277–285.

Svensson, M. Y., Lovsund, P., Haland, Y. and Larsson, S. (1996). The influence of seat-back and head-restraint properties on the head-neck motion during rear-impact. *Accident Analysis and Prevention*, **28**, 221–227.

Swanepoel, M. W., Adams, L. M. and Smeathers, J. E. (1995). Human lumbar apophyseal joint damage and intervertebral disc degeneration. *Annals of the Rheumatic Diseases*, **54**, 182–188.

Sward, L. (1992). The thoracolumbar spine in young elite athletes. Current concepts on the effects of physical training. *Sports Medicine*, **13**, 357–364.

Sward, L., Hellstrom, M., Jacobsson, B. and

Peterson, L. (1990a). Back pain and radiologic changes in the thoraco-lumbar spine of athletes. *Spine*, **15**, 124–129.

Sward, L., Hellstrom, M., Jacobsson, B. et al. (1990b). Acute injury of the vertebral ring apophysis and intervertebral disc in adolescent gymnasts. *Spine*, **15**, 144–148.

Swartzman, L. C., Teasell, R. W., Shapiro, A. P. and McDermid, A. J. (1996). The effect of litigation status on adjustment to whiplash injury. *Spine*, **21**, 53–58.

Swezey, R. L. (1996). Chronic neck pain. *Rheumatic Diseases Clinics of North America*, **22**, 411–437.

Swezey, R. L. (1996). Exercise for osteoporosis – is walking enough? The case for site specificity and resistive exercise. *Spine*, **21**, 2809–2813.

Szypryt, E. P., Twining, P., Mullhollnad, R. C. and Worthington, B. S. (1989). The prevalence of disc degeneration associated with neural arch defects of the lumbar spine assessed by magnetic resonance imaging. *Spine*, **14**, 977–981.

Takahashi, H., Suguro, T., Okazima, Y. et al. (1996). Inflammatory cytokines in the herniated disc of the lumbar spine. *Spine*, **21**, 218–224.

Takahashi, K., Miyazaki, T., Ohnari, H. et al. (1995). Schmorl's nodes and low back pain. Analysis of magnetic resonance imaging findings in symptomatic a symptomatic individuals. *European Spine Journal*, **4**, 56–59.

Takata, K. and Takahashi, K. (1994). Hamstring tightness and sciatica in young patients with disc herniation. *Journal of Bone and Joint Surgery*, **76B**, 220–224.

Tallroth, K. and Schlenzka, D. (1990). Spinal stenosis subsequent to juvenile lumbar osteochondrosis. *Skeletal Radiology*, **19**, 203–205.

Tamura, T. J. (1989). Cranial symptoms after cervical injury. *Journal of Bone and Joint Surgery*, **71B**, 283–287.

Tan, J. C. and Nordin, M. (1922). Role of physical therapy in the treatment of cervical disk disease. *Orthopedic Clinics of North America*, **23**, 435–449.

Taylor, J. A., Clopton, P., Bosch, E. et al. (1995). Interpretation of abnormal lumbar spine radiographs. A test comparing students, clinicians, radiology residents, and radiologists in medicine and chiropractic. *Spine*, **20**, 1147–1154.

Taylor, J. R. and Finch, P. (1993). Acute injury of the neck: anatomical an pathological basis of pain. *Annals of the Acadamy of Medicine, Singapore*. **22**, 187–192.

Taylor, J. R. and Kakulas, B. A. (1991). Neck injuries. *Lancet*, **1**, 338–343.

Taylor, J. R. and Twomey, L. T. (1986). Age changes in lumbar zygapophyseal joints. *Spine*, **11**, 739–745.

Taylor, J. R. and Twomey, L. T. (1993). Acute injuries to cervical joints: an autopsy study of neck sprain. *Spine*, **18**, 1115–1122.

Teale, C. and Mulley, G. P. (1990). Support collars: a preliminary survey of their benefits and problems. *Clinical Rehabilitation*, **4**, 33–35.

Teasell, R. W. and Marchuk, Y. (1994). Vertebro-basilar artery stroke as a complication of cervical manipulation. *Critical Reviews in Physical and Rehabilitation Medicine*, **6**, 121–129.

Teresi, L. M., Lufkin, R. B., Reicher, M. A. et al. (1987). Asymptomatic degenerative disk disease and spondylosis of the cervical spine. MR imaging. *Radiology*, **164**, 83–88.

Tertti, M., Paajanen, H., Kujala, U. M. et al. (1990). Disc degeneration in young gymnasts. A magnetic resonance imaging study. *American Journal of Sports Medicine*, **18**, 206–208.

Tertti, M. O., Salminen, J. J., Paajanen, H. E. et al. (1991). Low back pain and disk degeneration in children: a case-control MR imaging study. *Radiology*, **180**, 503–505.

Thiel, H. W. (1991). Gross morphology and pathoanatomy of the vertebral arteries. *Journal of Manipulative and Physiological Therapeutics*, **14**, 133–141.

Tillyard, M. W., Spears, G. F., Thomson, J. and Dovey, S. (1992). Treatment of post-menopausal osteoporosis with calcitriol or calcium. *New England Journal of Medicine*, **326**, 357–362.

Tini, P. G., Wieser, C. and Zinn, W. M. (1977). The transitional vertebra of the lumbosacral spine. *Rheumatology and Rehabilitation*, **16**, 180–185.

Torg, J. S., Pavlov, H., Genuario, S. E. et al. (1986). Neuropraxia of the cervical spinal cord with transient quadriplegia. *Journal of Bone and Joint Surgery*, **68A**, 1354–1374.

Transfeldt, E. E., Robertson, D. and Bradford, D. S. (1993). Ligaments of the lumbosacral spine and their role in possible extraforaminal spinal nerve entrapment. *Journal of Spinal Disorders*, **6**, 507–512.

Trevor-Jones, R. (1964). Osteo-arthritis of the paravertebral joints of the second and third cervical vertebrae as a cause of occipital headache. *South African Medical Journal*, **38**, 392–394.

Triano, J. T., McGregor, M., Hondras, M. A. and Brennan, P. C. (1995). Manipulative therapy versus education programs in chronic low back pain. *Spine*, **20**, 948–955.

Troillet, N. and Gerster, J. C. (1993). Metabolic alterations in patients with diffuse idiopathic skeletal hyperostosis; a prospective controlled study in 25 patients. *Review of Rheumatism*, **60**, 239–244.

Troup, J. D. G. (1976). Mechanical factors in spondylolisthesis and spondylolysis. *Clinical Orthopaedics and Related Research*, **117**, 59–66.

Tsitsopulos, P., Fotiou. F., Papakostopulos, D. et al. (1987). Comparative study of clinical and surgical findings and cortical somatosensory evoked potentials in patients with lumbar spinal disc protrusion. *Acta Neurosurgica*, **84**, 54–63.

Tuite, G. F., Stern, H. D., Doran, S. E. et al. (1994). Outcome after laminectomy for lumbar spinal stenosis. Part 1: clinical correlations. *Journal of Neurosurgery*, **81**, 699–706.

Tunks, E., Crook, J., Norman, G. and Kalaher, S. (1988). Tender points in fibromyalgia. *Pain*, **34**, 11–19.

Turk, Z. and Ratkolb, O. (1987). Mobilization of the cervical spine in chronic headache. *Journal of Manual Medicine*, **3**, 15–17.

Turner, J. A., Ersek, M., Herron, L. and Deyo, R. (1992). Surgery for lumbar spinal stenosis. Attempted meta-analysis of the literature. *Spine*, **17**, 1–8.

Twomey, L. and Taylor, J. (1985). Age changes in the lumbar articular triad. *Australian Journal of Physiotherapy*, **31**, 106–112.

Twomey, L. and Taylor, J. (1995). Exercise and spinal manipulation in the treatment of low back pain. *Spine*, **20**, 615–619.

Twomey, L., Taylor, J. R. and Taylor, M. M. (1989). Unsuspected damage to lumbar zygapophyseal (facet) joints after motor-vehicle accidents. *Medical Journal of Clinical Nutrition*, **151**, 210–217.

Tyrrell, A. R., Reilly, T. and Troup, J. D. G. (1985). Circadian variation in stature and the effects of spinal loading. *Spine*, **10**, 161–164.

Uden, A., Johnsson, K. E., Johnsson, K. et al. (1985). Myelography in the elderly and the diagnosis of spinal stenosis. *Spine*, **10**, 171–174.

Ulrich, C. M., Georgiou, C. C., Snow-Harter, C. M. et al. (1996). Bone mineral density in mother–daughter pairs: relations to lifetime exercise, lifetime milk consumption, and calcium supplements. *American Journal of Clinical Nutrition*, **63**, 72–79.

Underwood, M. R. and Dawes, P. (1995). Inflammatory back pain in primary care. *British Journal of Rheumatology*, **34**, 1074–1077.

Urban, J. P. G. and McMullin, J. F. (1988). Swelling pressure of the lumbar intervertebral discs: influence of age, spinal level, composition and degeneration. *Spine*, **13**, 179–187.

Vallfors, B. (1985). Acute, subacute, and chronic low back pain. *Scandinavian Journal of Rehabilitation Medicine*, **11** suppl 11, 1–98.

Valojerdy, M. R., Salsabili, N. and Hogg, D. A. (1989). Age changes in the human sacroiliac joint: joint fusions. *Clinical Anatomy*, **2**, 253–261.

van der Heijden, G. J. M. G., Beurskens, A. J. H. M., Koes, B. W. et al. (1995). The efficacy of traction for back and neck pain: a systematic, blinded review of randomized clinical trial methods. *Physical Therapy*, **75**, 93–104.

van Duersen, L. L. J. M., Patijn, J., Ockhuysen, A. L. and Vortman, B. J. (1990). The value of some clinical test of the sacroiliac joint. *Manual Medicine*, **5**, 96–99.

van Herwaarden, G. M., Anten, H. W., Hoodgduin, C. A. et al. (1994). Idiopathic spasmodic torticollis: a survey of the clinical syndrome and patient's experiences. *Clinical Neurology and Neurosurgery*, **96**, 222–225.

Van Holsbeeck, M., van Melkebeke, J., Dequeker, J. and Pennes, D. R. (1992). Radiographic findings of spontaneous subluxation of the sternoclavicular joint. *Clinics in Rheumatology*, **11**, 376–381.

van Linthoudt, D. and Revel, M. (1994). Similar radiologic lesions of localized Scheuermann's disease of the lumbar spine in twin sisters. *Spine*, **19**, 987–989.

Vandertop, W. P. and Bosma, N. J. (1991). The

piriformis syndrome: a case report. *Journal of Bone and Joint Surgery*, **73A**, 1095–1097.

Vanharanta, H. (1994) The intervertebral disc; a biologically active tissue challenging therapy. *Annals of Medicine*, **26**, 395–399.

Vanharanta, H., Sachs, B. L., Spivey , M. A. et al. (1987). The relationship of pain provocation to lumbar disc degeneration as seen by CT-discography. *Spine*, **12**, 295–298.

Vanharanta, H., Guyer, R. D., Ohnmeiss, D. D. et al. (1988a). Disc deteriation in low back syndromes: a prospective multi-center CT discography study. *Spine*, **13**, 1349–1351.

Vanharanta, H., Sachs, B. L., Ohnmeiss, D. D. et al. (1989). Pain provocation and disc deterioration by age. A CT discography study in low back pain population. *Spine*, **14**, 420–423.

Vanharanta, H., Floyd, T., Ohnmeiss, D. D. et al. (1993). The relationship of facet tropism to degenerative disc disease. *Spine*, **18**, 1000–1005.

Varlotta, G. P., Brown, M. D., Kelsey, J. L. et al. (1991). Familial predisposition for herniation of lumbar disc in patients who are less than twenty-one years old. *Journal of Bone and Joint Surgery*, **73A**, 124–128.

Varughese, G. and Quartey, G. R. (1979). Familial lumbar spinal stenosis with acute disc herniation: case report of four brothers. *Journal of Neurosurgery*, **51**, 234–236.

Vaz, M., Wadia, R. S. and Goklhole, S. D. (1978). Another case of a positive crossed-straight leg raising test (letter). *New England Journal of Medicine*, **299**, 779.

Vernon, H. (1991). Spinal manipulation and headache of cervical origin. *Journal of Manual Medicine*, **6**, 73–79.

Vernon-Roberts, B. (1994). Christian Georg Schmorl. Pioneer of spinal pathology and radiology. *Spine*, **19**, 2724–2727.

Vernon-Roberts, B. and Pirie, C. J. (1977). Degenerative changes in the intervertebral discs of the lumbar spine and their sequelae. *Rheumatology and Rehabilitation*, **16**, 13–21.

Vesterskold, L., Axelsson, B. and Jacobsson, H. (1994). A combined method for quantitative pertechnetate scinigraphy in the diagnosis of sacroiliitis. A controlled study. *Scandinavian Journal of Rheumatology*, **23**, 16–21.

Vidal, P., Roucoux, A. and Berthoz, A. (1982). Horizontal eye position-related activity in neck muscles of the alert cat. *Experimental Brain Research*, **46**, 448–453.

Videman, T., Nurminen,T., Tola, S. et al. (1984). Low back pain in nurses and some loading factors of work. *Spine*, **9**, 400–404.

Videman, T., Nurminen, M. and Troup, J. D. G. (1990). Lumbar spine pathology in cadaveric material in relation to history of back pain, occupation and physical activity. *Spine*, **15**, 728–740.

Videman, T., Sarna, S., Battie, M. C. et al. (1995a). The long-term effects of physical loading and exercise lifestyles on back-related symptoms, disability and spinal pathology among men. *Spine*, **20**, 699–709.

Videman, T., Battie M. C., Gill, K. et al. (1995b). Magnetic resonance imaging findings and their relationships in the thoracic and lumbar spine. *Spine*, **20**, 928–935.

Viitanen, J. V., Kautiainen, H., Kokko, M. L. and Alapeijari, S. (1995a). Age and spinal mobility in ankylosing spondylitis. *Scandinavian Journal of Rheumatology*, **24**, 314–315.

Viitanen, J. V., Lehtinen, K., Suni, J. and Kaitiainen, H. (1995b). Fifteen months follow-up of intensive inpatient physiotherapy and exercise in ankylosing spondylitis. *Clinical Rheumatology*, **14**, 413–419.

Vleeming, A., Stoeckart, R., and Snijders, C. J. (1989). The sacrotuberous ligament: a conceptual approach to its dynamic role in stabilising the sacroiliac joint. *Journal of Biomechanics*, **4**, 201–203.

Vleeming, A., Stoeckart, R., Volkers, A. C. W. and Snijders, C. J. (1990a). Relation between form and function in the sacroiliac joint. Part I: clinical anatomical aspects. *Spine*, **15**, 130–132.

Vleeming, A., Volkers, A. C. W., Snijders, C. J. and Stoeckart, R. (1990b). Relation between form and function in the sacroiliac joint. Part II: biochemical aspects. *Spine*, **15**, 133–135.

Vleeming, A., Van Wingerden, J. P., Dijkstra, P. F. et al. (1992). Mobility of the sacroiliac joints in the elderly. *Clinical Biomechanics*, **7**, 170–176.

Vogler, J. B., Brown, W. H., Helms, C. A. and Genant, H. K. (1984). The normal sacroiliac joint: a CT study of asymptomatic patients. *Radiology*, **151**, 433–437.

Vucetic, N., Maattanen, H. and Svensson, O. (1995). Pain and pathology in lumbar disc hernia. *Clinical Orthopaedics and Related Research*, **320**, 65–72.

Wada, E., Ohmura, M. and Yonenobu, K. (1995). Intramedulllary changes of the spinal cord in cervical spondylotic myelopathy. *Spine*, **20**, 2226–2232.

Waddell, G. (1987a). Clinical assessment of lumbar impairment. *Clinical Orthopaedics and Related Research*, **221**,110–120.

Waddell, G. (1987b). A new clinical model for the treatment of low back pain. *Spine*, **12**, 632–644.

Waddell, G., McCulloch, J. A., Kummel, E. and Venner, R. M. (1980). Nonorganic physical signs in low back pain. *Spine*, **5**, 117–125.

Walheim, G. G. and Selvik, G. (1984). Mobility of the pubic symphysis: in vivo measurements with an electromechanic mehod and a roentgen stereophotogrammetric method. *Clinical Orthopaedics and Related Research*, **191**, 129–135.

Walker, J. M. (1986). Age related differences in the human sacroiliac joint: a histological study – implications for therapy. *Journal of Orthopedic and Sports Physical Therapy*, **7**, 325–331.

Walker, J. M. (1992). The sacroiliac joint: a critical review. *Physical Therapy*, **72**, 903–916.

Wallis, B. J., Lord, S. M., Barnsley, L. and Bogduk, N. (1996). Pain and psychologic symptoms of Australian patients with whiplash. *Spine*, **21**, 804–810.

Walsh, N. E. and Schwartz, R. K. (1990). The influence of prophylactic orthoses on abdominal strength and low back injury on the workplace. *American Journal of Physical Medicine and Rehabilitation*, **69**, 245–250.

Walsh, T. R., Weinstein, J. N., Spratt, K. F. et al. (1990). Lumbar discography in normal subjects. A controlled prospective study. *Journal of Bone and Joint Surgery*, **72A**, 1081–1088.

Walsh, W., Huurman, W. and Shelton, G. (1985). Overuse injuries of the knee and spine in girls' gymnastics. *Orthopedic Clinics of North America*, **16**, 329–349.

Watanabe, R. and Parke, W. W. (1986). Vascular and neural pathology of lumbosacral spinal stenosis. *Journal of Neurosurgery*, **64**, 64–70.

Watkinson, A., Gargan, M. F. and Bannister, G. C. (1991). Prognostic factors in soft tissue injuries of the cervical spine. *Injury*, **22**, 307–309.

Watters, W. C. and Levinthal, R. (1994). Anterior cervical discectomy with and without fusion. Results, complications, and long-term follow-up. *Spine*, **19**, 2343–2347.

Watts, R. W. and Silagy, C. A. (1995). A meta-analysis on the efficacy of epidural corticosteroid in the treatment of sciatica. *Anaesthesia and Intensive Care*, **23**, 564–569.

Weatherley, C. R., Mehdian, H. and Vanden Berghe, L. (1991). Low back pain with fracture of the pedicle and contralateral spondylolysis. *Journal of Bone and Joint Surgery*, **73B**, 990–993.

Webb, F. W. S., Hickman, J. A. and Brew, D. StJ. (1968). Death from vertebral artery thrombosis in rheumatoid arthritis. *British Medical Journal*, **2**, 537–538.

Weber, H. (1994). The natural history of disc herniation and the influence of intervention. *Spine*, **19**, 2234–2238.

Wedel, D. J. and Wilson, P. R. (1985). Cervical facet arthrography. *Regional Anesthesia*, **10**, 7–11.

Wehling, P., Cleveland, S. J., Heininger, K. et al. (1996). Neurophysiologic changes in lumbar nerve root inflammation in the rat after treatment with cytokine inhibitors. Evidence for a role of interleukin-1. *Spine*, **21**, 931–935.

Weinberg, S. and Lapointe, H. (1987). Cervical extension-flexion injury and internal derangement of the temporomandibular joint. *Journal of Oral and Maxillofocial Surgery*, **45**, 653–656.

Weinberger, L. M. (1977). Traumatic fibromyositis: a critical review of an enigmatic concept. *Western Journal of Medicine*, **127**, 99–103.

Weinreb, J. C., Wolbarsh, L. B., Cohen, J. M. et al. (1989). Prevalence of lumbosacral intervertebral disc abnormalities on MR images in pregnant and asymptomatic nonpregnant women. *Radiology*, **170**, 125–128.

Weinstein, J. (1991). Neurogenic and nonneurogenic pain and inflammatory mediators. *Orthopedic Clinics of North America*, **22**, 235–246.

Weinstein, S. M., Herring, S. A. and Derby, R. (1995). Epidural steroid injections. *Spine*, **20**, 1842–1846.

Weisz, G. M. and Lee, P. (1983). Spinal canal stenosis. Concept of spinal reserve capacity: radiologic measurements and clinical applications. *Clinical Orthopaedics and Related Research*, **179**, 134–140.

Werneke, M. W., Harris, P. E. and Lichter, R. L. (1993). Clinical effectiveness of behavioral signs for screening chronic low-back pain patients in a work-oriented physical rehabilitation program. *Spine*, **18**, 2412–2418.

Wertheim, S. B. and Bohlman, H. H. (1987). Occipitocervical fusion. Indications, technique and long-term results in thirteen patients. *Journal of Bone and Joint Surgery*, **69A**, 833–836.

Wesley, A. L., Gatchel, R. J., Polatin, P. B. et al. (1991). Differentiation between somatic and cognitive–affective components in commonly used measurements of depression in patients with chronic low back pain. Let's not mix apples and oranges. *Spine*, **16**, S213–S215.

Whitcomb, D. C., Martin, S. P., Schoen, R. W. and Jho, H. D. (1995). Chronic abdominal pain caused by thoracic disc herniation. *American Journal of Gastroenterology*, **90**, 835–837.

White, A. and Punjabi, M. (1990). *Clinical Biomechanics of the Spine*, 2nd edn. pp. 38–79, Lippincott.

White, K. P., Harth, M. and Teasell, R. W. (1995). Work disability evaluation and the fibromyalgia syndrome. *Seminars in Arthritis and Rheumatism*, **24**, 371–381.

Wiesel, S. W., Tsourmas, N., Feffer, H. L. et al. (1984). A study of computer-assisted tomography. 1. The incidence of positive CAT scans in an asymptomatic group of patients. *Spine*, **9**, 549–551.

Wilder, D. G., Frymoyer, J. W., and Pope, M. H. (1985). The effect of vibration on the spine of the seated individual. *Automedica*, **6**, 5–35.

Wilder, D. G., Pope, M. H. and Frymoyer, J. N. (1980). The functional topography of the sacroiliac joint. *Spine*, **5**, 575–579.

Wilder, D. G., Woodworth, B. B., Frymoyer, J. W. et al. (1982). Vibration and the human spine. *Spine*, **7**, 243–254.

Wilke, H. J., Wolf, S., Claes, L. E. et al. (1995). Stability increase of the lumbar spine with different muscle groups: a biomechanical in vitro study. *Spine*, **20**, 192–198.

Wilkinson, R. H. and Hall, J. E. (1974). The sclerotic pedicle: tumor or pseudotumor. *Radiology*, **111**, 683–688.

Willburger, R. E. and Wittenberg, R. H. (1994). Prostaglandin release from lumbar disc and facet joint tissue. *Spine*, **18**, 2068–2070.

Williams, R. W. (1991). Microdiscectomy—myth, mania or milestone? An 18-year experience. *Mount Sinai Journal of Medicine*, **58**, 139–145.

Willis, T. A. (1931). The separate neural arch. *Journal of Bone and Joint Surgery*, **13**, 709–721.

Willner, S. (1985). Effect of a rigid brace on back pain. *Acta Orthopaedica Scandinavica*, **56**, 40–42.

Wilson, L. F., Chell, J. and Mulholland, R. C. (1992). Adolescent disc protrusions: a long term follow up of chymopapaine therapy. *European Spine Journal,*. **1**, 1–7.

Wilson, P. R. (1987). Thoracic facet joint syndrome – a clinical entity? *Pain*, Suppl **4**, 87.

Wilson, P. R. (1991). Chronic neck pain and cervicogenic headache. *Clinical Journal of Pain*, **7**, 5–11.

Wiltse, L. L. and Rothman, L. (1989). Spondylolisthesis: classification, diagnosis, and natural history. *Seminars in Spine Surgery*, **1**, 78–94.

Wiltse, L. L., Widell, E. and Jackson, D. (1975). Fatigue fracture: the bone lesion in isthmic spondylolisthesis. *Journal of Bone and Joint Surgery*, **57A**, 17–22.

Wiltse, L. L., Newman, P. H. and Macnab, I. (1976). Classification of spondylolysis and spondylolisthesis. *Clinical Orthopaedics and Related Research*, **117**, 23–29.

Wing, L. W. and Hargrave-Wilson, W. (1974). Cervical vertigo. *Australian and New Zealand Journal of Surgery*, **44**, 275–277.

Winter, R. B. and Siebert, R. (1993). Herniated thoracic disc at T1–T2 with paraparesis. Transthoracic excision and fusion. Case report with 4-year follow-up. *Spine*, **18**, 782–784.

Wipf, J. E. and Deyo, R. A. (1995). Low Back Pain. *Medical Clinics of North America*, **79**, 231–246.

Wise, C. M. (1994). Chest wall syndromes. *Current Opinion in Rheumatology*, **6**, 197–220.

Wise, C. M., Semble, E. L. and Dalton, C. B. (1992). Musculoskeletal chest wall syndromes in patients with noncardiac chest pain: a study in 100 patients. *Archives of Physical Medicine and Rehabilitation*, **73**, 147–149.

Withrington, R. H., Sturge, R. A. and Mitchell, N. (1985). Osteitis condensans ilii and its differentiation from ankylosing spondylitis. *Scandinavian Journal of Rheumatology*, **14**, 163–166.

Wittram, C., Whitehouse, G. H., Williams, J. W.

and Bucknall, R. C. (1996). A comparison of MRI and CT in suspected sacroiliitis. *Journal of Computer Assisted Tomography*, **20**, 68–72.

Wolf, E. and Stern, S. (1976). Costosternal syndrome. Its frequency and importance in differential diagnosis of coronary heart disease. *Archives of Internal Medicine*, **136**, 189–191.

Wolfe, F. (1988). Fibrositis, fibromyalgia, and musculoskeletal disease: the current status of the fibrositis syndrome. *Archives of Physical Medicine and Rehabilitation*, **69**, 527–533.

Wolfe, F. (1994). The epidemiology of fibromyalgia. *Journal of Musculoskeletal Pain*, **1**, 137–148.

Wolfe, F. and Cathey, M. A. (1985). Epidemiology of tender points: prospective study of 1520 patients. *Journal of Rheumatology*, **12**, 1164–1168.

Wolfe, F., Cathey, M. A. and Kleinheksel, S. M. (1984). Fibrositis (fibromyalgia) in rheumatoid arthritis. *Journal of Rheumatology*, **11**, 814–818.

Wolfe, F., Smythe, H. A., Yunus, M. B. et al. (1990). The American College of Rheumatology 1990 criteria for the classification of fibromyalgia: report of the multicenter criteria committee. *Arthritis and Rheumatism*, **33**, 160–172.

Wolfe, F., Simons, D. G., Fricton, J. et al. (1992). The fibromyalgia and myofascial pain syndromes: a preliminary study of tender points and trigger points in patients with fibromyalgia, myofascial pain syndrome and non-disease. *Journal of Rheumatology*, **19**, 944–951.

Wood, E. G. and Hanley, E. N. (1992). Types of anterior cervical grafts. *Orthopedic Clinics of North America*, **23**, 475–486.

Wood, K. B., Garvey, T. A., Gundry, C. and Heithoff, K. B. (1995). Magnetic resonance imaging of the thoracic spine. *Journal of Bone and Joint Surgery*, **77A**, 1631–1638.

Wood, K. B., Popp, C. A., Transfeldt, E. E. and Geissele, A. E. (1994). Radiographic evaluation of instability in spondylolisthesis. *Spine*, **19**, 1697–1703.

Wooden, M. J. (1981). Pre-screening of the lumbar spine. *Journal of Orthopedic and Sports Physical Therapy*, **3**, 6–10.

Woodring, J. H. and Goldstein, S. J. (1982). Fractures of the articular processes of the cervical spine. *American Journal of Roentgenology*, **139**, 341–344.

Wright, J. T. (1980). Slipping rib syndrome. *Lancet*, **2**, 632–633.

Wynne-Davies, R. and Scott, J. H. S. (1979). Inheritance and spondylolisthesis. *Journal of bone and Joint Surgery*, **61B**, 301–305.

Wysenbeek, A. J., Mor, F., Lurie, Y. and Weinberger, A. (1985). Imipramine for the treatment of fibrositis: a therapeutic trial. *Annals of the Rheumatic Diseases*, **44**, 752–753.

Yamamoto, I., Ikeda, A., Shibuya, N. et al. (1991). Clinical long-term results of anterior discectomy without interbody fusion for cervical disc disease. *Spine*, **16**, 272–279.

Yamane, T., Yoshida, T. and Mimatsu, K. (1993). Early diagnosis of lumbar spondylolysis by MRI. *Journal of Bone and Joint Surgery*, **75B**, 764–768.

Yamashita, T., Cavanaug, J. M., El-Bohy, A. A. et al. (1990). Mechanosensitive afferent units in the lumbar facet joint. *Journal of Bone and Joint Surgery*, **72A**, 865–870.

Yang, K. H. and King, A. I. (1984). Mechanism of facet load transmission as a hypothesis for low back pain. *Spine*, **9**, 557–565.

Yarnell, P. R. and Rossie, G. V. (1988). Minor whiplash head injury with major debilitation. *Brain Injury*, **2**, 255–258.

Yates, D. A. H. (1981). Spinal stenosis. *Journal of the Royal Society of Medicine*, **74**, 334–342.

Yates, D. W. (1978). A comparison of the types of epidural injection commonly used in the treatment of intervertebral disc herniation. *Rheumatology and Rehabilitation*, **17**, 181–186.

Ylinen, J. and Ruuska. J. (1994). Clinical use of neck isometric strength measurement in rehabilitation. *Archives of Physical Medicine and Rehabilitation*, **75**, 465–469.

Yoganandan, M., Larson, S. J., Pintar, F. A. et al. (1994). Intravertebral pressure changes caused by spinal microtrauma. *Neurosurgery*, **35**, 415–421.

Yonezawa, T., Tsuji, H., Matsui, H. and Hirano, N. (1995). Subaxial lesions in rheumatoid arthritis. Radiographic factors suggestive of lower cervical myelopathy. *Spine*, **20**, 208–215.

Yoo, J. U., Zou, D., Edwards, W. T. et al. (1992). Effects of cervical spine motion on neuroforaminal dimension of the human cervical spine. *Spine*, **17**, 1131–1136.

Yoshizawa, H., O'Brien, J. P., Smith, W. T. and Trumper, M. (1980). The neuropathology of intervertebral discs removed for low back pain. *Journal of Pathology*, **132**, 95–104.

Young, S., Veerapen, R. and O'Laoire, S. A. (1988). Relief of lumbar canal stenosis using multilevel subarticular fenestrations as an alternative for wide laminectomy: preliminary report. *Neurosurgery*, **23**, 628–633.

Yu, S. W., Haughton, V. M., Sether, L. A. and Wagner, M. (1989b). Criteria for classifying normal and degenerated lumbar intervertebral discs. *Radiology*, **170**, 523–526.

Yu, S. W., Haughton, V. M., Lynch, K. L. et al. (1989b). Fibrous structure in the intervertebral disc: correlation of MR appearance with anatomic sections. *American Journal of Neuroradiology*, **10**, 1105–1110.

Yunus, M. B. (1992). Towards a model of pathophysiology of fibromyalgia: aberrant central pain mechanisms with peripheral modulation. *Journal of Rheumatology*, **19**, 846–850.

Yunus, M., Masi, A. T., Calabro, J. J. et al. (1981). Primary fibromyalgia (fibrositis): a clinical study of 50 patients with matched normal controls. *Seminars in Arthritis and Rheumatism*, **11**, 151–171.

Yunus, M. B., Kalyan-Raman, U. P., Kalyan-Raman, K. and Masi, A.T. (1986). Pathological changes in muscle in primary fibromyalgia syndrome. *American Journal of Medicine*, **81**, suppl 3A, 38-42.

Yunus, M. B., Kalyan-Raman, U. P. and Kalyan-Raman, K. (1988). Primary fibromyalgia syndrome and myofascial pain syndrome: clinical features and muscle pathology. *Archives of Physical Medicine and Rehabilitation*, **69**, 451–454.

Yunus, M. B., Ahles, T. A., Aldag, J. C. and Masi, A. T. (1991). Relationship of clinical features with psychologic status in primary fibromyalgia. *Arthritis and Rheumatism*, **34**, 15–21.

Zamami, M. H. and MacEwen, G. D. (1982). Herniation of the lumbar disc in children and adolescents. *Journal of Pediatric Orthopedics*, **2**, 528–533.

Zapletal, J., Hekster, R. E. M., Straver, J. S. and Wilmink, J. T. (1995). Atlanto-odontoid osteoarthritis. Appearance and prevalence at computered tomography. *Spine*, **20**, 49–53.

Zeidman, S. M. and Ducker, T. B. (1994). Rheumatoid arthritis neuroanatomy, compression, and grading of deficits. *Spine*, **19**, 2259–2266.

Ziran, B. H., Pineda, S., Pokhama, H. et al. (1994). Biomechanical, radiologic, and histopathologic correlations in the pathogenesis of experimental intervertebral disc disease. *Spine*, **19**, 2159–2163.

Zlatkin, M. B., Lander, P. H., Hadjipavlou, A. G. and Levine, J. S. (1986). Paget's disease of the spine: CT with clinical correlation. *Radiology*, **160**, 155–159.

Zoma, A., Sturrock, R. D., Fisher, W. D. et al. (1987). Surgical stabilization of the rheumatoid cervical spine. A review of indications and results. *Journal of Bone and Joint Surgery*, **69B**, 8–12.

Zucherman, J., Derby, R., Hsu, K. et al. (1988). Normal magnetic resonance imaging with abnormal discography. *Spine*, **13**, 1355–1359.

Zylbergold, R. S. and Piper, M. C. (1981). Lumbar disc disease: comparative analysis of physical therapy treatments. *Archives of Physical Medicine and Rehabilitation*, **62**, 176–179.

Index

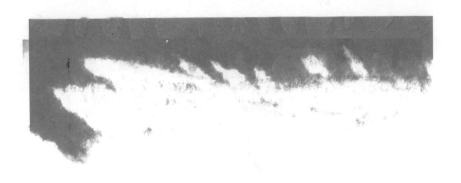